ADVANCED
BACH FLOWER
THERAPY

ADVANCED
BACH FLOWER
THERAPY

A SCIENTIFIC APPROACH
TO DIAGNOSIS
AND TREATMENT

GÖTZ BLOME, M.D.

Healing Arts Press
Rochester, Vermont

Healing Arts Press
One Park Street
Rochester, Vermont 05767
www.InnerTraditions.com

Healing Arts Press is a division of Inner Traditions International

First English Language edition published by Healing Arts Press 1999

Copyright © 1992 by Verlag Hermann Bauer, Germany, published under arrangement
Translation copyright © 1999 by Inner Traditions International

*Note to the reader: This book is intended as an informational guide. The remedies,
approaches, and techniques described herein are meant to supplement, and not to be a
substitute for, professional medical care or treatment. They should not be used to treat a
serious ailment without prior consultation with a qualified health care professional.*

Library of Congress Cataloging-in-Publication Data

Blome, Götz.
    [Neue Bach-blüten-buch. English]
    Advanced Bach flower therapy : a scientific approach to diagnosis and treat-
ment / Götz Blome.
      p.   cm.
    ISBN 0-89281-828-X (alk. paper)
    1. Flowers—Therapeutic use.   2. Homeopathy—Materia medica and thera-
peutics. I. Title.
RX615.F55 IN PROCESS
615'.321—dc21   99-30201
                                                              CIP

Printed and bound in the United States

10 9 8 7 6 5

Text design and layout by Virginia L. Scott
This book was typeset in Bulmer with Futura as a display face

CONTENTS

INTRODUCTION

There is no doubt that modern scientific medicine has had spectacular successes in the fight against physical illness. But it can do nothing against spiritual and emotional suffering; indeed, it even seems that the drastic measures of chemical-technical therapy have driven the pathogenic locus of illness from outside to inside and increased the incidence of mental and emotional problems. More than fifty years ago, the distinguished doctor and researcher Dr. Edward Bach developed his new form of "flower therapy," which focused on the mental and emotional factors as causes of illness. Given the results of modern treatments, it's little wonder that the popularity of Dr. Bach's flower therapy continues to grow by leaps and bounds.

Bach flower therapy does not seek the physical symptoms of an illness but instead looks to the underlying or predominant mental and emotional conditions and aims to treat the psychic, not the physical, symptoms. Bach flower therapy attempts to treat the patient's soul; physical problems are secondary. Dr. Bach had a sound basis for this unusual concept. In searching for a truly humane form of treatment, he stumbled across a phenomenon that has been largely unobserved in modern medicine: according to the structure of the personality and the emotional constitution, the same illness can cause very different psychic symptoms in different individuals. These manifestations, such as restlessness or apathy, openness or reserved behavior, fear of death or an attraction to death, grouchiness or gratitude, lend the objective physical symptoms their individual, personal meaning.

We normally describe a sick person something like this: he has such and such a temperature and runny stools, and he sweats profusely. Lab results are such and such, and the patient is apathetic and weak. We can, however, describe the physical symptoms brought about by the psychic ones, beginning like this: the patient's face has a sad, troubled expression; his voice is feeble; he is suffering the consequences of a great loss and gives the impression he wants to die. Or we can say he is unusually self-pitying and in need of consolation and sulks when someone is not paying constant attention to him. He's anxious and restless and also suffers from a fever, runny stools, and so on.

Although the physical symptoms are identical, we are dealing with two different illnesses. The first case stems from the tendency to want to end one's life owing to a great loss, while the second condition is, above all, a cry for attention. It is clear that the treatment must take into account the background of the illness. When we ignore the mental and emotional state of a patient, we are imposing treatment in an impersonal, objective, essentially senseless way, addressing only the symptoms and not the patient. If, however, we observe the psychic signs, we understand the illness in a larger context and can treat the patient as an individual, suffering being.

Dr. Bach described the connection between the mental and emotional state and illness as a conflict between the "personality" and the "higher self." In each individual traumatized by life, he also saw the core of an essentially good, healthy human being and was convinced that health can return only when the balance of the psyche is restored and the inner self is once again whole and revitalized. It is this premise, expressed differently, that informs today's psychosomatic medicine. While psychosomatic medicine attempts to resolve these conflicts mainly through conditioning or raising consciousness, however, Bach flower therapy goes about trying to minimize or treat precisely defined psychic conditions with thirty-eight floral essences, in ways that have still not been scientifically explained.

The positive effects of Bach flower therapy can be significantly bolstered through the patient's conscious work on her own sick "personality." This is where this book comes in, pointing out the deeper psychological connections. Often just by concentrating on the underlying mental and emotional conditions, we can untie our inner knots and begin the healing process, even without any kind of medication. This process can then be strengthened and promoted by using the appropriate flower essences. Despite its astounding success, Bach flower therapy does have its limits. Since healing, like illness, is a phenomenon that is very much dependent on fate and circumstance, we cannot always force it on our own. When the patient is determined to be healthy again, and when such crucial factors as timing, mental and emotional condition, and therapist and medication working together in an ideal manner all fall into place, we have the requisites for healing to take place. Sometimes one form of therapy will be called for and sometimes another. There is no such thing as a cure-all, and there never will be. When we are not as successful as we would like to be, we should be open to other methods of treatment. Homeopathy works especially well as a companion form of treatment to Bach flowers.

The strength of Bach flower therapy lies in the normalization of psychic disruptions and the resolution of inner conflicts as well as in the improvement of physical conditions that have recognizable psychic causes or symptoms. Bach flowers are particularly suitable for children. They are appropriate not just as a treatment that attempts to achieve a harmony of mind and body in all types of illnesses—even as a supplement to routine medical treatment—but also, because they can stabilize or eliminate psychic weak points, as a form of "preventive maintenance." For example, we can treat the eternally irritable, aggressive patient with Holly; a restless, nervous type with Impatiens; the patient with a pathological craving for recognition with Heather; a fearful patient with Mimulus; or a depressed type with Mustard. They will be plagued by their emotional and related physical problems less often or not at all.

Please note that not every psychic condition is treatable, nor is it necessarily the sign of an illness. Psychic manifestations can be a significant part of our personality and part of what makes us unique. Treatment is called for only when they cause us to suffer—for example, in the form of conflicts, frustrations, depression, self-denial, or difficulties in coming to terms with our everyday lives.

Structure and Use of This Book

This book is divided into three parts. In the first chapter you will find exact descriptions of the thirty-eight essences that form the basis of Bach flower therapy. Each essence (Bach flower) is associated with a typical psychic condition that can be expressed in groupings of various individual symptoms that, taken together, are known as "syndromes." With the help of a new kind of analysis, the various personality types of those who can be treated with Bach flowers will be explained clearly. The ideally developed personality of each type will be described, followed by the problems that become apparent when each is unfavorably developed. Each of us has a unique psychic structure that affects our emotions, thoughts, and actions. We can develop harmoniously or experience inharmonious manifestations that can cause illness or psychosomatic conditions. Being able to treat these pathological manifestations is the strength of Bach flower therapy. It can restore our balance and free us from physical manifestations of problems that are often psychic or emotional in origin. Bach flower therapy cannot, however, make a person into his ideal opposite.

The thirty-eight classic Bach flowers encompass nearly all of the important qualities of the human psyche; taken singly, however, they may not have sufficient complexity or strength. Because most illnesses arise from the interplay of various psychic or physical influences and particularities of personality and character, Bach flowers are normally administered by combining several essences. The most common and important combinations are listed in chapter 1 and described in detail in the second chapter, at the end of each individual flower description. These combinations allow for more precise and effective treatment—since each has its own area of efficacy—and open up a new perspective to understanding most personality and behavioral problems. Each combination can be found in chapter 2 under the name of the essence listed first: for example, you would find the Chicory/Heather combination (8/14) under the letter C or the number eight. The combinations are listed again in the repertory, where they are marked with an asterisk(*).

In the third chapter, the therapeutic lexicon, you will find—in alphabetical order—thorough advice on the practical application of Bach flowers that will allow you to become acquainted with their various qualities and facets. This chapter also contains many suggestions for understanding and solving most human problems. An arrow (—›) indicates that more information about the condition can be found under that entry. Essences linked together by a plus sign (+) should be taken together.

An asterisk (*) indicates that the particular combination described is mentioned in more detail in chapter 2.

The Thirty-eight Bach Flowers

1. Agrimony *(Agrimonia eupatoria)*
2. Aspen *(Populus tremula)*
3. Beech *(Fagus sylvatica)*
4. Centaury *(Centaurium umbellatum)*
5. Cerato *(Ceratostigma willmottiana)*
6. Cherry Plum *(Prunus cerasifera)*
7. Chestnut Bud *(Aesculus hippocastanum)*
8. Chicory *(Cichorium intybus)*
9. Clematis *(Clematis vitalba)*
10. Crab Apple *(Malus pumila)*
11. Elm *(Ulmus procera)*
12. Gentian *(Gentiana amarella)*
13. Gorse *(Ulex europaeus)*
14. Heather *(Calluna vulgaris)*
15. Holly *(Ilex aquifolium)*
16. Honeysuckle *(Lonicera caprifolium)*
17. Hornbeam *(Capinus betulus)*
18. Impatiens *(Impatiens glandulifera)*
19. Larch *(Larix decidua)*
20. Mimulus *(Mimulus guttatus)*
21. Mustard *(Sinapis arvensis)*
22. Oak *(Quercus robur)*
23. Olive *(Olea europea)*
24. Pine *(Pinus sylvestris)*
25. Red Chestnut *(Aesculus carnea)*
26. Rock Rose *(Helianthemum nummularium)*
27. Rock Water (water from rock springs)
28. Scleranthus *(Scleranthus annuus)*
29. Star of Bethlehem *(Ornithogalum umbellatum)*
30. Sweet Chestnut *(Castanea sativa)*

31. Vervain *(Verbena officinalis)*

32. Vine *(Vitis vinifera)*

33. Walnut *(Juglans regia)*

34. Water Violet *(Hottonia palustris)*

35. White Chestnut *(Aesculus hippocastanum)*

36. Wild Oat *(Bromus ramosus)*

37. Wild Rose *(Rosa canina)*

38. Willow *(Salix vitellina)*

The Practical Use of Bach Flower Therapy

Bach flower therapy is unusual not just from an intellectual standpoint but also because the manufacture of the essences is unique. All essences, with one exception (Rock Water, which comes from rock springs), are made from flowers. The essence (the soul, so to speak) of the plant is most clearly expressed in its flowers. The healing properties unique to each plant either are the result of the effects of the sun or are transferred through boiling in spring water. The tinctures are then mixed with alcohol and diluted into a final mixture, which is taken with a dropper. In addition, several complementary essences can be mixed together.

Dosages should be adjusted to the individual. With acute conditions or serious problems, place one to three drops of essence in a glass of water (boiled water, if possible) and drink from the glass during the course of a day; sometimes it is more effective to put a drop directly on the tongue. In the case of long-term treatment or with sensitivity to the essences, the essences can be diluted; put five drops (sometimes only two will suffice) in $^1/_3$ ounce of water and add approximately 10 percent alcohol for sterilization. It is best to use a small bottle with a dropper. Take five drops of this dilution daily. Combinations are made in the same way: put the chosen essences in water or a dilution.

In order to achieve the desired success with Bach flower therapy, you must proceed carefully. Familiarize yourself with all the essences or at least read all the descriptions carefully and attentively. Do not be content to choose the first essence that seems right to you. Try continually to select the correct essence of the thirty-eight. It is often advisable to combine several essences (three to six), and for many specific problems or complaints, there are special combinations described in chapter 2. Chosen correctly, Bach flowers can have remarkable results. But you should be aware that each of the thirty-eight essences acts in some way on every individual, and there is the danger of trying to accomplish too much at one time.

Bach flowers work primarily on the psyche, the disturbances of which can take many forms, including physical illness. For this reason it is important to consider the causes and contributing factors when choosing an essence. We should ask several questions: How and why has this particular condition come to be? What is the reason for this pathological behavior? What does this illness mean, and what is the psyche trying to tell us? At best, you should proceed as follows when choosing the proper essences. First, you should be sure which *psychic condition* is the dominant one. The first question is, "How do I feel?" (sad, exhausted, irritated, discouraged, restless, driven, bitter, and so on). Even with physical illnesses we must first take note of the mental and emotional state, since this is a deciding factor in choosing the appropriate essence. In this way, you will find the essence to treat the superficial causes of your condition.

Next you must find out the underlying causes for your condition with the following questions: "Why do I feel so bad? Which factors have played a role in creating my problem?" (For example, because I become too angry, because I rush, because I've experienced something terrible, because I can never give up, because I'm under too much strain, because I have no self-confidence, because I'm afraid, and so on.) In this way, you will find an essence that will address the underlying causes or bad habits and have deeply working effects.

You must also take your personality into account. Here you can ask: "What kind of person am I? Which characteristics or qualities make me what I am?" (that is, dominant, afraid, unfocused, dreamy, self-confident, acquisitive, shy, dishonest, afraid of conflict, pessimistic, uncertain, easily influenced, disciplined, and so on). In this way you will find an essence that is appropriate for your personality type and, in the long term, bring about positive change for your entire being.

For best results, take one or two essences from each of these three categories (superficial symptoms and causes, underlying factors, and personality type) and try to concentrate on the problem that is causing you to suffer. In terms of the essences from the third category (personality), the connection with the dominant condition or illness is not always easily recognizable. Take the essence anyway when the characteristic factors are very pronounced. Essences in this category work indirectly and will be effective not just in improving the situation temporarily but in leading you on the path to permanent improvement as well.

If you don't know how or where to begin, first look in the repertory (chapter 3) for your symptoms, read the appropriate descriptions in chapter 1 thoroughly, and then check for the recommended individual essences and combinations (chapter 2). If the selection seems too large and you have difficulty selecting an appropriate essence, begin with Wild Oat and Agrimony. Soon you'll notice some improvement, and you'll be able to see your problem more clearly. If you have absolutely no starting point for choosing an essence, take Agrimony, which is an important Bach flower and nearly always used to begin a therapy.

If treatment is successful and you notice improvement, turn your attention to the problems that come to the foreground. You will be able to rejuvenate your entire personality; it is entirely possible that certain essences will be used more than once. For problems that have only recently appeared and that are not deep-seated, the effects will be faster than for chronic or constitutional problems. Sometimes these long-term symptoms must be treated for months while the inner psychic structure is being healed. One of the unique features of Bach flower therapy is that its effects are decidedly organic and gentle. Often, one doesn't connect the Bach flowers with the improvement, which almost seems as if it just happened on its own.

If, after a few weeks, you notice no clear improvement—normally you'll notice a difference in hours or a few days—you have either not chosen the proper dosages (try higher dosages or a more potent dilution) or your choice has been too superficial. Naturally, it could be that Bach flower therapy is not the correct choice for your condition or should be combined with another form of therapy. Homeopathic (or naturopathic) treatments lend themselves especially well to such combination. In the case of a serious or long-lasting illness, you should consult an experienced, qualified doctor.

Do not throw in the towel too early. If something goes wrong, it is usually because of a problem in diagnosis. Look again in the repertory under the terms given there for those conditions that have the most in common with yours. List all the possible symptoms and conditions that should be treated and the appropriate essences used to treat those conditions. Any essence that appears more than once on your list will probably be helpful. You can also let the flower essences come into contact with the skin. Rescue Remedy salve is one example (see chapter 2). If a patient cannot take the essences orally, place a few drops on the lips or massage into the forehead or the afflicted area.

ONE

MEANING AND USE OF INDIVIDUAL BACH FLOWERS

1: Agrimony

Characteristics

Agrimony is the essence for people who cannot recognize the truth and who go out of their way to avoid conflict. Out of the need to avoid painful conflict (both internal and external), they try to keep their true feelings (fears, aggression, or sorrow) hidden from their consciousness and hidden from everyone else by maintaining a feigned carefree, happy demeanor.

AREA OF USE

Agrimony is used as a basic treatment for fear of conflict, deception and artificiality, hidden inner discord and emotional anguish, psychic complexes, tendency to repress, glossing over of personal problems, tension, and an inclination toward alcoholism and drug abuse. Used to treat any conditions related to tension, inhibitions, fear of conflict, dishonesty, artificial behavior, or oversensitivity. In daily life, used to treat phoniness, playacting, the "tears of a clown" syndrome, insincerity, embarrassment, inhibitions, tension, inner restlessness, oversensitivity to pain, and dependence on barbiturates or alcohol.

Causes and Symptoms of Agrimony Syndrome

This condition is characterized by a pronounced sensitivity and a strong need to be happy. Harmoniously developed, the Agrimony type instinctively avoids unhappiness of all kinds. He does this the most natural way possible: he defuses problems by accepting them as part of life and by making the best of them. (Problems are created when we try to ignore reality, fight against it, or create a false one.) Spontaneous, natural, and unfit for confrontation, the harmoniously developed Agrimony type does not try to cover up or falsify the unpleasant or repress or avoid difficulties. When faced with life's problems, he does not become lost or betray himself; when necessary, he bends with the blows like reeds in a windstorm—with a flexible, natural grace, without breaking or being damaged. Critical situations that can be catastrophic for negative individuals float harmlessly past him. He's always natural, genuine, spontaneous, and full of life. Because his special strength (even in times of trouble or need) is always being able to recognize and hold on to the positive ("chocolate-covered") side of life, he is always happy. It often seems as if his role on the stage of life is that of a carefree, happy character. Actually, he has a talent for acting, but every "role" he plays is an expression of his own happy self and is never a strange, artificial role. Because of his naturalness, his carefree and affable demeanor, and his optimism, he is welcome everywhere.

Unfavorably developed, the Agrimony type's sensitivity can change to oversensitivity, his ability to love life can become a flight from reality, and his talent for acting can become mere hypocrisy. The Agrimony person cannot and will not suffer. Life can be especially difficult for him because his sensitive nature makes every unpleasant experience so incredibly painful. Out of fear of suffering, he cowardly steps out of the way of all unpleasantness, every conflict, and every argument, even when only an honest and forthright confrontation is called for. If he is not up to such a confrontation, he ignores his problems and carries on as if everything were just fine.

To avoid the conscious confrontation of problems, fears, and conflicts (even though he continues to repress them in his subconscious), he tries to replace them with the illusion of a make-believe, happy world. He wears the eternally happy mask of a carefree companion, always pretends to be optimistic and in a good mood (even though the reality can be totally different), is always joking around even though he suffers inside, bolsters the spirits of others, and pretends to be nonchalant after a doctor's diagnosis even when he knows himself to be very ill. He tries, like a miscast actor, to fool everyone, himself included. The happy face he always shows hides his tears. He is always trying to distract himself and can never dwell on reality. He keeps smiling and doesn't show his true inner feelings. This works, of course, only on a superficial level, while his very real problems eat away at him constantly, like rust on an old piece of iron. Even though he seems happy, he suffers from anxiety and depression. The more he tries to seem peaceful and happy on the outside, the more he loses those same qualities on the inside, and his behavior becomes that much more forced and unnatural. With time, to provide at least temporary relief, he can turn to various addictions: mindless entertainment and distraction, binge eating, work, alcohol, or drugs. (Alcohol, by the way, makes many people seem carefree, uncannily sociable, and funny and, at the same time, totally unable to engage in any real, meaningful contact.) In addition, he often suffers from sleep disorders, restlessness, cramps, and tension or aches and pains.

The Effects of Agrimony

Agrimony is the essence of choice to promote honesty and natural behavior. It works against the habit of not taking our problems seriously and awakens the desire for more honesty with ourselves and others. With Agrimony, we are more open and relaxed and also more able to engage in conflict, so that, when necessary, we can be strong enough to face unpleasant situations. Agrimony is one of the most important Bach flowers and can be used by just about everyone. It should be taken as an accompaniment to any form of psychotherapy because it strengthens the patient's will to be truthful, to come to know himself better, and to be more open with his therapist.

Owing to the breakdown of normal psychic defense mechanisms, it often happens that suppressed fears and anxieties can become more intense with treatment and trigger an unconscious counterattack: we feel naked and defenseless. In such a case, the patient might break or spill bottles of essence—accidentally, of course—or discontinue therapy. This reaction can be corrected with the help of Walnut, which serves to strengthen the camouflage instincts of the negative Agrimony type. In general, regardless of the type of condition, Agrimony has a positive influence on the course of an illness if the patient wants to downplay it or keep it secret. This essence can resolve anxiety and tension, rheumatic complaints, constipation, sleep disorders, or inner restlessness.

Psychotherapeutic Notes

Agrimony is connected with two very important psychic functions that help ensure our survival: repression and lies. Repression protects us from the consequences of our own all-too-human shortcomings and weaknesses. If we did not ignore the greater part of our perceptions and impressions, we would be unable to think clearly and make intelligent decisions. And if we were to be consciously aware of the whole truth about ourselves, we would quite simply shatter. That is why our psyche constantly filters countless bits of information, impressions, and perceptions that influence us. It takes note only of those that we can process in any given moment and stores the great majority in the archive of the subconscious, where they stay until we are ready to use them.

Lies, on the other hand, protect us from resentment and misunderstanding. At a very young age we learn to lie and be hypocritical in order to survive, or in other words, to behave ourselves, be respectable, and run with the pack. If we were to act as we truly are, say openly what we mean, or do whatever we wanted without thinking of the consequences, we would have a slim chance of survival in our world, where jungle rules are the norm. People who think that nothing ever bothers them and who are in a perpetually good mood are not being truthful to themselves about how they really feel.

Nevertheless, as helpful as repression and lies can be under certain circumstances, at bottom they also signify a betrayal of the truth. Our spirit, which is always seeking the truth, allows us to be dishonest when absolutely necessary, but not out of mere convenience. We must continually seek out a compromise that we can live with—only enough self-deception so that our external life is not threatened and sufficient honesty that our spirit allows us to go on living. The main thing is that we do not betray our personal truth, that we understand and can be responsible for our actions. When we continue to wear the mask that we normally wear only in times of danger or out of personal weakness, when we act hypocritically or lie without reason, or when we even begin to believe our own lies, our spirit resists, and this resistance causes us to suffer.

As everyone knows from experience, this suffering consists of a certain discontentment, if we are again unnecessarily fooling ourselves or pretending that our emotions are not what they really are. The Agrimony type, however, nearly always represses to minimize conflicts or deceives himself or those around him. This approach can lead to severe frustration, depression, loneliness, or a hidden mental and emotional anguish. Most Agrimony types, however, will do something about their condition only if they are under great pressure or are suffering tremendously. They commonly need psychotherapeutic help, which makes them aware of their behavior and puts them in the position to consciously steer their own course. When they can clearly and objectively evaluate their life situation, they can decide freely if and when they should disguise or repress unpleasantness. And they can also learn not to do so. The more decisively they act in this regard, the stronger they will become. Despite their supposed weaknesses and shortcomings, being able to make this conscious decision will provide them with more strength and security than all the masks they've been hiding behind.

Common Combinations with Other Essences

Aspen (1/2): repressed fears or anxieties due to repression

Beech (1/3): artificial tolerance

Centaury (1/4): pathological cheerfulness

Cherry Plum (1/6): dangerous psychic pressure caused by repression

Chestnut Bud (1/7): learning difficulties or immaturity due to shirking

Larch (1/19): repressed inferiority complex

Mimulus (1/20): repressed fears and anxieties

Red Chestnut (1/25): repressed, secret worries

Rock Rose (1/26): frozen in panic

Star of Bethlehem (1/29): psychic wounds concealed behind the happy facade

Walnut (1/33): total self-alienation

Water Violet (1/34): human contact problems due to a lack of openness

Wild Oat (1/36): lack of self-awareness

2: Aspen
Characteristics

Aspen is for people who are tormented by unpleasant ideas or vague, indefinite anxieties or fears.

AREA OF USE

Aspen is used as the basic treatment for fears and phobias, general or unexplained anxiety, panic, horror, bizarre ideas, terrifying fantasies, and delusion in relationships. Used to treat all pathological conditions related to terrifying fantasies or unexplained fears. In daily life, used to treat general anxiety, strange feelings and premonitions, fear of the future, and fearful worries.

Causes and Symptoms of Aspen Syndrome

This condition is characterized by a well-developed sensitivity and an active imagination. Harmoniously developed, the Aspen type is a sensitive and sensible person who possesses a kind of sixth sense. Intuitively, she knows more than the average person and can often predict future events or developments or divine secret connections unnoticed by others. She pays attention to the signs that life offers, such as dreams and inspirations or unusual occurrences and miracles, and she can interpret their meanings with uncanny intuition and imagination. She goes through life with an almost sleepwalking kind of security. She knows no fear, and her deep-rooted sense of a higher power gives her the knowledge that we are all safe and fills her with an unshakable sense of optimism. When faced with problems, dangers, or suffering (which often happens, owing to her great sensitivity), she doesn't try to avoid them but uses them as opportunities to gaze ever deeper into the secret of her existence and to affirm her confidence in life and fate. Her life is an ongoing process of developing awareness, a relentless search for personal truth, and inspiring proof that we can have a fearless, instinctive trust in the natural order of things.

Unfavorably developed, the Aspen type is not able to deal with her feelings and inspirations and cannot translate them into intuitive knowledge or clear awareness. If her strong sensitivity becomes oversensitivity, it can create overwhelming, vague, nebulous fears that can be a never-ending source of torment.

This can sometimes lead to sudden panic attacks that rip her out of sleep or fall on her suddenly at work. Generally, the Aspen type will try to neutralize these vague fears and attempt to direct them to everyday occurrences. For example, she may suffer from an irrational fear of being mugged, the house burning down, a family member being involved in a serious accident, or someone wanting to hurt her. The worst is the uncertainty that is accompanied by a sense of helplessness. The Aspen syndrome can also be caused by exposure to toxic substances (such as drug use or abuse) or physical illness—for example, waking up in the middle of the night from heart palpitations, panic attacks through hormonal disruptions, or inexplicable anxieties due to a frail constitution.

The Effects of Aspen

Aspen is the essence of courage. It is effective against anxiety, foreboding, and vague and irrational fears and improves our ability to guide subconscious material into our consciousness, to deal sensibly with intuition, and to interpret anxieties and fears. Aspen can also help improve any physical conditions accompanied by anxiety, such as a frail constitution, sensitivity to changes in the weather, cardiac insufficiency, or hormonal imbalances. It should normally be combined with Mustard.

Psychotherapeutic Notes

The Aspen type has an especially sensitive, intuitive nature and can perceive much that stays hidden for most of us stuck in our daily grind. She resembles the artist who takes the material for her work out of the essential truths of life that are inaccessible to most of us. Unlike the artist, the Aspen type cannot always make sense of these intuitions or incorporate them in her life's art. She suffers from a deep-seated mistrust of life and is too sensitive to its painful experiences and lessons.

Her mistrust prevents her—mostly unconsciously—from concerning herself with perceptions or feelings, and this can result in mental and emotional burdens. These are components of her exceedingly rich emotional life and important messages shared from the deepest recesses of her unconscious. They cannot simply be pushed away but are constantly trying to rise up to consciousness and will become more and more unbearable and anxiety-ridden the more she tries to shake them out of her thoughts. She can, to some extent, try to keep them in check by projecting them onto concrete phenomena. For example, she might predict a certain accident or accuse someone of holding ill will against her. These worries cannot, however, be controlled so easily. They lurk like wild animals in the nether regions between the conscious and subconscious, and as soon as she relents in her watchfulness, they take the form of inexplicable, generalized anxieties. This is the central problem of the Aspen syndrome.

The Aspen type's fear shows that she has lost a part of her fundamental trust in life. This consists of an instinctive belief in a divine order and in the knowledge that despite so much pain and suffering, our world is inherently good. None of us can live without trust. We develop it in early childhood, when we are brought helpless into the world. Trust comes from the fundamental experience of being loved, especially by our parents. The knowledge that there is someone willing to make a place for us in the world, who will give us warmth and sustenance and is happy with our mere presence, is so basic and essential that it becomes forever ingrained into the psyche of a child. It is this knowledge that allows all children (animals and humans) to follow their parents with complete trust into an unknown life.

Receiving the benefits of parental care and attention (especially from the mother in a child's infancy) is an enduring element of the human psyche. Without it, we would not know the meaning of love, security, or well-being, and it is this that opens our eyes to the good and beautiful in life and, when we become adults, gives us the knowledge that a benevolent force or being ("God the Father") leads us through this life. People who have not developed this fundamental trust owing to a lack of parental love, or who have lost it as the result of too many negative experiences, find life to be nothing more than something that must be endured. Life no longer fills them with awe and a sense of adventure but seems only horrible and dangerous—a terrifying affair from which they always expect some sort of harm.

The Aspen type's fears can be overcome only by maintaining a positive, optimistic attitude. At best, an improvement in her relationship with her parents is necessary, perhaps through a conscious reexperiencing of the childlike feelings of trust and love (which do not necessarily need to be directed at the people the parents have become). What is most important is that the pleasant memories of childhood are awakened and that the happy feelings lying hidden in the memory are released. Even if we no longer know our parents, or if we hate them, we have all found some substitute (grandparents, relatives, neighbors, sometimes even animals or plants) that helps us survive and has reawakened our hope and touched our hearts. The more positive memories we have of the past, the more optimism we can expect from our attitude toward the future.

Artistic, religious, or spiritual influences are also helpful in allowing us to rekindle our fundamental trust in life. Eternal beauty, the incommunicable truth of a work of art, the compelling grandeur of a great idea, or the delightful humility of a good deed can restore our hope and contentment, and they help remind a person full of fears and anxieties that, in spite of all that he has suffered and cannot comprehend, there is also an unending source of good in this life.

Anyone suffering from the Aspen condition should try seriously to confront what he feels, perceives, or believes and attempt to build a trusting, hopeful attitude. Life is constantly offering us proof of the rightness of all we experience. It is up to us to sharpen our view of the truth and beauty and learn to nurture an inner voice that speaks to us out of our inner courage and trust.

Common Combinations with Other Essences

Agrimony (1/2): repression of anxieties or anxieties due to repression

Cherry Plum (2/6): sudden panic attacks or irrational behavior

Mimulus (2/20): total fear

Mustard (2/21): anxiety-ridden depression

Red Chestnut (2/25): generalized anxiety-related worries

Rock Rose (2/26): absolute panic

Rock Water (2/27): anxiety-induced self-abuse

Scleranthus (2/28): indecisiveness provoked by vague fears and anxieties

Star of Bethlehem (2/29): mental and emotional injuries due to anxieties; anxieties brought about by trauma

Water Violet (2/34): problems with human contact due to vague fears and anxieties

White Chestnut (2/35): mental block due to vague fears

3: Beech

Characteristics

Beech is for people with a deep-seated, unconscious intolerance disguised as an excessive sense of tolerance and empathy.

AREA OF USE

Beech is used as the basic treatment for excessive tolerance that serves as a compensation for and repression of a deep-seated intolerance; internalized, repressed intolerance (organic); allergies; denial of our own natural aversions and dislikes; and an inner conflict between emotional intolerance and intellectual tolerance. Used to treat all pathological conditions related to false, excessive tolerance, deeply rooted intolerance, or allergies. In daily life, used to treat allergies, a tendency to trivialize or gloss over problems, false empathy, exaggerated generosity, and aversions.

Causes and Symptoms of Beech Syndrome

Beech syndrome is characterized by an emotional intolerance at odds with intellectual tolerance. Harmoniously developed, the Beech type can accept his own natural aversions and dislikes but will not be ruled by them. He has an open, generous, tolerant spirit and can see the good in everything. If he judges something, which he is very capable of doing, he does so not frivolously or hastily but with the knowledge that there are "good" and "bad" sides to everything and that any judgment can only be relative. He tries to reject as little as possible and accept as much as he can. His sure instinct, great wisdom for life, and pronounced openness toward others allow him to find the best compromise between two conflicting choices in any situation. He is very popular because he is willing (within limits) to "live and let live" and he manages to find a positive element when others will only be able to judge and criticize.

Manifested negatively, the contradictory nature of his condition—on the one hand, the very individual, sensitive emotions that bring with them many dislikes and aversions and, on the other, an open spirit that understands and accepts everything—can lead to internal conflict. Essentially, there are two possibilities in this situation: either his inborn aversions begin to conflict with his mental and emotional openness and generosity, or (and this is the great problem with the Beech type) his tolerant nature compels him to be critical of his own intolerance. Because he possesses an open spirit and shies away from conflict, he would rather downplay or ignore his personal aversions, even when they are justified, than give up his often excessive tolerance. Better to be at odds with himself than with people around him. Thus he forces himself to see only the positive, even when it is obviously not appropriate. The Beech type irritates almost no one, understands nearly everyone, puts up with anything, and can always find a justification for everything that happens around him. Because this great facade of tolerance is merely an overcompensation for an equally strong inner intolerance and springs from a fear of conflict, it does not ring true. We never feel quite comfortable with his tolerant nature because we sense instinctively that something is not right, that he's not expressing himself freely, and that pressures and fears are motivating his behavior. Only those of us who are very superficial, insecure, or self-centered feel comfortable with someone who finds everything about us to be just fine.

The Effects of Beech

Beech is the essence of choice in promoting a natural balance between tolerance and intolerance. Since we normally think of tolerance as a positive quality, this condition is often difficult to understand. Some "good" qualities that we display outwardly serve above all to neutralize their "bad" counterparts, of which only we are aware. Beech is used to treat decidedly tolerant, generous, understanding, positive people but in reality works against their underlying, deep-seated, unconscious, and, one could say, inbred intolerance.

Beech should be used as a means of treating the mental and emotional constitution, especially for people who naturally have a minimal range of tolerance. It is also used for those who are in constant fear of stepping on someone's toes, who are never able to engage in conflict or to criticize, or who never allow themselves to have negative feelings. Beech is not used just for mental and emotional conditions but is also effective in treating allergies, which are a kind "cellular intolerance."

Psychotherapeutic Notes

In a nutshell, Beech syndrome is characterized by a falsely understood tolerance and a denial and repression of our own intolerance. Tolerance is the ability or willingness to accept something or someone, and it is normally thought of as a positive quality. We all find it agreeable to be tolerated, and we tend to tolerate only what is pleasant. Intolerance, on the other hand, is typically considered in negative terms: we find intolerant people unpleasant, and we try to protect ourselves from unpleasantness.

Tolerance and intolerance are important, meaningful principles in the natural world. In nature, everything exists in very exactly defined conditions—in so-called limits of tolerance. These can be external as well as internal phenomena (such as a physical structure, physiological reactions, and a psychic constitution) and have evolved to ensure that each living thing has the best possible chances for survival. In certain circumstances, these tolerance limits can be so drastically altered that specific conditions or influences, which were previously useful or tolerable, suddenly become harmful or intolerable. We can even develop an intolerance to ourselves rather than toward the outside world, as, for example, when our organism has an allergic reaction to its own cells or when we develop self-destructive tendencies.

The Beech type's central problem lies in this perversion of the relationship between tolerance and intolerance. He rejects—even if, to some extent, unconsciously—his own protective intolerance and aversions and develops an unnatural and unwarranted tolerance toward all shortcomings and negativity in his environment and the people around him. If this attitude were dependent on self-awareness and wisdom, it would be very possible to overcome our own small-minded intolerance through the conscious practice of generosity. The Beech type is acting unconsciously, however, out of personal weakness, a shortage of self-esteem, and moral pressures. And while these qualities are all very endearing, they are of little value. They serve only to create confusion and stunt our personal growth and development.

While many of us feel a certain amount of alienation toward ourselves, we all seek an inner truth. Such a contradiction places the Beech type in a constant and profound state of discontent. He feels intuitively that something is wrong, and his body tells him in the form of an allergic reaction that his balance of tolerance and intolerance is out of whack. He must recognize clearly that his own natural dislikes and aversions, which he constantly displaces with an excessive and false sense of tolerance, are essential conditions of his personal self-realization. Only then can he avoid the people or situations that are not good for him and proceed more confidently on his way in life. His relationships will also become more clear and honest; he will take each person as he or she really is and attribute to no one qualities that really don't exist.

Common Combinations with Other Essences

Agrimony (1/3): false friendliness and tolerance

Heather (3/14): opportunistic tolerance

Holly (3/15): allergic shock reaction

Larch (3/19): tolerance stemming from a lack of self-confidence

Mimulus (3/20): tolerance provoked by fear

Pine (3/24): tolerance on moral grounds

Rock Water (3/27): generosity with others and stinginess with oneself

Vine (3/32): total intolerance

Water Violet (3/34): distant, yet excessively tolerant and accepting

4: Centaury
Characteristics

Centaury is for people who are excessively cheerful or for obsequious people who allow themselves to be used too often.

AREA OF USE

Centaury is used to treat weak personality, lack of self-assertiveness, servility, dependence, fretful selflessness, self-deception, or self-deprivation. Used to treat all conditions related to pathological cheerfulness or servility. In daily life, used to treat shyness, excessive cheerfulness, or excessive willingness to accommodate the needs of others.

Causes and Symptoms of Centaury Syndrome

This condition is characterized by an excessive tendency to devote oneself to others and a pronounced sense of altruism. Harmoniously developed, the Centaury type is an altruistic, cheerful, empathic human being. Because he can sense if others are happy, and his own happiness is dependent on the well-being of others, he is always ready to serve others or be of assistance in times of difficulty. His behavior entails what is often meant by the best sense of the word *selflessness,* and because it is so natural and guileless, it is taken advantage of not just by others but also by the Centaury person himself: in his selflessness he gives full expression to his devotion, follows his inner purpose in life, and finds self-realization. This self-realization is an essential component for a fulfilling, happy life and includes developing and making full use of all of our talents and possibilities.

The well-developed Centaury type serves others without being a servant, helps himself by helping others, and is selfless in order to fulfill the needs of his self. The love his behavior inspires is increased all the more because he gives of himself so freely and with no strings attached. Unfavorably developed, the Centaury selflessness can lead to a loss of self, and his sense of devotion can result in a sense of resignation. His good-natured service serves no good and helps create inhumane relationships marked by thoughtless exploitation: the Centaury type simply allows himself to be used.

Sick Centaury types have no strength for self-assertiveness and fulfill with devotion all wishes or orders that are imposed on them. They become weak, frustrated, or depressed and are unable to lead their own meaningful, independent lives. They are like animals whose will has been broken, and their goal in life is to be used and abused. It often happens that they waste their lives in self-sacrifice, caring for egotistical, thoughtless family members, or that they are used by institutions or are subjugated by anyone who appears to wield some kind of authority.

As pure as this behavior may seem, and as pleasant as it can be for anyone who enjoys living off others, it is very damaging to the Centaury type himself. On the surface, it makes it easier for him to give in to his pathological compulsions, but in the deepest recesses of his being, it can create an inability to address his own legitimate needs and develop his own personality, which in turn leads to discontentment and depression.

The false morality that he commonly calls upon to replace his lost happiness can do nothing to rectify the situation. Seemingly pleasant, ready to be exploited, and never daring to undertake self-realization, he resembles a plant growing in an unfavorable location—which is also the result of his existing weakness or disrupted development. The weak or totally broken personality, the general lack of strength, and the fundamental absence of joy and happiness show that something is not right and that a force is working counter to life's basic principles of growth and development. It is common for people in the company of a typical Centaury person to feel sympathy at most, but never joy.

The Effects of Centaury

Centaury is the essence of choice in treating self-resignation and pathological denial. It restores personal strength and promotes consciousness, the awareness of self-worth, and a sense that we have the right to lead our own lives. Centaury should be given to dependent, shy, or excessively cheerful people—especially children. It enables them to claim their rightful place in society. It is often used in family therapy for relationships that are dependent or exploitative. Centaury promotes the sexual development of children with colorless personalities and can also be useful in treating spinal problems of servile individuals.

Psychotherapeutic Notes

The natural ability of Centaury types to devote themselves to others, combined with their selflessness, makes it difficult for them to oppose the demands placed on them by others. They just can't say no. For any acquisitive, demanding person, the Centaury is easy prey. Sensitive, altruistic children are often turned into slaves at an early age by egocentric, arbitrary parents or guardians. These children hardly dare to have their own wishes and needs, let alone to express them. In order to survive, they learn to defer to the wishes, needs, and demands of others while rewarding themselves very little, if at all. This behavior will become second nature as the child matures and will not allow him to develop his own personality. Even his environment will allow him no opportunity, since every human relationship has some kind of influence on us. As R. Wilhelm wrote in the I Ching, "Truthfulness against subversive elements is dangerous. Even the best of men allow themselves to come in contact with dangerous elements. Once we allow ourselves this contact, the subversive influence works, slowly but surely, and drags its dangers along with it." When we behave badly, it provokes in those around us a sort of behavior that is equally negative. Surprisingly, this is also the case with the typical, seemingly exemplary, Centaury behavior. Just as a victim's fear inspires aggressiveness in one who preys on others, the Centaury's unnaturally compulsive and passive behavior provokes an opposite need to dominate. Anyone who has ever had any contact with a Centaury type has come to expect the Centaury's automatic good-humored tractability, selfless need to accommodate, and inability to look after his own needs and desires.

This pathological element does not entirely consist of putting his own interests on the back burner to be helpful to others but stems from an unreflective, inner compulsion. The good-natured, selfless, self-sacrificing behavior is the expression of a neurosis brought about by the life-threatening pressure of an overpowering environment and is put into practice mechanically and without any conscious positive motivation. It is of utmost importance for the "thin-skinned," sensitive, and harmony-seeking Centaury type to remain on good terms with his environment. His behavior is not the spontaneous "innocent" expression of his constitution but its distorted image, which has developed out of negative pressures. These consist not just of people with whom he comes in contact but also the mental and cultural milieu into which he is born—above all, Christian morality, which is based on guilt, renunciation, and self-denial.

According to the Christian ideal, we live to serve our neighbors. If our own needs and desires are not compatible with this view, they should be repressed or eliminated. These demands are essentially part of an unrealizable theory that runs contrary to the laws of nature (and, by the way, are hardly practiced by the Church itself), but such views are so deeply ingrained in anyone brought up in a Christian environment that we find even the smallest amount of self-realization accompanied by guilt feelings.

The good Christian develops a guilty conscience if things are going well for him and seeks immediately to atone for his happiness by replacing it with the bitter poison of the suffering of others. Absurdly, he believes that the world will be a better place if he suffers with others: suffering shared is suffering halved. In truth, however, shared suffering is suffering doubled, because two must suffer instead of one.

The tragic thing about this situation is that a totally just and decent principle is being perverted. Naturally, it is beautiful and humane to want to increase happiness and diminish suffering in the world, but we cannot achieve it by taking on a part of the suffering for ourselves. In fact, the opposite is true: we add our own voluntary suffering to the suffering of others. A Christian upbringing denies people the fundamental knowledge that only joy and happiness can create more happiness and only when we are happy ourselves can we begin to make others happy. In trying to follow a good impulse, we take the wrong path; instead of being healers, we become false healers.

The Centaury type places himself at the service of others not so much out of a personal, spontaneous, responsible motivation but rather out of a pathological inner compulsion and a dishonest self-deception. He is not happy and strong when he is serving others at sacrifice to himself, but instead frustrated in the very depths of his soul. It's as if an iron band were constricting his heart. He knows that he needs a life of his own, and yet his heart provokes in him a negative inner voice that compels him to sacrifice his own life and deny himself happiness.

It is extremely important to take note of this spiritual crippling. The Centaury should recognize that his behavior, far from being the expression of high moral character that he has been told and believes it to be, is merely the pathological result of a suppressed personality. Moreover, he caves in to the thoughtless, selfish demands of others. He must understand that he has a right to his own life and that to whatever end his nobler, kinder tendencies drive him, he can accomplish what he needs only with his entire "egotistical" self intact.

If he learns to recognize his own needs, if he can live according to his own sense of morality and not cave in to the pressures and dogma of others, he will know what to do. One time he may refuse to help someone in need, even if that person is suffering, and another time he will place himself selflessly at the service of another, not thinking of any advantage for himself. Then he will know that he is responsible for himself and not for the rest of the world. Once we follow our inner call to selflessly stand by another, it is not simply self-resignation but a joyous fulfillment of the self.

Common Combinations with Other Essences

Agrimony (1/4): pathological good-natured behavior
Cerato (4/5): dependence due to a weak personality
Chicory (4/8): selfish self-sacrifice
Gentian (4/12): weakness of the personality and will
Gorse (4/13): compliance and tractability due to hopelessness
Hornbeam (4/17): feelings of stress and overwork due to dependence
Larch (4/19): readiness to help from an inferiority complex
Mimulus (4/20): obsequiousness due to fear
Pine (4/24): self-sacrifice due to guilt
Red Chestnut (4/25): worried, anxious selflessness
Walnut (4/33): dependent and easily influenced
Wild Rose (4/37): resignation from a weak personality

5: Cerato
Characteristics

Cerato is for insecure people who do not know how to do things and constantly seek the advice and counsel of others.

AREA OF USE
Cerato is used for the basic treatment of underdeveloped self-confidence, insecurity, lack of independence, dependence, and lack of instinct. Used to treat all pathological conditions related to insecurity, helplessness, or a lack of self-confidence.

Causes and Symptoms of Cerato Syndrome

The condition is characterized by the wish to make everything right and—because of a lack of self-esteem—the need to be dominated by others. Harmoniously developed, the Cerato type places high demands on herself and is always concerned with doing the right thing. She enjoys the good favor of her friends, superiors, and guardians. She is very conscientious and undertakes nothing without having studied and checked it thoroughly; she seldom makes mistakes. If she should err, no one can find fault with her because no one could have done the job better. She also has the ability to fit into any existing power structure without rocking the boat. She is attentive and has a sure instinct for not upsetting the status quo and for fulfilling the expectations of those in power. If she has religious tendencies, her higher spiritual values are an important part of her personality.

Negatively developed, the desire to make everything right can lead to a strong sense of insecurity. The Cerato type doesn't know what she should do, doesn't trust her opinions and instinct, always asks for advice, allows herself to be sent on wild goose chases, does everything halfheartedly, and loses her self-confidence by degrees. In this condition she has lost her mental and emotional orientation. Instead of following her inner voice and intuition, she hooks up with stronger, more self-confident people and refuses to take herself seriously. She is deeply frustrated because she doesn't feel that she is capable of mature judgment and because she must learn again and again (the hard way) that she's been following advice that runs counter to what she believes and that takes her down the wrong path.

The Effects of Cerato

Cerato is the essence of choice to treat insecurity. It improves our relationship with our "inner voice" and allows us to trust our own opinion, so that we can do what we really want. Cerato promotes the maturing process and mental and emotional independence in people (especially children) who, instead of solving problems by themselves, immediately seek the help and advice of others. It improves our ability to distinguish between good and bad as well as right and wrong.

Psychotherapeutic Notes

The basic motivation of the Cerato person is the desire to always do the right thing. Her problem is that she doesn't know what the right thing is, and the mistake she often makes is that she believes that others *do* know and can tell her. Instead of listening to herself and trusting her own judgment, she asks everyone around her what she should do, and then becomes frustrated when she realizes that she has followed the wrong advice.

How else could it be? The "right thing" (or the "truth") is not a universal fact that we can learn from others. It is a totally personal phenomenon that we can perceive only by listening to our inner voice, which constantly tries to guide us down the path that is right for us. The Cerato type, however, does not trust this inner voice. She is easily influenced and wants to be liked. The good thing about her disposition is that everyone likes her; she has no enemies. But her disadvantage is that she loses her sense of proportion and, in the end, has no idea how to act.

A so-called normal upbringing that teaches us to uphold the status quo and discourages us from asserting our individuality only accentuates these tendencies. Even the smallest child must learn to sacrifice her own personal needs to those of the general good and replace her own values with someone else's. To add to the problem, Christian morality (which propagates a belief in self-denial and in our inherent guilt and brands us all as moral scoundrels) instills in her such a profound self-doubt that she can hardly dare to find good in anything that makes her happy, let alone avoid those things that make her suffer.

Despite her need for the goodwill of those around her, however, the Cerato person possesses a well-developed sense of individuality that, to a certain extent, allows her to follow her own path and puts her in conflict with what is thought to be normal and expected of her. Thus, she is often insecure and dares to do what she wants only when she is encouraged to do so, but this happens very seldom. Generally she is thwarted in her wishes, and her insecurity causes her to follow what she believes to be the best advice (which, more often than not, turns out to be the worst).

At heart, Cerato types are seekers of the truth. Their only mistake is that they look for it in the wrong place—in other people instead of in themselves. They need to trust in their own feelings, intuition, and instinct and should always make it clear to themselves that "good" and "right" are merely relative terms and make sense only if we consider them in relation to ourselves. The decisive question of our lives is not "How do I do the right thing?" or "What is the absolute right?" but "What is right for me, and how do I find it?" The more closely we pay attention to the things that speak to our bodies and souls in the form of happiness and sadness, the more clearly we will recognize the truth when it comes to us.

Receiving advice is useful only as a last resort and when we know where to look for it. Cerato types, however, tend to seek advice without really needing it and without ascertaining whether the person giving the advice is competent to do so. It is better to try to overcome this habit and risk failure. Our own mistakes are especially instructive, because they speak to both our reason and our emotions. Furthermore, we build character when we learn from our mistakes, but suffering the consequences of bad advice inflicted on us by other people is merely frustrating.

It is noteworthy that in the vicinity of the Cerato person, you will often find her opposite—the notorious know-it-all (the Vervain or Vine type), who loves to become involved in other people's lives. Their advice (well intended, of course) is harmful to the Cerato type because it strengthens her inability to listen to her instinct or insight. Cerato types who are constantly asking for advice should, whenever possible, refuse to listen to it. This will encourage them to learn from their own mistakes. "What doesn't kill us can only make us stronger!"

Common Combinations with Other Essences

Centaury (4/5): dependence due to a weak personality

Chestnut Bud (5/7): helplessness due to carelessness and inattentiveness

Larch (5/19): insecurity due to feelings of inferiority

Mimulus (5/20): anxious insecurity

Pine (5/24): insecurity stemming from guilt

Rock Water (5/27): mental dependence and self-abuse

Scleranthus (5/28): insecurity and indecisiveness

Star of Bethlehem (5/29): insecurity due to a shocking experience

Walnut (5/33): insecurity that leads one to be easily influenced

Wild Oat (5/36): insecurity due to the lack of a worldview

6: Cherry Plum
Characteristics

Cherry Plum is used to treat people who are in danger of committing irrational acts or of losing their reason.

AREA OF USE

Cherry Plum is used for the treatment of mental or emotional pressure, obsessive behavior, hysteria, suicidal tendencies, and irrational actions. Used to treat all pathological conditions related to hysteria, obsession, or psychotic behavior. In daily life, used to treat hysterical conduct, being too tightly "wound up," uncontrollable emotions, and emotional problems.

Causes and Symptoms of Cherry Plum Syndrome

This condition is characterized by compulsive, imaginative emotions on the one hand and a disciplined sense of reason on the other. Harmoniously developed, the Cherry Plum type is an internally rich, resourceful person whose emotions and reason work together very well. He feels first, then thinks, and then acts. Because he understands his emotions, drives, motivations, and feelings, they do not lead him to hysteria or destructive behavior but manifest themselves in a distinctively creative manner and a rich, lively life. Anything the Cherry Plum type undertakes is always characterized by deep, lively emotions and a clear mind. In this he can be compared to the prudent operator of a dam, who oversees the transformation of a torrent into electricity and, by diverting the flow in times of high water, ensures that the dam doesn't break.

Unfavorably developed, the contradictory nature of the Cherry Plum type can lead to a conflict between reason and its opposite, between letting go and staying in control, instead of living a merely creative, lively life. In addition, moral or rational pressures can prevent him from giving full expression to his feelings, emotions, and drives in a sensible, yet vibrant manner. The pressure from these tormenting inner struggles can build up dangerously, like the steam in a kettle, creating a highly explosive psychotic potential that threatens the mental balance. Thus, the Cherry Plum type can face a total breakdown.

People in this condition feel a catastrophe looming ominously ahead and fear (justifiably) that their sense of reason is about to explode. When these psychic pressures pile up uncontrollably, Cherry types believe they have to do something drastic, such as make a fool of themselves, break societal rules or deep-seated taboos, or even attempt suicide or run amok. As these mental and emotional torments continue to increase and a liberating/destructive eruption approaches, the Cherry Plum types strengthen their defenses. Sometimes they can seek help in time or find a way out of danger themselves. Often, however—especially when they lead relatively unenlightened lives—they will be so dominated by the approaching breakdown that they are no longer open to good advice and seem obsessive to anyone who observes them. One has the feeling that they will fall apart at any minute.

The Effects of Cherry Plum

Cherry Plum is the essence we use to treat the buildup of excessive psychic pressure. It can minimize internal tension in emotionally charged situations or prevent psychoses. Cherry Plum works to resolve internal conflicts by reducing moral or rational pressures and the intensity of emotions and compulsions. It is always helpful when the Cherry Plum type is in danger of losing his reason because of some emotionally charged situation, when he can no longer control his feelings, or when he is capable of doing something he really doesn't want to do and may later live to regret. In such cases, Cherry Plum should be taken frequently and, if it does not achieve adequate results, should be tried in stronger potencies.

Psychotherapeutic Notes

As children of an age predominantly characterized by reason, we often tend to emphasize our rational faculties and downplay our emotions, feelings, and drives. Since these emotions (and not logic and reason) are really the things that guide our lives and provide our motivations, there arises an inner conflict that becomes more serious the more personally important the suppressed compulsions and drives are. This is the problem of the Cherry Plum type, who tends to be very tightly wound. On the one hand, he possesses a finely developed sense of reason and, on the other, a strong emotional intensity.

Under the influence of an upbringing that places order over happiness and reason over emotions, he can consistently downplay every motivation and drive that serves to lead to his self-fulfillment: his sexuality, his acquisitiveness and desire for power, and his need for freedom. These drives, however, are very strong in the Cherry Plum type and are so fundamental and powerful that when they are suppressed, the result is a dangerous inner pressure that, in unfavorable conditions (especially additional emotional setbacks), can break down the control of reason like a raging stream crashing through a dam and destroy a healthy mental and emotional balance. It can also lead to hysteria, deterioration of awareness, or psychosis.

The goal of therapy for Cherry Plum types should be to loosen the control of reason while making clear that he is entitled to experience and give full expression to his emotions, feelings, and impulses. The most important thing is that he learn to distinguish between his own morality and that which is imposed on him by others. Once he learns to make this distinction, he will be able to shape his own life as it best suits him. In the end, we are all ultimately responsible for ourselves, and our own true morality does not always jibe with popular opinion.

When we find ourselves under strong emotional pressure, we must find a way to let off steam. Cherry Plum types do this instinctively for the most part. From time to time, they can go a little bit crazy, have attacks of hysteria, or fits of rage or crying. These fits provide them with some relief and will continue to do so until the next crisis arises, but they certainly do not serve as a cure. For a cure, a change of the basic makeup is necessary. This means either a breakdown of rational control or a reduction of emotional impulses. Such fundamental changes happen very seldom, however, which is why Cherry Plum types remain temperamental individuals. Once they become conscious of their inborn conflict between emotions and intellect, however, they can achieve a certain amount of stability and begin to build a self-concept that integrates both components. They must always keep in mind the needs of mental and emotional independence and their own sense of morality and be ever on guard for disruptions of the inner balance and able to take timely action to restore that balance.

The emotional life of the Cherry Plum person is like an effusive, bubbly spring that floods everything if it can't find a sufficient outlet. Cherry Plum people should be aware of the need for an artistic outlet to allow for expression of their emotions and avoid an inner mental and emotional blockage. Sometimes they can see themselves through an impending crisis by expressing an unclear inner impulse or an inexplicable tension in a work of art that serves as a key to resolving their fundamental conflict.

Common Combinations with Other Essences

Agrimony (1/6): displacement causing dangerous psychic pressure

Aspen (2/6): sudden anxiety with a danger of irrational behavior

Elm (6/11): at the end of psychic and physical resilience

Holly (6/15): uncontrollable fits of rage

Impatiens (6/18): prepsychotic restlessness

Mimulus (6/20): serious anxiety conflicts

Oak (6/22): overwork resulting in reaching the emotional breaking point

Red Chestnut (6/25): rage due to excessive worries

Rock Water (6/27): psychosis as a result of self-imposed pressures

Star of Bethlehem (6/29): psychosis as a result of mental and emotional injury

Sweet Chestnut (6/30): despair caused by emotional stress

White Chestnut (6/35): mental obsession

7: Chestnut Bud
Characteristics

Chestnut Bud is for people who have difficulties learning or who continually make the same mistakes.

AREA OF USE
Chestnut Bud is used to treat learning difficulties, undeveloped awareness, and all pathological conditions related to carelessness, learning disabilities, or pathological distracted and absentminded behavior. In daily life, used to treat carelessness and absentmindedness.

Causes and Symptoms of Chestnut Bud Syndrome

This condition is characterized by a serious inability to concentrate or to become engaged in activities. Harmoniously developed, the Chestnut Bud type is completely engaged in her experiences and activities and learns valuable lessons from them. Life is a constant learning process that broadens her intellectual horizons and helps her mature. All this is possible only when she doesn't get bogged down in trivial details and tangents but always concentrates on the important aspects of the task at hand. Because she is uniquely predisposed or possesses special talents, many things that are important to others have virtually no meaning for her. She hardly acknowledges these things, even if they can bring her great advantage or fortune. She chooses the path that is right for her, and engages herself only with those things that make her happy. Even in school, she will excel in those subjects that engage and interest her. Some Chestnut Bud types become great scholars or sought-after experts in a unique and valuable field and don't seem to mind that they lack knowledge in fields outside their own.

Unfavorably developed, this ability to concentrate so intensely on one specialized area can lead to losing interest in other facets of life. The Chestnut Bud type will be inattentive to reality and unable to benefit from her experiences. She will not learn from her mistakes but will make them again and again and will often find herself stuck repeatedly in the same situations. Chestnut types are often plagued with learning difficulties: she simply cannot learn from life. Or she will be unable to take notice of many things, such as certain information or an everyday event, even though she might come across them time after time; she seems to have a kind of mental block that keeps certain things from registering. Her personality is unable to develop sufficiently, she gains no experience or wisdom, and, in some respects, she remains childlike, clumsy, and undeveloped. A well-known variety of the Chestnut Bud syndrome type is the "absentminded professor": she is a master in her area of expertise but a failure in the simplest life situations, and she repeats the same laughable mistakes again and again. By concentrating her energies so intently on complex problems, she has nothing left over for the banalities of everyday life. This is often a characteristic of students with special talents: they excel in what they know but fail miserably at everything else.

The Effects of Chestnut Bud

Chestnut Bud is the essence for mental maturity and experience. It improves our ability to learn, not in connection with specialized knowledge but in general areas. It helps us remember and learn from our experiences and cope with life in general. Our spirit is more open, we are more ready and able to take things in, and our interest in things outside our narrow area of expertise increases. Chestnut Bud is for children with difficulties in school as well as for people who are not making enough progress in their lives and find themselves always dealing unsuccessfully with the same problems. Naturally, any organic conditions that can accompany Chestnut Bud syndrome, such as vitamin deficiencies or chronic exhaustion, must be treated appropriately.

Psychotherapeutic Notes

The learning difficulties of the Chestnut Bud syndrome are mainly determined by a very self-centered personality. The Chestnut Bud type is interested only in those things that concern her personally or speak to her special talents or tendencies. General, theoretical knowledge or impersonal facts are virtually meaningless to her, and she ignores them for the most part. It is very difficult for her to occupy herself with anything with which she does not have a personal relationship. Her learning difficulty is not so much pathological as extremely characteristic of her personality.

Learning is a very subjective process. We retain what seems important to us and toss aside all other information, impressions, and insights that flow into our mind and awareness. The ideal subject matter is anything that has meaning for us and that speaks to our emotions. Lifeless, meaningless knowledge that is incessantly hammered in and learned by rote is, at best, only useful in preparing us for an automated, spiritless occupation. Such lifeless learning is also harmful because it leads to a bloodless life without emotions.

Theoretically, if the Chestnut Bud type learns properly, she retains only those things that touch and interest her personally. Her problem is only that while she has significant interest in one particular topic, the rest (the stuff that most of our lives are made of) does not receive sufficient attention. Often the cause is that such a person has been raised in a milieu that is intellectually too narrow, or that she has negative experiences associated with learning; in this situation her spirit will become flat and one-dimensional. This is especially common with children; often an unpleasant teacher or a frustrating failure will cause the psyche to close itself off to the events and attempt to repress the memories. Learning must be enjoyable if it is to make sense and be successful. We fight against anything taught to us in an unpleasant manner, and our teachers too often respond by trying to hammer things into us, often with little success.

The first objective of Chestnut Bud treatment is the fostering of intellectual openness, the broadening of general interests, and an increasing overall awareness and attentiveness. In addition, we attempt to understand the emotional memories that cause this mental block or replace them with happier memories (of success, for example). Children who are having difficulties in school sometimes simply need a change of subject matter, the learning process, the teacher, or the school in order to remember how to enjoy learning. Adults who are not successful in their work or who encounter the same problems over and over again should ask themselves if there might not be something better for them or if the conditions in which they are living and working are right for them.

Common Combinations with Other Essences

Agrimony (1/7): learning difficulties or immaturity due to shirking

Cerato (5/7): helplessness due to inattentiveness

Clematis (7/9): carelessness from daydreaming

Gentian (7/12): lack of attentiveness leading to a relapse

Honeysuckle (7/16): carelessness caused by nostalgic daydreams

Scleranthus (7/28): distraction leading to learning difficulties

Water Violet (7/34): closed-mindedness

White Chestnut (7/35): carelessness caused by persistent distracting thoughts

Wild Oat (7/36): lack of a clear concept of life due to carelessness

Wild Rose (7/37): careless resignation

8: Chicory

Characteristics

Chicory is the treatment for greedy people who sacrifice themselves for others in order to get affection and cling to them.

AREA OF USE

Chicory is used as a basic treatment for conditional love and attention, an excessive need for emotional relationships, egotism, excessive greed, selfish self-sacrifice, a tendency toward inflicting emotional tyranny and terror on others, and exaggerated sympathy and self-pity. Used to treat all pathological conditions related to an unusually strong need for love or self-pity. In daily life, used to treat excessive (insincere) caring for others, mothering, helpless child feelings, excessive devotion, selfish jealousy, readiness to take offense, and self-pity.

Causes and Symptoms of Chicory Syndrome

This syndrome is characterized by the need for intense emotional relationships, the joy of helping and caring for others, and great personal strength. Harmoniously developed, the Chicory type is warmhearted and full of life and has a strong need to help other people. In caring for those he loves, he can use his great strength and satisfy his need for intensive emotional relationships. As long as he takes a personal interest in the well-being of those around him, he remains internally lively and content. He stands by the people close to him, takes care of them, takes on their problems, and tries to cheer them up and make their lives easier. Since he invests a lot of himself in everything he does, he gets something out of the relationship as well. As long as he can make someone happy, he will be just as happy, and when he is able to ease someone else's pain, he, too, is free from the pain that he feels just as deeply. What makes his kind of love and caring so special is not just his open, friendly, easygoing spirit but also his sensitivity and need to be happy. He makes sure that he does not arbitrarily force his good deeds upon anyone or live a life of self-sacrifice and self-denial but that his help is given in a way that will benefit all parties. His behavior is distinguished by a very life-affirming, idealistic form of love that makes both the giver and the receiver happy. He helps others to help himself, gives others joy and feels joy himself, and shows compassion in order to receive it: in short, he loves and is loved in return.

Unfavorably developed, on the other hand, the Chicory type loses sight of his limits and instead of an innocent kind of helping and attention, he offers his love with strings attached. He still looks after those he loves and offers them affection, help, or self-sacrifice, but he expects that they will return in kind. He demands that they be thankful, be always at his disposal, and basically be willing to give up living their own lives. On the surface, the Chicory type appears to love intensively, but in reality he's very selfish and wants to make others dependent on him and exploit their feelings. Anyone who is on the receiving end of the typical Chicory type's conditional "affection" learns very quickly that she must pay for it in the form of an intense connection, obligation, and gratitude. If she tries to free herself, she will be treated to an exhibition of reproaches, insulted behavior, threats of the withdrawal of love, and self-pity.

What should be a natural need for emotional relationships is transformed into a sorrowful obsession. Instead of helping joyfully, and giving selflessly (which is his nature), the Chicory type loves conditionally and shows an attentiveness that makes the object of his affection dependent, afraid, and needing more. Naturally, this behavior is not always so blatant, but this egotistical addiction to relationships and attachments is more common than we might think and only gets stronger when it goes unsatisfied. It leads to excessive self-sacrifice, pity or self-pity, emotional blackmailing, or base jealousy. Any sort of lightness or unconditional love is lost. Typically, we see this syndrome at work in the overbearing mother who makes her children dependent and unable to cope with life by showering them with excessive attention and constantly fussing over them; in children who have a constant, insatiable need for proof that they are loved; or in selfish spouses who dominate the object of their "love" and cause them to be dependent.

The Effects of Chicory

Chicory is the essence for true love. It helps restore human relationships by breaking down pathological egotism, emotional dependence, emotional terror and blackmail, and self-pity and fosters the ability to exist in a free, loving relationship. It is an important essence for treating partners and is often used in healing neurotic parent-child relationships.

Psychotherapeutic Notes

The salient characteristic of the Chicory type is a strong need for love. Because the Chicory type has great personal strength, it often happens that he puts his partner in the passive role of a taker. When he gives and receives love freely, he's happy. In spite of his generous nature, the Chicory person is by no means a selfless, self-denying individual but has a natural form of egotism. A musician feels pleasure when she is able to produce a beautiful sound with her instrument, and the harmoniously developed Chicory type takes great pleasure in making other people happy.

With a pathological manifestation of the Chicory syndrome, however, this is not the case. In thinking too much of his own benefit, the Chicory type has lost touch with what it means for two hearts to be united. He loses his liberating sense of generosity and exchanges love in a kind of transaction in which each instance of giving is offered with a demand for repayment. He works tirelessly for his love and takes care of him or her, but he demands a high price in return: the object of his love must show gratitude and forever be in his service.

His motive is the perfectly understandable desire for love, but he forgets that love is a matter of the heart and can exist only if it is given joyously, unselfishly, and unconditionally. It cannot be bought, sold, earned, or forced upon someone. Above all, it must awaken within us before we can encounter it outside us, and we can find only what we carry within us; doing and experiencing are expressions of being and feeling. We are mistaken when we think that love depends upon external conditions. Love is an expression of the spirit, a feeling that begins within and is projected outward. Only when we are full of love in ourselves can we shower love on those around us, and if we are not ready to love ourselves, we are deaf and blind to it.

If we are not loved, we cannot love, and if we feel unloved, we cannot see the love that exists around us in multifarious forms. It is life—the great, divine entity—but it reveals itself to us where and how it wants, not where and how *we* want. When we think that love must take this form or that and be related to this or that person or situation, and when we try to tie it down with preconceptions, conditions, or demands, it leaves us and appears transformed as sorrow to make us aware of our mistakes.

In Chicory syndrome, we think that we can earn love by doing good deeds or that we can force it through psychological terror. If this doesn't work, we react with pity or self-pity, passivity or helplessness, or self-sacrifice or emotional blackmail or by being offended, hurt, jealous. When we recognize these symptoms in ourselves (we all have a little bit of Chicory in our blood), we should be attentive and recognize them as signs of an internal disruption. We need only look in the mirror that those who love us hold up to us; our love is only beneficial when the objects of our love can come to us freely and are free to go when they wish.

Parents who believe that their children don't want to be seen with them should immediately start looking for the fault in themselves, instead of making accusations. No child leaves parents who love them and treat them well. It is always the parents who drive their children out of the house, by giving love only under certain conditions or by spoiling their children's lives by scolding, bellyaching, or dominating them. Children who become emotional tyrants and have an insatiable demand for attention are often the victims of a Chicory mentality. At best, these children can become free only when and if their parents change or if they cut off all contact with them.

Common Combinations with Other Essences

Centaury (4/8): selfish self-sacrifice
Heather (8/14): an addiction to loving and being loved
Holly (8/15): hate-love
Honeysuckle (8/16): sadness due to the loss of love
Mimulus (8/20): anxious clinging
Mustard (8/21): depression caused by unrequited love
Oak (8/22): overbearing attention and love
Red Chestnut (8/25): total self-sacrifice
White Chestnut (8/35): obsession with love
Willow (8/38): bitterness caused by rejection or ingratitude

9: Clematis

Characteristics

Clematis is for people who are susceptible to fantasies and daydreams and who lose their grip on reality.

AREA OF USE

Clematis is used as the basic treatment for a disjointed relationship to reality, daydreaming, uncritical optimism, illusions and fantasies, deteriorating consciousness, a tendency to fainting or unconsciousness, or the wish to die. Used to treat all pathological conditions related to absentmindedness or unconsciousness. In daily life, used to treat inattentiveness, sleepiness, and a susceptibility to fainting.

Causes and Symptoms of Clematis Syndrome

This syndrome is characterized by a visionary imagination, a strong need for happiness, and a general sense of optimism. Harmoniously developed, the Clematis type has a rich inner life. She takes emotions and intuition just as seriously as reason and logic. She understands how to shape a happy reality from her inspirations, dreams, and longings and can give them a sensible form in her clearheaded manner. She is perceptive and possesses a visionary talent that often enables her (as an artist, scientist, or philosopher) to predict future developments, to recognize connections between events, or to develop futuristic ideas. She is introverted and often seems a stranger to the world or a dreamer, but because of her optimism, she is often considered a transforming symbol of hope. She often gets along well in life and it frequently seems that she has a sixth sense for solving problems, but when her problems seem too great to overcome, she retreats into herself and waits patiently for better times.

Unfavorably developed—which is to say, in the case of sobering life conditions or mental and emotional strain—her intuitive, optimistic, emotional outlook can become fantasy-filled daydreaming and flight from reality. She increasingly loses her interest in everyday life and becomes inattentive, distracted, or eccentric. She begins to neglect herself and her obligations and to flee unpleasant reality in favor of a more pleasant fantasy world, to dream of a better future life, or even, if she is very unhappy, to yearn for redemption in death. She can also develop a tendency or inclination to fainting or losing consciousness. The lighter, less serious form of Clematis syndrome consists of the inability to concentrate on the here and now because the thoughts are always on vacation. While the Clematis type constantly has wonderful and interesting ideas, projects, or fantasies in mind, she is also unable to deal with practical matters that need attention. In severe cases, this syndrome is the culprit in children who make a cocoon out of their imagination and cannot develop a connection with real life, in romantic dreamers who think constantly of finding their great love, or in anyone who lives in a fantasy world. One will also find in this category the compulsive gambler who is always waiting for the next big jackpot, the religious zealot who is a stranger to life and lives in the hereafter, as well as the drug or alcohol addict who tries to substitute pleasant hallucinations for a frustrating and unsatisfying reality. These are all variations of the Clematis syndrome.

The Effects of Clematis

Clematis is the essence for a healthy relationship to reality. It addresses a tendency to distance oneself from reality and is appropriate not just in the case of severe daydreaming, fantasies, or even drug addiction but also for general carelessness, absentmindedness, or sleepiness. A susceptibility to fainting or unconsciousness is also an indication of trying to hide from reality. Clematis is a component of Rescue Remedy. Children with problems in school often need Clematis, especially when they have a hard life and try to escape through "internal emigration." Clematis should also be tried in cases of a death wish that arises during the course of a serious illness.

Psychotherapeutic Notes

Our lives are based upon the interplay between the rational and irrational, the here and now and the eternal. We need to keep an attentive, watchful eye on sobering reality as well as to be in touch with our dreamy, intuitive, visionary side to lead a rich, happy life. Life is essentially a work of art, or at least it should be, in that it allows us to translate our visions, impressions, and inspirations into an understandable, tangible form. Each of us is occupied with the task of making our dreams into reality and transforming our inner vision into a tangible form, and we do this in the way that comes most naturally to us. While the sober-minded realist concentrates on the practical and material elements, the Clematis type has a decidedly less practical orientation.

This personal mix of rational and emotional elements forms a fragile internal balance that constantly modulates to meet changing life conditions. If we become too sentimental or unrealistic, our psyche takes charge and brings us back down to earth. If our life becomes too sobering or difficult, our psyche provokes us to change the circumstances by calling forth an irresistible yearning for the beautiful and fantastic. It also gives us dreams, inspirations, and signs in the form of symbols, which we need only decipher and integrate into our lives in order to find our way back to the right path.

Clematis types tend to be very romantic and have a constant need to be happy. They are not fighters but instead tend to withdraw into their own dreamworld, which they can fashion as they like. There is always the danger, under circumstances that are too heavy for them—such as an unhappy family life or an unsatisfying career—that they will loosen even further their already tenuous grip on reality and replace the unpleasant here and now with pleasant fantasies and positive expectations. This provides some relief and helps them get by temporarily, but it actually intensifies their problems in the long run. The more the Clematis type withdraws from an uninspiring or unhappy life situation, the more she loses her motivation for a rejuvenating change of life.

Instead of fleeing unhappiness by seeking out pleasant fantasies and daydreams, we must address reality with a clear eye and an open heart. Any emotions that have been ignored or glossed over must be consciously experienced, confronted, and seriously worked through. Only then will it become clear that improvement must start from within. Only then can we stop substituting dreams for reality and start trying to make dreams become reality. Instead of waiting to be saved, we realize that we must save ourselves; instead of waiting for a prince (or princess) to come and save us from a wretched marriage, we will search ourselves; instead of taking a wild gamble, we learn to earn our own way; instead of seeking relief for a frustrating life through alcohol or drugs, we will try to make positive changes in our own lives; instead of waiting with a kind of lifeless patience for paradise in the hereafter, we can try to seek and create paradise in this life.

When the Clematis type has found what she needs within, she no longer goes to the cinema of her illusions to wile away a few pleasant hours (only to wake up sober in the here and now); she strives instead to use the strength of her intuitive knowledge and yearning to create a truly interesting, fulfilling, and beautiful life. Clematis children, who do not have the possibility to consciously shape their lives, must depend on the ability of their parents, guardians, or teachers to observe in which direction the child's dreams and wishes are taking her. They should try seriously to recognize and understand the symbols that are working to make themselves understood in the child's spirit, and attempt to determine down which path they should encourage the child to go.

Common Combinations with Other Essences

Chestnut Bud (7/9): absentmindedness and daydreaming

Gentian (9/12): weak will and daydreaming

Honeysuckle (9/16): total daydreaming

Olive (9/23): drowsiness, absentmindedness, hallucinations, or loss of consciousness caused by exhaustion

Rock Rose (9/26): tendency to faint in a panic situation

Scleranthus (9/28): indecisiveness and daydreaming

Star of Bethlehem (9/29): loss of consciousness due to a shocking experience

White Chestnut (9/35): persistent daydreaming

Wild Rose (9/37): resignation and suicidal thoughts

10: Crab Apple

Characteristics

Crab Apple is for people who feel impure or poisoned—physically or spiritually.

AREA OF USE

Crab Apple is used for the basic treatment of compulsive cleanliness; compulsive obsession with character, morality, impurity, or poisoning; external or internal toxic damage; skin conditions; and chronic illnesses. Used to treat all pathological conditions related to a pathological need for cleanliness or order. In daily life, used to treat pettiness in matters of cleanliness, nausea, infections, and skin conditions.

Causes and Symptoms of Crab Apple Syndrome

This condition is characterized by an excessive need for cleanliness and order and a certain dependence and tendency to be easily influenced. Harmoniously developed, the Crab Apple type is decidedly pure and loyal and generally respects and does what is good and right and is an upstanding member of society. He is not just clean in external matters but is also internally pure and uncompromising in his values and morals. He is normally very healthy because he avoids impurities of any type (such as in food, illness-causing bacteria, or unclean, unwholesome people), which might cause illness.

Negatively developed, the Crab Apple type has a compulsive, excessive attention to inner and outer cleanliness and order that, in extreme cases, can become an obsession with filth. In such cases, cleanliness has lost its true life-affirming function. It is practiced for the most part without any justification and serves, above all, as an outlet for psychic compulsions. People with Crab Apple syndrome see, or think they see, filth everywhere they look. They clean frantically and unnecessarily, and they can also tyrannize others with their excessive demands for cleanliness or even begin loathing themselves because of imagined uncleanliness. They are often tortured with pathological nausea or a groundless fear of filth. This can manifest itself in fear of possible infection through contagion, fear of being poisoned, or even fear of immoral behavior. Sexuality brings up special difficulties—Crab Apple types often find sex filthy and repugnant and seldom develop an open, positive attitude toward it. When their energies are directed inward, they can often elaborate a life-negating pseudomorality, which they use to tyrannize themselves or to get on the nerves of those around them. Occasionally, this attitude can escalate to a neurotic desire for spiritual purity that makes it impossible for them to lead a normal life.

The Effects of Crab Apple

Crab Apple is the essence for a healthy attitude toward physical and spiritual cleanliness and purity. It reduces pathological obsessions with impurity or shame, nausea, fear of uncleanliness, and an excessive sense of "morality." It is also good for purifying the blood. It can help protect against impurities of the skin, eczema, chronic inflammation, and infection and is useful in keeping contagions in check. Anyone who has any contact with sick people should take Crab Apple as a preventive.

Psychotherapeutic Notes

Crab Apple types are relatively dependent and easily influenced. They have difficulty standing up to dominating or intolerant parents, guardians, or authority figures. As early as childhood, they have norms and preconceptions forced upon them, and then for the rest of their lives they try desperately to live up to the expectations and demands that have been forced upon them. Since these demands stem from an outside source, however, they cannot take them to heart, but can make only a superficial, halfhearted attempt to fulfill them. This has two tragic consequences: first, a compulsive pettiness and a need to emphasize structure that is totally devoid of meaning, and second, a constant fear of failure and punishment, which manifests itself in the form of feelings of guilt or inadequacy. The need for cleanliness is a basic component of the Crab Apple type's psyche and can often progress to a neurotic compulsion for cleanliness that can focus on outer appearances or inner behavior or, as is usually the case, on both, depending on the extent of spiritual development. Instead of living by his organic and innate needs, he tries obediently and as faithfully as possible to live by norms forced upon him by others, which will often include a component of cleanliness, purity, or order.

To free himself of these compulsive drives, he must get to know his own needs better. He should become used to taking responsibility for himself and scrutinizing the opinions, rules, traditions, or dogmas of others before deciding whether they have relevance for him. Only then can he live with the integrity, correctness, and purity that are in his nature. Above all, he needs to develop a concept of cleanliness that is appropriate for him. The main point is that when cleanliness and order exist to bring happiness and improve the quality of life, they are just fine; if, however, they arise from a compulsive need and self-abuse, or as psychic countermeasures against insecurity and anxiety, they are pathological and pathogenic. The same rule applies to all forms of morality that represent an inner form of cleanliness.

Although many kinds of "morality" can address many people in a universal way, they can be harmful if they do not speak to us or our personality directly. They can disrupt the normal psychic balance, and the effects will last longer the earlier they are embodied in the psyche of a child. Finally, only a personal morality that begins within each individual can be a free and healthy expression of our being. There are times, of course, when being true to ourselves can bring us into conflict with prevailing societal mores.

Common Combinations with Other Essences

Larch (10/19): feelings of uncleanliness and self-loathing

Mimulus (10/20): excessive fear of uncleanliness

Pine (10/24): morally tinged compulsion concerning cleanliness

Rock Water (10/27): excessive cleanliness and discipline

Star of Bethlehem (10/29): pathological nausea

Vine (10/32): petty, fanatical cleanliness

White Chestnut (10/35): tormenting thoughts of impurity

11: Elm

Characteristics

Elm is for those who suddenly feel unable to carry out an important mission or responsibility.

AREA OF USE

Elm is used for the basic treatment of an acute crisis related to achievement and goals, uncontrollable ambition, inappropriate behavior due to stress, and acute illnesses. Used to treat all pathological conditions related to sudden fear of failure or acute feelings of stress and overwork. In daily life, used to treat work-related stress, sudden feelings of stress and overwork, impending breakdown, and acute illnesses.

Causes and Symptoms of Elm Syndrome

This condition is characterized by a great feeling of responsibility and the need for achievement with a tendency to push oneself past one's limits. Harmoniously developed, the Elm type is a decidedly capable, confident person who feels she is on a mission or taking on an important responsibility. She is goal- and achievement-oriented, and her goals can be social, athletic, or spiritual in nature. We often find her in an important or highly visible position. Examples would be a mother who is always there for her children, the boss on whose performance the fortunes of the entire company depends, or the politician who has spent her life serving her constituents but has also fought alone and put all of her strength into her self-imposed mission. Although she is unsparing toward herself, she is also wisely, acutely aware that we should not expect of someone more than he or she can achieve. Therein lies the secret of her success.

Unfavorably developed, the Elm type loses all sense of proportion in her desire for achievement and pushes herself, without thinking of consequences, to such a point that her reserves are exhausted and she begins to break down. When the Elm syndrome kicks in, she becomes weak, and she realizes with a certain amount of desperation that she can no longer continue. This has to do less with her physical than with her psychic abilities. She simply has no more inner strength to bear the stress that she has piled upon herself. This is a defining moment that can have serious consequences and compares with the phase of an illness in which the body suddenly loses its strength and seems on the verge of collapse. Since the Elm type has a strong constitution, however, she is soon ready to pick up the pieces and start again. She learns from her experience only seldom; normally, she just continues as she did earlier and sooner or later falls again into the same trap.

The Effects of Elm

Elm is an essence used in extreme situations, when a collapse (usually psychic) is imminent. It reduces psychic stress or pressures related to performance and releases blocked energy so that we can continue the struggle. Taken in a timely manner during a time of great exertion, it can prevent us from overextending ourselves or placing ourselves under excessive stress while increasing our ability to achieve. For serious illnesses, especially those with a sudden onset, it should always be given to mobilize additional strength.

Psychotherapeutic Notes

Favorably developed, the Elm state is characterized by our ability to use our energies and strength at their maximum limits and to stretch those limits as well. This is the principle of growth, without which life itself is impossible. A growing organism dissolves its various forms and replaces them with newer, better, more advanced ones. The tendency of all beings is to want to stay in a stable state forever. To change and overcome our natural sluggishness, we must apply a certain amount of force or energy. The more energy we supply, the greater the potential for change, growth, and development.

Here lies the strength of the Elm type. Where others stay sluggish in their habits and seldom really push themselves, the Elm personality forces the Elm type to constantly push herself beyond her limits. This is the secret of her great achievements and personal growth. Strength, however (like everything else in this world), has a negative effect when given in the wrong dose. We can waste away when it is lacking, but it can also create stress or disrupt us when there is too much. Stress arises when the body mobilizes more energy than it can safely put into play. Stress creates harmful inner pressures (such as high blood pressure, stroke, or heart attack) or can lead to inappropriate, senseless behavior. At bottom, it derives from a miscalculation: when faced with an extreme challenge or danger, we lose perspective on how much energy we need to overcome it, and we overreact.

The primary cause is fear, which makes the danger seem worse than it is and prevents an appropriate response. Negatively developed Elm types have an exaggerated sense of ambition and drive in which they lose their perspective and proportion and are overcome by stress. Like settlers in the jungle with a boundless desire for possessing, they try to take on too much. Their strength becomes exhausted in a desperate and pointless fight against the forces of nature, and they stand in danger of losing everything. The very thing that serves to make their lives positive—their great strength and readiness to take action—can ruin them.

All of us are familiar with the stressful Elm condition in one form or another. Normally, we think that external factors are to blame. In fact, the primary cause is our own inability to keep the realities of life in mind when using our ability to achieve. We become stressed because we cannot properly estimate a situation, we take on too much, or we allow ourselves to undertake a fight against fate that simply cannot be won. Suddenly we find ourselves at the point where we realize that we have defeated ourselves, that our "eyes were bigger than our stomachs," and we try to drop the whole project. These feelings of failure are very strong and vehement in Elm types. They are similar to the lightning that precedes a brewing storm, but they do not signal the coming of a final catastrophe. They are the warning signs of a psyche that is accustomed to success and falls into a panic at the first signs of difficulty (and not at the signs of a total breakdown). This psyche tends to exaggerate the extent of the danger in order to ensure a timely about-face. In this way, the Elm type gets a whiff of impending breakdown well beforehand and has thereby the possibility of a timely change of her course of action. Only seldom does a calamity actually occur. At most, her feeling of powerlessness helps her redefine more realistic goals or outline a more successful strategy. In the end, she battles on, undeterred; she has vast reserves of strength. Since these stressful conditions can drain our strength, the Elm type needs to examine more critically her ambitions and drives, be more aware of her limits, and learn to be content with what life will allow.

When Elm types pay attention to the signs accompanying stress and overwork—fear, desperation, difficulties with concentration or sleeping, tension, lack of enthusiasm, feelings of inadequacy, irritability, fear of failure, and oversensitivity—they can give up their plans before it's too late or begin to find another way to achieve them. At the very least they should consider taking time out to reassess the situation. The human organism can withstand nearly any kind of stress, as long as it has time to recover. After periods of intense stress and overwork, it needs a chance to regenerate and rest, such as with meditation or yoga or other similar methods.

It would be best for the Elm type to limit her self-imposed compulsion to achieve so that she can grow into her challenges gradually, much the way a long-distance runner paces herself to save enough strength to finish the race. Her happiness hinges on pursuing her goals with her entire being and with all her energy, but she must be careful not to feel any bitterness or disappointment when things appear out of reach.

Common Combinations with Elm

Cherry Plum (6/11): at the end of physical and psychic endurance

Gentian (11/12): feelings of stress and overwork, despondency

Gorse (11/13): sudden feeling of hopelessness due to stress and overwork

Hornbeam (11/17): acute crisis due to one's sense of achievement

Larch (11/19): sudden loss of self-confidence

Mimulus (11/20): sudden fear of failure

Oak (11/22): excessive demands and compulsive achievement

Olive (11/23): severe physical/spiritual exhaustion

Rock Rose (11/26): stress-induced panic

Star of Bethlehem (11/29): breakdown due to spiritual shock

Sweet Chestnut (11/30): desperation caused by stress and overwork

12: Gentian

Characteristics

Gentian is for people with a weak will and a tendency to be easily discouraged.

AREA OF USE

Gentian is used to treat weak will, lack of endurance, reactive depression, insufficient determination, and a tendency toward relapse. Used to treat all pathological conditions related to a weak will or a tendency to be easily discouraged. In daily life, used to treat discouragement, depression caused by failure and difficulties, giving up prematurely, pessimism, and relapses in the healing process.

Causes and Symptoms of the Gentian Syndrome

This condition is characterized by tractability and a great talent for adaptability. Harmoniously developed, the Gentian type is free of false desires, envy, or ambition because he is convinced that fate brings each of us what is best for us. Without frustration or regret, he can let go of goals or expectations that cannot be realized. When something does not go his way, he is not disappointed but instead realizes that fate has chosen another path for him and optimistically follows the signs that come his way. Because he possesses a thoughtful, introspective manner, he never falls into petty arrogance but believes that a clever person will need to give in and admit to being wrong on occasion. He artfully avoids insurmountable problems and continues along his personal path unimpeded. Because of his cheerfulness, indulgence, and serenity, he is well liked by those around him.

Unfavorably developed, the Gentian type's ability to compromise and defer to others can lead to a habit of giving up too easily, and his acceptance of fate can manifest itself in pessimism. When faced with difficulties or challenges, the negative Gentian type will often say, "I knew it would turn out like this!" or "I'll never be able to do it," instead of trying to find out how he can better solve his problems. Hindrances and setbacks do not challenge his creativity and his will but instead serve as signs that something simply was not meant to be. Thus, he passes up many opportunities—often without justification—withdraws into himself, and becomes despondent when his plans cannot be realized without resistance. Because of his weak will, lack of determination, and pessimism, he often helps bring about failure himself; indeed, it frequently seems as if he's looking for an excuse to give up. Because this deference and self-denial is pathological and runs counter to his natural desire for success and self-realization, he can become unhappy and depressed.

Depression arises when urgent desires are unfulfilled or when important needs are suppressed. We speak of "endogenous" depression when the cause is unclear, and "reactive" when the cause is known (as in the case of Gentian syndrome). In this case, the cause is failure brought about by the Gentian type's own weak will and lack of resolve. The Gentian type suffers not simply because of his own pathological weaknesses but because of their consequences. Gentian syndrome can also manifest itself in the healing process of physical illness; we see it in a relapse or delay in the healing process after an initial improvement. It seems as if the organism does not possess the strength to completely overcome the illness.

The Effects of Gentian

Gentian is the essence for strength of will. It is appropriate for people who are weak willed, despondent, and eager to give up. It strengthens the will, increases our resolve and endurance, and helps instill an optimistic attitude. Because it generally improves the ability to overcome setbacks or to achieve a desired goal, Gentian is also helpful when relapses or delays interrupt the healing process.

Psychotherapeutic Notes

Success means achieving our goals. This can take place in one of two ways: either we fight to reach our goals, forcefully overcoming any obstacles that may get in our way, or, from the beginning, we choose a path that has no difficulties. The secret of the successful person is going after only what can be realistically achieved. Which of these strategies is appropriate depends on the individual's mentality. Certainly the second, when seen in relation to costs and benefits, is the more effective and simple of the two.

The harmoniously developed Gentian type is the ideal prototype of the successful person. He understands how to reach his goals, without facing opposition or loss of strength, by not allowing himself to become caught up in hopeless ventures and skillfully avoiding all obstacles. His strengths, however, can become fatal weaknesses if people with an insensitive and combative disposition influence him (especially in childhood) and induce him to go against the tide, instead of taking the path of least resistance. In this case, the difficulties that appear cannot be dealt with simply, but must be overcome forcefully, which is not a natural part of his sensitive constitution. It is no wonder, then, that in the face of inevitable failures encountered during this process, he will lose his optimism and courage and throw in the towel at the first sign of difficulties or resistance. He becomes desperate, easily discouraged, and weak willed.

Experiencing success is an essential ingredient for further success. Anyone who has achieved a goal has programmed himself for future success. A Gentian type who has failed needs reprogramming. He needs to realize, in principle, that he can achieve anything he wants, and then he needs to prove to himself that he can, in fact, succeed. When it becomes clear to him that he possesses a sensitive, prudent personality that avoids conflict, and when he learns to understand that these qualities are not signs of weakness or cowardice (as others have tried to convince him), he can begin again to live life in his way. This attitude will, as he will doubtless be quick to notice, bless him with all the success he desires. His successes are simply not so obvious, bold, or glitzy as those of more extroverted individuals.

Success is not an objective, constant fact, but a subjective matter that can be measured only by our own well-being. One outcome can be crucial for one individual and might prove quite harmful for another. Likewise, the many types of courage cannot be measured with an impersonal yardstick. Courage can be extroverted and spectacular or internal and absolutely personal. All that it really means is that we are ready to meet and overcome challenges in our own way. As long as the Gentian type admits to his sensitivity and realizes that his well-being is the measure of his success, he will avoid difficulties and failure so straightforwardly and instinctively that it will seem as if he can achieve anything he sets his mind to.

Common Combinations with Other Essences

Centaury (4/12): weak will and personality

Chestnut Bud (7/12): lack of attentiveness leading to reversion
to old habits

Clematis (9/12): weak will and a tendency to daydream

Elm (11/12): dejection and a feeling of pressure from stress
and overwork

Gorse (12/13): weak will and hopelessness

Honeysuckle (12/16): weakness due to nostalgia

Hornbeam (12/17): pessimism and weak will

Larch (12/19): weak will and lack of self-confidence

Mimulus (12/20): yielding, deferential, and fearful

Mustard (12/21): bad moods and depression

Olive (12/23): exhausted and discouraged

Scleranthus (12/28): relapse in recovery

Star of Bethlehem (12/29): weak will due to psychic trauma

Walnut (12/33): despair caused by a major change in life

Wild Rose (12/37): resignation and weak will

13: Gorse
Characteristics

Gorse is for people without hope.

AREA OF USE

Gorse is used as the basic treatment for a pessimistic attitude, loss of hope, and serious illnesses with negative prognosis. Used to treat all pathological conditions related to hopelessness. In daily life, used to treat pessimism.

Causes and Symptoms of Gorse Syndrome

This condition is characterized by ambivalence—an especially positive and hopeful attitude tempered by a tendency to live without desires or expectations. Harmoniously developed, the Gorse type has such a fine balance of these two attributes that she is decidedly positive and optimistic, but at the same time she is prepared for self-denial, hopelessness, and lack of desire. These exist not as negative qualities but more in keeping with the Asian view that "nothing" must be a prerequisite for "everything." In the optimistic cheerfulness of the harmoniously developed Gorse type, there is always a bit of serenity and seriousness; one has the impression that she has a deep, unconscious knowledge and that she can experience and accept life in all its "positive" as well as "negative" manifestations. For those around her, she serves as a symbol of hope, which is all the more valuable because this particular variety of hope is not the everyday, superficial kind but a deeply felt, profound knowledge and assurance that all is right with the world.

In unfavorable circumstances, this complicated makeup can lose its subtle balance and manifest itself negatively. Just as her desires for happiness can turn to an equally strong sadness when they are not fulfilled, the very optimistic attitude of the Gorse type can transform into its opposite when her expectations are disappointed. Her self-denial displaces her more hopeful, life-affirming self, and the result is a life-negating hopelessness. Renunciation no longer means a willingness to accept the greater dimensions of life but is something more akin to being closed up in a dark room. The Gorse syndrome becomes pessimism and resignation. Anyone finding herself in this position has given up any thread of hope; resignation to fate is no longer part of an invaluable process of discovery but instead a process of inner destruction.

This condition can affect our physical health, in particular; it is characterized by severe, chronic ("hopeless") illnesses and the transition into a phase from which there is generally no hope of recovery. Gorse types who become ill do not want to go on anymore; their goal becomes the ultimate "cure" through death. If they still undertake treatment or therapeutic measures, they do so only because of the pressure of a friend or family member.

The Effects of Gorse

Gorse is the essence used to fight hopelessness. It stimulates our will to live. It braces us against loss, disappointments, or defeats and helps restore our positive, sensible attitude. For severe, hopeless illnesses, it can promote a positive change, especially when a downward trend has become evident. Gorse is especially important in cancer treatment, since cancer, when it is incurable (which, by the way, is true only in the rarest of cases), means that the organism has given up hope of overcoming the pathological cause of the illness.

Psychotherapeutic Notes

Gorse syndrome normally develops during a prolonged battle (such as an illness or the achievement of an important life goal) that is plagued with misfortune and failure. It is the expression of internal exhaustion, a disruption of the balance between taking and giving. Granted, the symptoms that characterize this condition are common; we all find ourselves susceptible to losing hope in the face of failure or bad luck. It is very important in our love for life and our optimism that we always remember that all life's beauty and its transitory desires and joys are merely the more superficial manifestations of a deeper, more meaningful dimension and that everything that happens has meaning and occurs for a reason. It is exactly this subtle trace of the transitoriness of all earthly manifestations and joys that also provides us with a fleeting glimpse of a profound and unknowable eternity.

There is a phrase sometimes used by religious people that goes something like this: "You can't fall deeper than into the hand of God." All of our losses, disappointments, and suffering are, in the end, trivial when seen in the greater and more profound context of our existence. Everything that we encounter has a deeper meaning and serves our divine self, of which we comprehend so little yet which is the ultimate goal of our existence. When we lose this intuitive knowledge, we find ourselves desperately enmeshed in the meaninglessness and wrongness of the world. In the Gorse syndrome, we are without positive expectations. Without hope, however, we cannot survive; we cannot face a new day, think, breathe, or act. We persistently hope that everything will be all right, that life circumstances will turn out for the better. When there is no more hope, life is finished.

As long as even one person is alive, however, there will be a hopeful element that allows us to look toward the future and fan the flame of life. We must find out at which point the lever of destruction was switched on and where the "life nerve" of the Gorse type was hit. Sometimes the reasons can seem banal and meaningless to outsiders, but for the person affected, they can speak to her very being. If we can, at this point, reopen the door that has been shut, put the fulfillment of our desires in perspective, or instill in ourselves the desire to pursue other dreams or wishes, then hope can return and, with it, life.

Common Combinations with Other Essences

Centaury (4/13): passivity caused by hopelessness

Elm (11/13): sudden hopelessness through too much stress and overwork

Gentian (12/13): weak will and hopelessness

Mustard (13/21): depression caused by hopelessness

Olive (13/23): hopelessness caused by exhaustion

Star of Bethlehem (13/29): hopelessness due to severe trauma

Sweet Chestnut (13/30): absolute hopeless desperation

Wild Rose (13/37): total resignation

14: Heather
Characteristics

Heather is for egocentric people who need recognition, who cannot be alone, and who speak constantly of themselves.

AREA OF USE

Heather is used as the basic treatment for egotism, vanity, pathological self-love, craving for recognition, an inferiority complex, and fear of being alone. Used to treat all pathological conditions related to severe egocentrism, talkativeness, or an abnormal need to be in the company of others, brought about by humiliation or rejection. In daily life, used to treat boasting, need for attention, fear of not being acknowledged, talkativeness, feeling left out, and loneliness.

Causes and Symptoms of Heather Syndrome

This condition is characterized by positive but insecure behavior and an excessive need to communicate. Harmoniously developed, the Heather type is a positive person, and he carries that attitude over to those around him. He embodies self-love in its pure, innocent form—somewhat in the sense of loving our neighbors as we love ourselves. Because he loves himself, he can love others and is worthy of being loved in the true sense of the word. He is without malice and has no fear of others. He loves to be around other people, chatting and exchanging thoughts. It makes him happy to share his heart freely; he has a positive relationship to himself and to the world, and he has nothing to hide. Life is a game for him, and he is happy to have others play along—if he has someone he can turn to and in whom he can find himself. If the bond to those around him is broken, he becomes lonely and unhappy, but this happens very seldom because he behaves so admirably.

Under negative circumstances, in the seriousness of the competition of life, this condition can lose its playful, lovable aspect and manifest itself in an egocentric, overbearing form of self-assertiveness. The Heather type's naive happiness becomes contorted into a pathological need for recognition and a constant questing for one's own worth in relation to others. The innocent talent for communication becomes an incessant chattiness, which is often a kind of naive self-eulogizing. Instead of loving his neighbor as he loves himself, his new motto might be "How can I love you if you won't love me first?" More than anything, the Heather wants to be liked and needs others to affirm his worth. He speaks only of himself and his own problems or, if his condition is severe, pushes himself in the spotlight everywhere he goes. He gets on everyone's nerves with uninterrupted reports of his own merits, talents, and deeds. One senses clearly his unsatisfied need for recognition or admiration—the so-called inferiority complex. The Heather syndrome is often very strong in children, such as those who make themselves very conspicuous in playing or being too loud when guests come to visit. Such behavior often has the exact result that the Heather type fears the most—isolation, loneliness, and humiliation. With his constant talking about himself, he is very annoying to those around him. He wants to use them as a sounding board for his own importance, without taking any actual interest in them. They feel no great need to be with him and, on the contrary, avoid him. He takes this as rejection—usually with good reason—or even humiliation, which puts him in even more isolation and makes him egotistical to a greater extent. His contact grows more superficial, and by degrees he becomes ill, often with problems in the lungs and heart.

The Effects of Heather

Heather is the essence used to treat vanity and the need for recognition. It helps instill a natural feeling of self-worth and minimizes feelings of inferiority. Heather promotes the ability to acknowledge and pay attention and works against boasting and arrogance. Overbearing chattiness is a special symptom. This essence should also be used to treat any illness that is the result of a humiliating experience.

Psychotherapeutic Notes

Heather syndrome is a product of unfavorable conditions in which competition causes an unconscious, instinctive self-love to develop into vanity and an excessive need for attention. The Heather type who has already confronted envy, vanity, or the craving for power in his childhood notices very quickly that someone is after the position he is steering toward and that he must constantly assert or defend himself. Because his tendency is to strive toward harmony and agreement, however, he does not incline toward an active show of strength but tries to gain popularity in a roundabout, passive manner, through the blatant, unsubtle demonstration of his merits. The Heather principle can be seen in the animal kingdom in the form of the peacock, who in its beauty (accentuated by its own vanity) leaves all others in the shadows. The peacock has to deal with very little competition, but people are faced with limitless competition. For this reason, Heather types, as long as they are unaware of their personal strengths, will always have the humiliating feeling that others are better, more attractive, more intelligent, or stronger than they are.

If the peacock were to engage in a test of strength against the lion, he would also suffer from an inferiority complex. In his unconscious being, however, he sees only himself. Human beings cannot behave similarly because they are conscious beings. We must learn to recognize our strengths and weaknesses and, at the same time, come to accept that we are as unique in our way as others are in theirs. Our uniqueness is the source of our own beauty and worth. Once the Heather type understands that no good is served by constantly comparing himself to others, he can better learn to accept and love himself as he is. His big mistake is that he pays too much attention to individual details—for example, eyes, legs, memory, muscle tone, genetics, family—and doesn't think about the whole of his personality. As unique individuals, we are all incomparable.

Heather types should also note that for any lack they may suffer, they will compensate for it in a strength. They should evaluate themselves not just in terms of superficial individual characteristics but as the sum total of their entire being. When we have developed an appropriate sense of self-confidence, we don't need to beg desperately for recognition and love; in fact, begging will only cause us to lose those things. We can, however, openly and straightforwardly approach those around us, like an innocent animal, without being overbearing or trying to humiliate them. We can also learn to acknowledge others, accept that in some areas they may be superior to us, and not be jealous of them—without anyone thinking less of us for it. A friendly, open, peaceful coexistence can take place only when both parties accept and acknowledge each other.

Common Combinations with Other Essences

Chicory (8/14): the need to be loved and liked

Honeysuckle (14/16): youthful vanity

Larch (14/19): boasting due to an inferiority complex

Mimulus (14/20): overbearing, pushy behavior caused by the
fear of being alone

Star of Bethlehem (14/29): psychic trauma caused by
humiliation

White Chestnut (14/35): persistent, compulsive vanity

15: Holly
Characteristics

Holly is for people who are inclined to behave in an unfriendly or aggressive manner.

AREA OF USE

Holly is used for the basic treatment of aggression, choleric or sanguine temperament, lovelessness, negative or destructive attitude, violence, and lust for revenge. Used to treat all pathological conditions related to irritability or aggression. In daily life, used to treat unfriendliness, rage, irritability, envy, hate, mistrust, and jealousy.

Causes and Symptoms of Holly Syndrome

This condition is characterized by very vital, animal-like reactions and defensiveness. Harmoniously developed, this is a person who is ready to react forcefully and, when necessary, aggressively to anything that stands in the way of her self-realization. Because she is always ready to defend herself when necessary and does not allow her emotions to become pent up, she is open, honest, and not hypocritical. Hate (which is the result of suppressed aggression) does not exist for her because she reacts to every attack spontaneously and directly. She always defends her rights with an innocent naturalness, and one always knows where one stands with her. Because you cannot come at her indirectly, there can be no underhandedness or falseness with her. Aggression has a meaningful, natural function for her. She is like a crusader who fights openly against any injustice without thinking of herself.

Under unfavorable circumstances, when her aggressiveness and spontaneity are taken away from her and her instinct for self-realization is suppressed, the Holly type can develop into a person who is very easily irritated and reacts with excessive belligerence. She cannot respond to problems calmly or with understanding but is immediately angered, becomes hateful, or flies into a rage. She is like a loaded gun with a hair trigger. Variations on these reactions are hate, envy, jealousy, lust for revenge, and mistrust. She has a lower threshold for potential threats than most people; competition loses its sporting character and takes on an underhanded, foul tone. The aggressive, hostile behavior of many Holly types is suppressed in childhood, through the influence of either parents with a gentle, defensive nature or moralistic, ideological, or selfishly motivated teachers. Because aggression is a natural, instinctive phenomenon that cannot be eliminated either by violence or reason, it seeks out other forms of expression when it cannot be expressed directly. A child who is forced to suppress her anger might vent her stifled emotions, for example, by torturing defenseless animals or by tearing up flowers. The Holly syndrome has many variants: petty, everyday anger; a bad mood for absolutely no reason; excessive irritability; and inexplicable unfriendliness. It can be especially strong in people who are normally indulgent and gentle but lose it and suddenly see red when they are faced with unusual external pressure. An illness with an aggressive nature, such as high fever, strong allergic reactions, sudden serious infection, or an unusual irritation at the beginning of an illness are also indications of the Holly syndrome.

The Effects of Holly

Holly is the essence used against negative emotions. It can lessen aggression, irritability, anger, rage, lust for revenge, resentment, and jealousy; it promotes the control of aggression and makes us friendlier, more able to compromise, more patient, gentler, and more able to love. Naturally, Holly cannot simply turn rage and hate into their opposites. It should be used with other appropriate substances when unusual irritability shows itself at the beginning of an illness or when that illness runs its course very violently or aggressively.

Psychotherapeutic Notes

There would be no life without aggression. Life means growth, development, and self-realization, and these, in turn, all exact a cost on other beings. Every cell acts so that it can become larger, every plant tries to grow, every animal strives to flourish, every race or people seeks to expand. In each case, some form of aggression against other cells, plants, animals, or people is necessary in order to claim needed nourishment, space, or even existence. The territory on Earth is limited, and not all creatures can expand their size or territory to the extent they require. All beings are condemned to battle. While this means "eat or be eaten" for many living things, it also ensures that life in general may continue.

In addition to the limitations on resources and territory, we are also instilled with a natural desire to want to maintain all that we have and all that we are. The corollary is that others, who as yet have nothing, should not get anything. Naturally, they take this as a hostile stance, as we would if we were in their shoes. Who is right? We could discuss this subject and philosophize about it endlessly. Life itself answers this question simply and irrefutably, by compelling us to satisfy our needs for food or safety directly, aggressively when necessary, and at the expense of other beings.

This attitude is a function of the basic elements of life, but giving up a part of our abundance is an equally widespread natural phenomenon: trees share their fruit, springs let their water flow, even humans will share with their neighbors when they feel that they have sufficient material or spiritual resources. When we have strength, fearlessness, and self-confidence, our aggression can find an honest, direct outlet. Otherwise, it will develop into an inner pressure that we will release at the first opportunity in the form of groundless hostility, irritability, rage, hate, envy, lust for revenge, mistrust, jealousy, or other similar manifestations. In the case of Holly syndrome, we are no longer in control of our emotions. Even if we want to, we cannot be friendly or approachable, make our rage disappear, transform our hate into love, or let go of our jealousy—with some exceptions, of course.

To overcome the Holly syndrome, we need a deep understanding of the workings of our psyche. Aggression is basically an instinctive reaction that can generally be diminished with personal conditioning. We react aggressively because we feel threatened or under attack, whether or not that is actually the case. It depends on our ability to get to know our own fears and the sensitivities that create our aggression and to change them so that we can react appropriately and sensibly. Theoretically, it is entirely possible to find attitudes and values that can enable us to rise above the level of primitive life and not see a potential enemy in every person or a threat in every activity. We all have borders we must defend; how tight these limits are depends on our character and our spiritual awareness.

As conscious human beings, we have the opportunity for mental and spiritual growth as well as physical growth. The more highly developed our self-awareness and our awareness of the world, the more generous and tolerant and stronger we will be. The existence of other people will seem less of a threat to us. A true Holly type will never become an absolute pushover, but she can learn to consciously control her combative personality. She can recognize that she has a tendency to inflict violence or injustice upon others and that she can also hurt herself through her sometimes too wild behavior (her enemies can defend themselves, too). Likewise, she can learn to feel that her raging negative emotions can poison her. After all, who is happy when she is feeling envious, full of rage, jealous, ready for revenge, or steeped in hate? When this becomes clear to her, it will be in her own interest to bring her internal source of toxins into check through an honest developing of self-awareness or through the clarity that will result when she directly confronts her own worst tendencies.

Common Combinations with Other Essences

Beech (3/15): allergic shock reaction

Cherry Plum (6/15): uncontrollable attacks of rage

Chicory (8/15): hate/love

Impatiens (15/18): impatient and irritable

Mimulus (15/20): anxious irritability

Star of Bethlehem (15/29): aggression due to a mental or emotional shock

Vervain (15/31): irritable do-gooder

Vine (15/32): rage at the sign of opposition or the mistakes of others

Water Violet (15/34): irritable misanthrope

White Chestnut (15/35): aggressive thoughts

Willow (15/38): bitterness with rage or hate

16: Honeysuckle
Characteristics

Honeysuckle is for people who cannot let go of the past.

AREA OF USE
Honeysuckle is used for the basic treatment of disruption in the relationship to reality, flight from reality, lack of interest in the present, melancholia, and excessive nostalgia. Used to treat all pathological conditions related to melancholic memories. In daily life, used to treat memories, homesickness, and sadness caused by loss.

Causes and Symptoms of Honeysuckle Syndrome

This condition is characterized by a dreamy sensitivity, a great need for happiness, a good memory, defensive timidity, and passive behavior. Favorably developed, the Honeysuckle type is romantic and emotional. He is generally happy and understands how to get the best out of life. To some extent, he sees the world through rose-colored glasses that emphasize the positive and minimize the negative. He doesn't falsify reality, but his naturally optimistic nature simply accentuates the sunny perspective. He is a master of the art of never losing touch with reality (which itself is always a mixture of the positive and negative) and understands in his predominately happy reality that even the smallest hint of annoyance, distress, and grief, like the yeast in dough, allows us the opportunity to expand and develop and offers us a deeper look into the profound connections of our existence. Even (superficial) unhappiness will ultimately make him happy because it allows him to reach a more meaningful, valuable perspective. But he doesn't experience only reality as beautiful; he also possesses the ability to view his memories with happiness, memories that are so lively that they penetrate his entire being. Artists who understand how to distill the essence of eternal beauty from a fleeting moment possess this temperament. The harmoniously developed Honeysuckle type is very popular because he revives in others the awareness of beauty and wonder that is normally lost to most of us in our everyday lives and because he has little interest in material competition.

Unfavorably developed, the Honeysuckle type's overwhelming need to be happy, his vivid talent for remembering pleasant events, and his relative weakness can create in him the habit of fleeing the difficult present in favor of a happier past. Sensitive and passive as he is, the Honeysuckle type believes, almost as a matter of principle, that life used to be much better and easier. He achieves this view in part by glossing over his memories. In pleasant dreams and memories, he constructs soothing antidotes to an unpleasant and painful reality. Children suffering from homesickness or people who cannot recover from a loss often react in such a way that they cannot come to terms with their new circumstances. They flee the present by seeking out romantic memories and find themselves longing for the "good old days." Poets who pine longingly for lost happiness are representative of this syndrome. The Honeysuckle syndrome makes a person largely unable to come clearly to terms with life. He sinks into sadness, homesickness, or dreaminess and loses contact with the demands of daily life. It can even lead to the development of addictions, because addictions are essentially a search for happiness and wonder through artificial means.

The Effects of Honeysuckle

Honeysuckle is the essence against pathological nostalgia. It awakens an interest in the present and in reality and allows pleasant and persistent memories to fade away. It is helpful in cases of homesickness, nostalgic passions, and especially for sadness or mourning (which itself is a sign that we cannot accept a new reality because we believe the older one to be better). It improves our ability to come to terms with new, seemingly unhappy situations (homesickness) and can reduce the tendency for addictions that are triggered by a refusal to accept things as they are.

Psychotherapeutic Notes

Typical Honeysuckle behavior is the result of a hard, unhappy life. The Honeysuckle type, especially as a child, is very sensitive and needs to be happy. He lives in a protective cocoon, which he has woven out of pleasant experiences and in which he comforts and hides himself. When he is taken quickly or forcefully out of this cocoon, when he is confronted abruptly or brutally with an unpleasant reality, or when his poetic sensibility is singled out by less than sympathetic teachers, he can retreat into his own imaginary world—more out of an instinctive defensive reaction than out of defiance—and become unfit for "normal life."

There are, however, Honeysuckle types who are able to appropriate a certain clear-eyed efficiency from life's pressures, but these people generally develop only a very brittle shell and can plunge into an inconsolable sadness or mourning at the first sign of a deep loss or drastic change in life circumstances. They can even lose all touch with reality. We don't do the Honeysuckle type (adult or child) any favors by trying to rid him of his "poetic" disposition to make him "fit for life." If he is allowed to shape a life according to his own tendencies and in which his artistic self plays a major role, he can have one foot planted solidly in the "real world" and the other in a place where dreams and wonder make their home.

Anyone who has a clear case of Honeysuckle syndrome, such as in the form of an inconsolable homesickness or an unending sadness, needs empathy and understanding to help him adapt to his present reality when the fulfillment of his most urgent desires is impossible. He must be allowed to exercise and satisfy the dreamy, unreal elements of his character. We don't help him very much by suggesting he pull himself together or by making him aware of the benefits of some external, alternate way of looking at the world. It is better to find out what his soul most craves, even if it seems incomprehensible or foolish. Only then can he begin to find the trust and courage he needs to make his way in life.

Common Combinations with Other Essences

Chestnut Bud (7/16): distractedness and nostalgic dreaminess

Chicory (8/16): sadness and mourning due to the loss of love

Clematis (9/16): persistent daydreams

Gentian (12/16): nostalgia and a weak will

Heather (14/16): vain youthfulness and immaturity

Hornbeam (16/17): flight into the past due to stress and overwork

Larch (16/19): flight into the past due to a lack of self-confidence

Mimulus (16/20): flight into the past due to timidity
Mustard (16/21): depression caused by loss
Olive (16/23): inconsolable loss
White Chestnut (16/35): compulsive, persistent memories
Wild Rose (16/37): nostalgic, melancholic resignation
Willow (16/38): bitterness due to loss

17: Hornbeam
Characteristics

Hornbeam is for people who find the demands of everyday life too difficult, even though they are perfectly capable of fulfilling them.

AREA OF USE

Hornbeam is used as the basic treatment for fear of failure, a chronic feeling of being overwhelmed, groundless pessimism, and frustration. Used to treat all pathological conditions related to a constant feeling of overwork or exertion. In daily life, used to treat "blue Mondays," morning frustration, lack of interest in work, weakness, and flight into illness.

Causes and Symptoms of Hornbeam Syndrome

The Hornbeam type is characterized by a strong need for achievement and perfection combined with a tendency toward caution, self-criticism, and modesty. Harmoniously developed, the Hornbeam type is an achiever, but she is always careful not to overestimate her own abilities. She is almost always successful because she can allot her strengths sensibly and takes on only those tasks that she is sure she can handle. She has a tendency toward cautious understatement and always makes sure to keep a reserve in any project. This prevents her from failing and also gives her a sense of security. She is greatly valued by those around her because of her combination of natural modesty and secure circumspection, with a healthy desire to achieve. One gets the feeling that her caution and her constant striving to do her work flawlessly both arise out of an innate sensitivity. When she criticizes herself, she is not just fishing for compliments; this tendency is proof that she has a sensitive insight into the complexities of life. She goes on her way confidently but cautiously, critical of herself but not overly so, modest but sure of herself.

Unfavorably developed, this combination of natural modesty and a great drive to succeed can lead the Hornbeam type to an unconscious, compulsive drive for perfection with a need to push herself to the limit. Excessive caution can foster pessimism, and the striving for perfection can result in a fear of failure. The typical Hornbeam type feels stressed and overworked both in her everyday life and at work. She is pessimistic and feels every morning that she has insurmountable tasks to accomplish. Typical variants are the Monday morning depression or the funk caused by starting the day knowing that one has to achieve the impossible. What is most notable about these conditions is that they are all produced in the head; these feelings of stress and overwork are not based on reality but arise from pessimistic expectations. They are the way that the Hornbeam type prepares herself for failure. Normally, the Hornbeam type uses her challenges as a means for personal growth; she tries to do a good job despite her own expectations. Her problem is that despite her successes, she still feels under the gun and is plagued with a fear of failure. She feels she has failed before she has even begun. Although she would like to just toss in the towel, she heaves a sigh and gets on with it—secretly, she probably knows that things are not as bad as they seem—and the more she works, the more able and active she feels. This phenomenon can often be observed in people with poor circulation: the more active they are, the better they feel.

The Effects of Hornbeam

Hornbeam is the essence that helps us overcome our day-to-day challenges. It is effective against fear of failure, promotes a healthy desire to achieve, and helps restore enthusiasm, self-confidence, and a positive, active attitude. It can also help prevent us from running away from our challenges by becoming ill. If we wake up in a morning funk that seems to lessen over the course of the day or if we are overcome with a weakness that seems to disappear when we become more active, Hornbeam is the ticket.

Psychotherapeutic Notes

Hornbeam syndrome arises when we have a need for perfection in all that we do but sabotage ourselves by being overly critical and cautious. The Hornbeam type has a tendency to overestimate the tasks that face her and underestimate her own abilities. This is a constant source of torment, overwork, and fear of failure. But when her abilities are truly challenged, it's easy to see that it's all in her head; she is capable of achieving anything she puts her mind to.

She miscalculates her abilities when she is called upon to do something that is not in her nature and that she is not up to. This is something similar to guilt feelings, which arise when we believe that we cannot meet the moral demands placed on us by our environment simply because it is not in our nature to do what is demanded. While guilt (see the section on Pine) is related to the somewhat theoretical feeling of mental/emotional self-worth, the feelings of inferiority related to the Hornbeam syndrome have more to do with practical physical and intellectual abilities. The pessimistic expectations that characterize the Hornbeam syndrome are actually a kind of defense mechanism used to try to prevent disappointment or failure and a passive means to bring about a change in life or the demands placed on us.

When she is challenged, the Hornbeam type is truly capable of achieving great things, but we should not take that as a sign of her true abilities. That she falls so often into a state of pessimism is a sure sign that something needs to be changed. Two things have to be addressed: first, any illnesses that make her more susceptible to depression, and second, a change in her life. She needs to feel happiness and self-realization instead of obligation and compulsion. When the Hornbeam type (and this holds true for nearly anyone) is able to fulfill her own true needs, desires, and potentials—which we also think of as self-fulfillment—she will be more optimistic and able to achieve her goals. Children who suffer the effects of the Hornbeam condition should be nurtured in a way that will allow them to flourish; otherwise they will wilt like a flower in the desert.

Common Combinations with Other Essences

Centary (4/17): feelings of stress and overwork due to dependence

Elm (11/17): acute crisis related to one's ability to achieve

Gentian (12/17): pessimistic and weak willed

Larch (17/19): feelings of stress and overwork due to a lack of self-confidence

Mimulus (17/20): fear of failure

Wild Rose (17/37): despondency due to feelings of stress and overwork

18: Impatiens
Characteristics

Impatiens is used for impatient, restless people who are always in a rush.

AREA OF USE

Impatiens is used for the basic treatment of excessively "driven" behavior, restlessness, nervous temperament, sleeplessness, and overactive metabolism. Used to treat all pathological conditions related to restlessness or nervousness. In daily life, used to treat impatience, restlessness, excessive haste, superficiality, sleep disorders, itchiness, and fidgetiness.

Causes and Symptoms of Impatiens Syndrome

This condition is characterized by "driven" behavior, restlessness and nervousness, and a compulsive need to have everything done immediately. Harmoniously developed, the Impatiens type can think and act more quickly than most. He needs only one word to start a chain reaction of thoughts, doesn't waste his time, and usually has finished a job as soon as he's thought of doing it. As soon as he has an idea, he begins immediately and without hesitation to see that it is put into effect. He is nimble and typically finishes his work when others are just getting around to starting.

Under less than favorable conditions, the Impatiens type loses all sense of proportion. Instead of a positive, sensible quickness, he charges into everything full bore, without thinking of any possible setbacks. In this circumstance, speed becomes not just a means to achieving a result expediently but an end unto itself, a pathological symptom of the Impatiens syndrome. People in this condition are hasty, impatient, rushed, and very driven. Everything must proceed as quickly as possible for them, even when haste is not necessary. Every delay makes them nervous and irritable, and often the relative pokiness of those around them (even if it is only imagined) gets on their nerves and makes them intolerant and unjust.

When he becomes impatient with the slowness or slow-wittedness of others, he may try to do everything himself and thus isolate himself. His nervous energy leads to frustration at work, he doesn't have the time to be thorough or careful, his thoughts are often not fully formed, and his decisions are made in haste. His unrestrained speed allows for only mental superficiality, and he has no opportunity to explore himself. Behind the facade of constant activity and restlessness, he is often unhappy and lonesome. Even the body reacts consistently. His movements are nervous, fidgety, and often uncoordinated, and he suffers from all manner of nervous disorders, twitches and ticks, sleeplessness, cramps and tension, lack of concentration, high blood pressure, or itchiness (especially in the case of neurodermatitis).

The Effects of Impatiens

Impatiens is the essence for treating nervousness and restlessness. It fosters patience, circumspection, prudence, and thoroughness and helps us develop our own rhythms or succeed when we must live under the pressure of constant deadlines. Impatiens is useful for all conditions related to nervousness and restlessness, such as nervous tension before important appointments or interviews, hectic behavior when a deadline nears, nervous itchiness, or trembling or overstimulation accompanying a shock. Impatiens is an ingredient in Rescue Remedy.

Psychotherapeutic Notes

The essential problem for the Impatiens type lies in his need for speed. It is not just the speed in itself that is the problem but the inability to adapt that speed to different situations. He is like a coachman who constantly pushes his horses to the limit regardless of the road conditions. He can overshoot his destination and end up somewhere he never intended to be. His haste can cause him to make errors that must be put right, and he stands to ruin his nerves over unnecessary delays. With certain kinds of pressure (for example, an important appointment or job-related stress), these symptoms can appear in anyone, not necessarily just an Impatiens type. The Impatiens type could always reach his goals if he could learn to use his speed sensibly and harmoniously. Speed is fine when it is appropriate, but we also need thought and reflection. The Impatiens type, however, is compelled to put a specific idea immediately into action, to verbalize a thought too hastily, or to act so quickly that he can trip over his own feet and end up doing the opposite of what he intended.

We can try to improve the Impatiens type on two fronts: externally, by circumspectly avoiding any life situations that involve speed or deadlines and, internally, by allowing him a certain amount of time to incorporate his feelings, perceptions, realizations, experiences, and ideas into his actions. He needs a lot of conscious discipline to pull himself together after a painful experience. Even when this method is effective, the typical Impatiens type still works quickly; reflection, a slow pace, and patience are not naturally part of his character. He needs to find his own sense of perspective and keep everything in balance.

This is especially true of Impatiens children, who, because of their natural tendency toward jitteriness and hasty behavior, should not be put under pressure but should be given the chance to find their own rhythm. We should be careful not to demand of them any task requiring exactness or patience but allow them the opportunity to harmoniously and leisurely develop their own special talents. Modern computer games have an especially harmful influence by placing people under merciless pressure in a "game" context. Children who play them too often can shatter their nerves and throw their inner balance out of whack. Certain nutritional habits can also trigger serious nervous conditions, which should be kept in mind when planning a child's diet.

Common Combinations with Other Essences

Cherry Plum (6/18): prepsychotic restlessness
Holly (15/18): impatience and irritability
Mimulus (18/20): anxious restlessness
Red Chestnut (18/25): anxious restlessness
Rock Rose (18/26): panicky, driven behavior
Scleranthus (18/28): erratic, impatient behavior
Vervain (18/31): stressed and in a rush
White Chestnut (18/35): mentally driven behavior

19: Larch

Characteristics

Larch is for people who lack self-confidence.

AREA OF USE

Larch is used as the basic treatment for lack of self-confidence and problems with self-worth, tendency toward unnecessary self-denial, and an inclination to give up hastily. Used to treat all pathological conditions related to a lack of self-confidence or feelings of inferiority. In daily life, used to treat shyness and timidity.

Causes and Symptoms of Larch Syndrome

This condition is characterized by being easily influenced, a defensive attitude, and natural modesty. Harmoniously developed, the Larch type has an instinctive knowledge of the relative nature of all values and has a loving respect for all people. It would never occur to her to overestimate her own abilities and knowledge or to think of herself above others. Her sensitive wisdom and her need for the truth make it impossible for her to be caught in brazen boasting, to deal with obligations that she cannot fulfill, or to take on projects that are beyond her capabilities. Her unaffected, honest modesty (which stems from a clever insight into reality), her inner security (which comes from a realistic awareness of her abilities), and her friendly manner in dealing with others make her very popular. She does not know failure because she keeps her sense of proportion and never puts more on her plate than she is able to handle.

Unfavorably developed, her inborn self-critical modesty can turn into a false self-belittling, lack of appreciation for herself, or a form of self-deception that can, with time, become an inextricable tangle of ungrounded fears, fantasies, self-condemnation, and validations—known as an inferiority complex. The Larch type loses the ability to judge herself clearly and rationally, trusts herself too little and others too much, shies away from more daunting projects out of fear, and avoids any situations that might put her into competition with others. The Larch type is convinced that she is not good enough, attractive enough, intelligent enough, or strong enough. She often gives up an undertaking well before the thing has begun; she is easily embarrassed and tends to shy away from other people. This can essentially happen to anyone who experiences a serious failure or who is under the pressure of intense competition. While many will give up only temporarily, however, the Larch type remains dejected for a longer time, and her bad posture is often a dead giveaway to others that she is down on herself.

Larch syndrome often leads to spinal problems and a tendency toward Scheuermann's disease, Bekhterev's arthritis, or osteoporosis, which can deform the spine and is a physical manifestation of what is happening internally. Scheuermann's disease can appear in shy or repressed children, Bekhterev's arthritis in adults with a distorted feeling of self-worth, and osteoporosis in women after menopause, which is a time when they often perceive themselves as less than whole. Even the so-called widow's hump (a hunchbacklike curvature of the spine), which used to be common, is the result of the loss of social position of a widowed woman.

The Effects of Larch

Larch is the essence for self-confidence. It minimizes inferiority complexes and promotes a feeling of security that arises within and is not dependent on the approval of others. It is often recommended for sensitive children who find themselves in a harsh, uncaring environment or who must grow up in surroundings outside their own social class. Larch also promotes the development of special talents that are somewhat unusual and often considered to be useless. In conjunction with psychotherapy designed to strengthen the personality, it can be used for long-term treatment of changes in the back or spine.

Psychotherapeutic Notes

Modesty is rightly considered a virtue, but modesty does not mean self-denial and excessive (and forced) restraint, as is often thought. It means knowing our limits and taking only that to which we are entitled—no more and no less. People with a natural modesty guard themselves from excess as much as from unnecessary denial. They know that too much or too little not only makes a proper order in our world impossible but also makes them unhappy. Our spirit reacts always with frustration, pain, or suffering if everything is not as it should be.

This is quite clear in people with the Larch mentality, who could be described as having a false modesty. They are frustrated or unhappy because they have no faith in their own abilities, because they unnecessarily pass up chances and opportunities when they arise. Timid and shy, they pull back from many potentially useful opportunities that could strengthen their feeling of self-worth. In trying to protect themselves from failure, they also rule out any chance of success. They must remember that you cannot win if you do not play.

Larch types tend to be unique, special individuals, but they are also readily influenced because they can easily allow their own special talents to come into conflict with prevailing norms. Under the influence of very assured people, Larch types can lose their self-confidence and their feelings of self-worth. Parents and teachers can play an especially damaging role if they lack insight into the relative nature of all things and the need for healthy and appropriate self-criticism. If they set down their opinions as a universally binding law to a child who may be of a different nature than they are, they can cause the child to feel worthless.

Feelings of inferiority are more dangerous than we might think: they undermine our ability to lead an independent life. Our self-confidence determines whether we can properly assess the opportunities life brings our way and exercise our rights to exploit them. Our survival depends on these abilities. Having the inner conviction that we are able to master the tasks set before us is a prerequisite for success. If we do not know in advance that we are able to do something, we've already lost. We can see in nature that a battle between two rivals often is decided not just on physical strength but psychically as well; any opponent who senses the superiority of the other will leave the field without a fight.

When we feel ourselves to be inferior, weak, or unempowered, we are filled with a fear of failure, which is also a fear of future, imagined events. In the Larch type, these fears are based on a lack of self-esteem. We should become more familiar with our abilities and their limits, have a clearer concept of our standing in the rat race, and develop a value system that makes sense to us. This building up of our self-worth can take place only by degrees and should also be promoted externally, because we are always engaged in some kind of social competition. Larch types must recognize that if we are in the right place and using our abilities in a manner appropriate to our character, we can be successful. We should also understand, however, that failure is always a possibility and that success and failure depend on the circumstances of each situation. We need to realize that the "inferiority" we feel is, for the most part, subjective and can hardly be addressed with reason or logic. The best cure is direct experience, which often helps a living truth come to light. Sometimes it takes only a single success to restore the Larch type's self-confidence.

The moral realignment or restoration of the Larch type must always keep the body in mind. The spine is one of the most important areas that affects and is affected by self-assurance. The belief that we are inferior or unable to do something prevents an upright posture, and, likewise, a healthy sense of self-confidence is impossible with a crooked back. An appropriate measure of physical awareness can also help support the psychic process. Also keep in mind that many seemingly self-confident individuals, especially family members, friends, therapists, or notorious "helpers," build up their own sense of worth at the expense of the weak personality of the Larch type. It would certainly be valuable if they were to scrutinize themselves in this respect and begin their own Larch therapy—or, at the very least, take care not to put others down to make themselves look strong. As the Chinese proverb says: "You don't need to extinguish the light of another to make your own shine!"

Common Combinations with Other Essences

Crab Apple (10/19): feelings of impurity and self-loathing

Elm (11/19): sudden loss of self-confidence

Gentian (12/19): weak will with a lack of self-assurance

Hornbeam (17/19): feelings of stress and overwork due to a
lack of self-confidence

Mimulus (19/20): anxiety due to a lack of self-worth

Olive (19/23): self-doubt due to exhaustion

Pine (19/24): feelings of moral inferiority

Rock Water (19/27): feelings of inferiority from idealistic
demands placed on oneself

Star of Bethlehem (19/29): loss of self-confidence due to mental or emotional trauma

Walnut (19/33): very impressionable due to a lack of self-esteem

Water Violet (19/34): human contact problems due to feelings of inferiority

Wild Oat (19/36): lack of direction due to a lack of self-confidence

Wild Rose (19/37): lack of drive due to a lack of self-assurance

20: Mimulus

Characteristics

Mimulus is for people who suffer from vague, generalized fears and anxieties.

AREA OF USE

Mimulus is used as the basic treatment for a tendency to fear excessively and too easily. Used to treat all pathological conditions related to fears and anxieties. In daily life, used to treat groundless fear, anxiety, timidity, and shyness.

Causes and Symptoms of Mimulus Syndrome

This condition is characterized by excessive sensitivity and feelings of vulnerability. Harmoniously developed, the Mimulus type is decidedly sensitive and vulnerable and feels happiness and pain more strongly than most. This finely tuned sensitivity causes him to scrutinize every situation instinctively and without interruption to look for possible sources of pain. As soon as anything threatens to become unpleasant, he will begin the most effective countermeasures he can muster or retreats skillfully. He manages skillfully and adroitly to avoid pain and suffering of all kinds. Because one hardly notices how carefully he examines everything with which he has the slightest connection, he generally gives the appearance of being brave. This impression is strengthened when he fights against the suffering of others—mostly in his own interest, since the suffering of others causes him as much pain as his own.

Unfavorably developed, this great sensitivity can turn into excessive anxiety and timidity. Instead of avoiding or neutralizing situations that could cause him suffering or unhappiness, he will often trigger them himself simply because an earlier incident that caused him pain leads him to imagine the same result. Over time, this pattern will serve to amplify his timidity, turning it into a generalized, groundless, and tormenting anxiety that his psyche tries to defuse by rationalizing and connecting his unhappiness with specific occurrences or objects. This reaction at least makes the situation somewhat manageable for the Mimulus type, but these fears are very distressing because they are excessive or simply unjustified. Typical Mimulus types are always afraid of something, which drastically limits their potential for self-realization. Adventures or risks of any sort are a horror to them; the prospect of anything new is absolutely terrifying. Their uncontrollable, lively imagination creates vivid new horrors or sorrows that hover before them or lurk in dark corners like a wretched apparition.

Sensitive children especially tend toward this condition because they possess neither the physical nor the mental strength to confront potential and unknown dangers. Sometimes the Mimulus type will try to ignore his fears by seeming self-assertive and self-confident, but normally he belongs to the group of people who say, "If you take a chance you could die from it" instead of "You cannot win if you do not play!" Even courageous people can find themselves in the Mimulus condition if they are not able to process a certain sorrowful experience. Their worldview then becomes so contorted that they become excessively cautious and fearful—at least on certain occasions. As the proverb says, "A baby burned will avoid a fire."

The Effects of Mimulus

Mimulus is the essence used against fear. It reduces real fears and anxieties, promotes the ability to assess dangers reasonably and properly, and makes us generally more courageous. Mimulus should always be given as a supplemental treatment in the case of any illness with fear as its cause or when an illness is strengthened by fear. It is especially appropriate for children who are afraid of new situations.

Psychotherapeutic Notes

Whenever a person is threatened, the organism mobilizes energy and enters into a state of tension, allowing him to defend or flee. Once this is done, the organism relaxes. Otherwise, an inner pressure would develop that would cause more inner tension and fear the longer it lasted and the stronger it grew. There are two forms of fear, depending on the nature of the threat. First, there is the immediate, unreflective, and overwhelming fear of death, which every organism experiences when faced with an acute, life-threatening situation and which stems from the fundamental knowledge of death that is innate in all living creatures. Second, there is the "theoretical" fear attached to expectation, which is caused when we anticipate or imagine potential pain or suffering. This fear has no basis in reality, since imagination and expectations can be only theoretical and unknown. It is a defensive reaction to still-active memories of earlier pain and suffering and serves to perpetuate those feelings.

The sensitive Mimulus types often suffer from the latter type of fear. The experience of suffering goes so deeply under their skin that all of their emotions are put into play, and, as with an allergy, they react to the smallest cause with groundless and excessive fear. It generally takes only the simple imagining of dangers or suffering to trigger such a reaction. This form of fear is so difficult to address because—in contrast to realistic fear—it cannot be countered with rational, practical measures. It is like a ghost that you can keep striking without actually hitting. It binds us and cripples us because it is irrational and can be countered (or at least minimized) only by striving for a conscious practice of clarity in our thinking and feeling.

There are several possibilities that we can pursue:

- We can neutralize the negative, anxiety-provoking expectations and counter them with positive ones. In this case, most suitable is a belief in a divine power or of release in the hereafter. The strength of most religions hinges on this tactic; once they have firmly planted fear in the souls of people, they offer salvation and release if one believes. Many frightened people latch on to this prospect of salvation and cannot live without it, but their fears are merely displaced and arise again when the power of belief abates.
- We can develop a habit of examining our fears and anxieties soberly and realistically, putting negative expectations under extreme scrutiny and exposing them as the nonsense they are. In this way, we replace irrational behavior with rational scrutiny, which can take place only with strict mental discipline.
- We do not run away from the situations that make us afraid but confront them and experience them consciously,

realizing that everything is not as bad as we thought and that the unhappiness we anticipated was only a figment of our imagination. This is possible only when we already possess a certain core of courage and our fears are not too deep-seated.

- We try to view the source of our fears in a different light, to assume a somewhat less defensive stance and face life with more openness and trust. This fundamental trust is the most effective antidote to fears and anxieties.

When we come to the realization that everything in our world is essentially good and that all pain and suffering pass and, ultimately, will bring us good, we can develop a positive basic attitude. We can also, as in the case of an operation, accept pain without truly suffering. It is also important to develop an acceptance of death, which, in essence, plays a role in fears of every kind. We fear death because it is the greatest, final loss, and we fear loss because we always connect it with suffering. Loss of health means illness, loss of property means poverty, loss of a partner means loneliness, loss of life means the absolute end. We must make it clear to ourselves that loss and death also mean growth and new beginnings—as with the phoenix rising from the ashes—*even if on another plane of existence.*

Courage does not mean rashly and daringly rushing into any adventure but rather having the willingness to confront our own fears. Courageous people dare to face their fears consciously. The (often superhuman) strength and grace they need arise in them from the trust in a powerful, eternal ideal, such as a great humanitarian idea, a life's calling, or the belief in an ultimately divine fate or an all-powerful and benevolent god. The Mimulus type, who tends toward fear owing to his sensitivity, can, when he is ready and willing, live his life without the constant need for validation and self-deception and develop an uncommonly strong courage. Once he learns how to make the transformation, his weakness will become his strength.

Common Combinations with Other Essences

Agrimony (1/20): secret fears

Aspen (2/20): total fear

Beech (3/20): tolerance due to fear

Centaury (4/20): fearful obsequiousness

Cerato (5/20): anxious insecurity

Cherry Plum (6/20): serious anxiety conflict

Chicory (8/20): anxious clinging

Crab Apple (10/20): excessive fear of filth and contagion

Elm (11/20): sudden fear of failure

Gentian (12/20): indulgent, yielding behavior and fear

Heather (14/20): pushy and overbearing due to a fear of loneliness

Holly (15/20): anxious irritability

Honeysuckle (16/20): flight into the past caused by fear

Hornbeam (17/20): fear of failure

Impatiens (18/20): anxious restlessness

Larch (19/20): fear due to a lack of self-confidence

Olive (20/23): terror and exhaustion

Pine (20/24): fear of guilt

Red Chestnut (20/25): anxious doting

Rock Rose (20/26): anxiety with a tendency toward panic

Scleranthus (20/28): anxiety-induced indecisiveness

Star of Bethlehem (20/29): anxiety due to psychic trauma

Walnut (20/33): easily influenced owing to fear

White Chestnut (20/35): anxiety-induced compulsive thoughts

21: Mustard
Characteristics

Mustard is for people who fall into depression, bad moods, or melancholia from time to time without any apparent reason.

AREA OF USE

Mustard is used for the basic treatment of endogenous depression, groundless depression, lack of joy and humor, melancholia, pessimism, and periodic world-weariness. Used to treat all pathological conditions related to sadness or depression. In daily life, used to treat lack of enthusiasm, bad moods of any kind, dejection, and sadness.

Causes and Symptoms of Mustard Syndrome

This condition is characterized by several components: an intensive need for happiness, a tendency to take things seriously, a general introversion, and a certain level of fluctuation in the emotional state. Harmoniously developed, the Mustard type has the enviable ability to combine happiness and gravity sensibly and harmoniously. This combination means that her happiness will never degenerate into mere superficial enjoyment, and her soberness will never descend into a depressive tendency to take matters too seriously. The central point of her emotional life hinges on a light, rhythmic movement between these two poles, the consequence of which is a certain flexibility in her emotional condition. The harmoniously developed Mustard type does not have a bubbly and cheerfully optimistic temperament but does have an inner balance and sense of responsibility. Her life is fulfilled with a quiet joy and a deep, clear knowledge of the meaning of all things. This causes her to have a tendency to internalize and to seek the answers to the basic questions of life through an inner dialogue more than through external communication.

Unfavorably developed, the changeable nature of her temperament can lead to an inclination toward negativity and gloom. Her normal gravity can turn into a humorless, depressive seriousness, and her inborn introversion can induce her to cut herself off absolutely from the outside world. The typical Mustard type is often plagued by melancholy, sadness, or despondency, which hangs like a dark veil over her thoughts and feelings. In such phases, she loses touch with all feelings of happiness or, at the very least, loses her enthusiasm or goes into a funk; she can no longer find any meaning in life and greets those around her grouchily and negatively or totally withdraws from the world. We all experience these moods from time to time; the Mustard condition is very widespread, though usually in a weaker form. The condition is often accompanied by weak circulation, lack of drive, susceptibility to infections, or excessive tiredness. These depressive moods eventually give way to a more "normal" state, which, in the case of the typical Mustard type, never totally resolves itself in a feeling of lightness or happiness. Sometimes the inner rhythms are so pronounced that these phases of depression will alternate with phases of excessive, unnatural optimism.

The Effects of Mustard

Mustard is the essence used to treat depression. It causes a general inner lightening and breaks down depressive moods, lack of enthusiasm, grouchiness and ill humor, joylessness, and pessimism. Mustard has an overall stimulating effect and promotes an open, optimistic, and communicative demeanor. It also has a positive influence on illnesses that are often accompanied by depression, and, as a supplemental treatment, it can help prevent a worsening of such conditions.

Psychotherapeutic Notes

In medicine, we distinguish between two distinct forms of depression—reactive and endogenous. Reactive depression is an understandably negative response to unhappy life circumstances. This negative reaction eventually disappears when the cause dissipates. Endogenous depression (which resembles Mustard syndrome), on the other hand, is neither understandable nor directly influenced. Its source lies in the innermost depths of the psyche. In medicine, *endogenous* means that one can find no external cause for a condition; it is often falsely linked to the word *groundless*.

Naturally, endogenous depression has its own valid causes, but they can be so deeply embedded in the consciousness that even the afflicted person has no access to them; they can be very serious. The psyche protects us by displacing any impressions, emotions, or insights that burden our soul and that can crush us when their real meaning is made clear to us. It allows us to process consciously only what we are ready for, while everything else gets pushed aside into the subconscious. Nonetheless, there is some psychic material that brings us to such important truths that we cannot displace it no matter how painful or injurious it may be. It tries incessantly to rise up into our consciousness to help us better our lives; when it is not allowed into our conscious life, or when we don't recognize it for what it is, depression can be the result.

To understand depression, we must understand its place in the development of an illness:

- When a person's life development or self-fulfillment is threatened, handicapped, or suppressed, he often uses aggression as a vigorous defense, which manifests in increased activity, heightened self-assertion, and even rash, forceful reactions. Spontaneity and a certain amount of unconscious behavior characterize this phase. The individual fights innocently, like a wild animal, for all that is due her, and this is a healthy, normal reaction.
- If this spontaneous, aggressive self-assertiveness is held back or suppressed, frustration sets in; the resulting strain provokes a more forceful defensive approach, the goal of which is to try to force a correction in negative life conditions or false attitudes. In this phase, which actually signals the onset of an illness, body and spirit have lost their natural harmony, and various psychosomatic conditions will arise. Healing demands an honest self-awareness and a conscious confrontation with the causes of the illness.
- If this frustration is ignored or suppressed, it can degenerate into depression, characterized by emotional strain, a draining of strength and vitality, reduction of the activity and effectiveness of the body's defense mechanisms and physical processes, or the beginning of organic degeneration. Healing is possible in this phase only if we seek with renewed vigor the answers to life's most basic

questions, answers that bring us to happiness and the potential for self-realization.

- If the depression is not overcome, it can degenerate over time into resignation. This resignation can be differentiated from depression (which is always the external expression of an internal struggle) by an increasing sapping of the life strength. We come to accept our unhappiness without finding any personal meaning in it. Depending on the intensity, this condition can lead to a chronic infirmity with occasional flare-ups but with an insufficient healing phase, or it can lead to death as the final expression of hopelessness. Healing in this dangerous phase takes place only through a miracle—which means a fateful change in life conditions or a powerful wake-up call—that arises from some irrational cause.

Depression is a dangerous condition that can lead to the loss of the will to live and through which the spirit sends its last warning sign before it retreats from life. What is a depression? The name says it—a suppression, or lowering of mood, which can call forth sadness and melancholia. And what can prevent sadness or melancholia? The answer is easy—happiness!

As we ask this question, we are reminded how little we pay attention to happiness and how little respect we have for it. Because it bears no heavy burden for us, because it cannot make us rich or famous or powerful, we walk all over it, sacrifice it without thinking, and think of it as something irrelevant or inferior. It is, in fact, the basis of our existence, and neither body nor soul could exist without it; it can transform into pain and suffering if we do not consider it of prime importance in our thoughts, feelings, and actions. If we do not do so, we are committing an unforgivable and fundamental crime against ourselves.

Perhaps such words sound pathetic, but we all know from painful experience that they are true. What do all of our pain and suffering signify if not the absence of happiness? Do not sadness and melancholy result when we don't let the sun shine in our lives? Whatever moral or philosophical thesis and ideological or idealistic slogans or excuses we use to banish happiness from our lives, the longings of the spirit will not allow us to be rid of happiness and joy. As long as happiness remains a promise unfulfilled, we are in for a life of far-reaching sorrow. This realization, which each of us has, is essential for understanding and overcoming depression. The recipe is simple: when we are depressed, it means that we are depriving ourselves of something that gives us happiness. Whatever it is, we must get it back.

Following this recipe often requires overcoming considerable, painful opposition—especially morals and guilt feelings—and it often seems impossible to many. They would rather anesthetize themselves with alcohol or drugs, distract themselves with entertainment or work, deceive themselves with high moral standards, or try to tolerate their unbearable lives—in short, instead of using their strength to make their lives worth living, they misuse it to make the prison that their lives have become inescapable. Depression is, however, a life-negating, violent phenomenon. It becomes even more serious the more radically we renounce our own happiness. When we see a burned-out, depressed person, we cannot imagine for how long they have subjected themselves to monstrous self-abuse (often for years). They wear themselves out in an exhausting, all-consuming inner struggle between forces that create happiness and self-realization and those that thwart them.

When we examine closely the source of these negative, satanic forces (Satan symbolizes any power that is torn from the great unity—call it God or life—and is then used against it), we recognize that they are the result of a violent conflict that one calls "education" or "upbringing." We are taught very early that we have no chance of survival when we follow too closely those urges that bring us happiness. We grow accustomed to suppressing our own need for happiness, and we find the threat of punishment normal. Eventually, we grow obedient, and self-denial becomes second nature to us. Yes, even our own happiness becomes suspect because it has been beaten out of us and we've been browbeaten and scolded into believing that the pursuit of our own happiness is selfish, immoral, and antisocial. With this perversion of values, our chances of a happy, fulfilling life disappear. It would often be better if we would mount some resistance, despite the difficulties. As long as we're fighting for what is important to us, we're happy.

With Mustard depression, the desire for happiness is strongly suppressed. It requires a long process of relearning to set free our burned-out, withered longings and become conscious of them. First, the Mustard type has to experience happiness again—she must, so to speak, "taste blood." In this way, any embers that have not been extinguished totally will flicker again, and her reawakened longings will lead her once more on the road to freedom. This work, however, she must do herself; no one can do it for her. She must also break loose of her inner bonds and free herself from her negative ideas, convictions, and habits.

In order to encourage her through our own good example, we must convince ourselves that we deserve to be happy. Most professional therapists emphasize obligation, property, propriety, reputation, power, or the morals of others as being of utmost importance, and they are not suitable to aid this process. Mustard types can best find help simply by being with people who have maintained a simple, unspoiled heart or in nature, whose plants and animals, colors, and scents can best show us the true way to joy.

Common Combinations with Other Essences

Aspen (2/21): anxious depression

Chicory (8/21): depression through unrequited love

Gentian (12/21): bad moods and depression

Gorse (13/21): depression through hopelessness

Heather (14/21): depression caused by rejection or loneliness

Honeysuckle (16/21): depression caused by loss

Olive (21/24): depression caused by exhaustion or exhaustion due to depression

Pine (21/24): depression due to guilt feelings

Red Chestnut (21/25): depression and worry

Scleranthus (21/28): frequent mood swings

Star of Bethlehem (21/29): depression caused by psychic trauma

Water Violet (21/34): serious depression caused by human contact

Wild Oat (21/36): depression caused by a feeling of the meaninglessness of life

Wild Rose (21/37): depressive resignation

Willow (21/38): depression caused by bitterness

22: Oak

Characteristics

Oak is for people who cannot give up.

AREA OF USE

Oak is used for the basic treatment of pigheadedness, excessive responsibility, uncompromising and unyielding behavior, a compulsive sense of obligation, a compulsive sense of self-sacrifice, and ambition. Used to treat all pathological conditions related to unyieldingness or a compulsion to achieve. In daily life, used to treat obstinacy, obsessiveness, strain, and long-term stress.

Causes and Symptoms of Oak Syndrome

This condition is characterized by strength of will and pressure to achieve and succeed. Harmoniously developed, the Oak type is a strong-willed person who has great powers of concentration and the ability to see a task through to its completion. He eagerly takes on difficult tasks or accepts challenges that allow him to use his formidable strength. In pressured situations or illness, he never gives up hope and presses on when others have long given up. He continues with renewed efforts until he has reached his goal. As a loner, he can achieve marvelous things, and in a position of social responsibility, he is the person who carries the whole load or pulls the cart out of the mud. He never thinks of rewarding himself and has the habit of working until the last. Once he has a goal in sight, he never gives up until he has reached it. He also acts as many successful people do, in not taking on more than he can successfully accomplish. He knows his own limits and weaknesses and plans accordingly.

Unfavorably developed, the Oak type's great ability to see a task through to its completion becomes an obstinate unyieldingness, his strength becomes mere stubbornness, and the happiness he feels in reaching his goals can become a pathological form of ambition. Oak syndrome is characterized by the inability to give up in the case of overwork or excessive pressure and stress. The Oak type resembles an arrow that misses its target and falls harmlessly to the ground. Despite being at the edge of cracking up, he cannot lighten his load; despite having undertaken too much, he cannot relieve himself of his responsibilities; and despite obvious signs that a goal cannot be reached, he will not give up. He goes off course, becomes obsessed, steels himself, and refuses to acknowledge that he has taken on too much, has been mistaken, or has deceived himself. It is no longer a question of reaching a sensible goal but instead becomes purely a question of winning, of gaining the feeling of having finished, without taking any losses into account—what matters to him is that he not give up. The Oak syndrome can even be found in everyday life—when we take on a job and find ourselves under unrelenting stress, when we ruin our health by pursuing a challenging sport, when we cannot let go of a responsibility even though we are not up to the task, and when we cannot restrain our compulsion to achieve even though we place ourselves under dangerous stress. Naturally, this condition can lead to long-term stress and has damaging effects on the body. Typical symptoms are gallbladder complications, high blood pressure, high fat levels, thyroid problems, stiffening of the joints and rheumatic complaints, lost of mental flexibility, and grinding of the teeth.

The Effects of Oak

Oak is the essence used for the treatment of intransigence, stubbornness, and pigheadedness. It makes us more flexible, yielding, and willing to compromise; reduces the compulsion to achieve and take on too much responsibility; promotes the ability to accept fate; and enhances our ability to relax. This essence can help remedy any conditions having to do with strong, deliberate, excessive, relentless exertion. Oak also helps prevent the degeneration of the circulatory system and, in favorable conditions, can improve high blood pressure and high fat levels.

Psychotherapeutic Notes

A strength of character becomes a weakness when it grows excessive or unreasonable. This is especially clear in the case of the Oak type. His naturally strong will and his goal-orientated nature can become perverted into inflexibility, a compulsive need to achieve, and closed-mindedness once these elements are allowed to become too strong in his character and overshadow the other elements. This perversion often occurs under the influence of egotistical, ambitious parents or teachers, who can place too much emphasis on the Oak child's natural desire to achieve and readiness for responsibility. This emphasis can result in the development of a one-sided person addicted to success and with no awareness of his own limitations and no understanding of the relative nature of all things. Such a person can no longer recognize that achievement and success always need reasonable limits to be meaningful, and he is unable to admit that he cannot do everything. He becomes accustomed to using any means to have his own way, without thinking about the consequences. He is incapable of giving up, even though a task is beyond his abilities, and he cannot let go of a goal once it is in his sights.

To admit to his own powerlessness would lead to frustration and shatter his feelings of self-worth. To accept fate as something that is beyond his control goes against his grain so much that he finds himself in permanent conflict and thus open to receive a fatal blow that can bring him to his knees. At that point, he is like a mighty old tree that is immovable even in the face of a raging storm, until one day its inflexibility causes it to snap.

It is difficult for us to determine whether the Oak type, once he has latched on to a task that will take him to the very limits of his abilities, is using his abilities sensibly or whether he has become a slave to his compulsions. The deciding factor is whether it causes him to suffer and makes him unhappy—this, we find, is true of most people in most situations. As long as he's fighting tenaciously and with all his heart, he'll be happy. As soon as he loses his sense of proportion or suppresses other, equally important needs, he becomes locked in an inner conflict. The unhappiness he feels is a sign that something is wrong. Speaking generally, his stress and unhappiness are the result of his inability to relax. He subjects himself to an uninterrupted form of stress that is damaging because he doesn't give his body time to regenerate or detoxify.

In times of stress, the organism normally mobilizes its strength to achieve a specific goal or avert a potential danger, thereby reducing all synthesis and detoxifying functions to a minimum, to be restored at a more opportune time. Healthy people experience stress and relaxation in shorter rhythms, such as day and night, and stay within a sustainable framework, but these rhythms can be thrown out of balance (with respect to duration and intensity) in times of extreme duress. Moreover, since all strength is put into play during times of stress, the regenerative abilities are reduced to the lowest levels possible. When a relaxation phase begins anew, the body's regenerative functions are restored, often with a vengeance. The body reacts with signs of exhaustion and symptoms that are often mistaken for physical illness.

The Oak type should try to remain in control of his energies and continually ask himself if whatever he is engaged in is worth the effort and makes him happy. As soon as he senses that he is not happy and the symptoms mentioned earlier begin to appear, it is time to let up on the reins and take things a little less seriously. It is extremely important for him to take all of his needs into account and not to become too one-sided. Even the typical Oak type has other interests and proclivities that can seem contradictory. He should find a common denominator among his interests and needs and attempt to fulfill the whole of his personality or, as a temporary measure, limit himself to fulfilling his most pressing momentary requirements.

Everything we undertake should have the goal of serving our happiness (whatever form it may take). If not, the result will be suffering, unhappiness, illness, and destruction—all of which can have a negative impact on our lives. A certain amount of playfulness is essential to see life in its best light and to regard life's constantly unforeseeable, changeable nature. When we take things too seriously, we single out an important element and experience it out of context with the rest of life. This seriousness then becomes the point around which all else revolves. In doing this, we dissect life and restrict its variety and vitality. There is perhaps a good reason that we use the phrases *dead serious* and *lust for life*. Parents should take note and not force their children to concentrate only on achievement and ambition; they may grow up to be successful, but they may not necessarily be happy.

Common Combinations with Other Essences

Cherry Plum (6/22): on the verge of breakdown caused by stress and overwork

Chicory (8/22): stubbornly insistent care or love

Elm (11/22): overexertion caused by a compulsion to achieve

Pine (22/24): uncompromising perfectionism

Rock Water (22/27): self-tormenting compulsion to achieve

Vervain (22/31): stress caused by a compulsion to achieve

Vine (22/32): dogmatic need to achieve

Water Violet (22/34): loneliness caused by ambition

White Chestnut (22/35): compulsive thoughts related to success

Willow (22/38): unrelenting lust for revenge

23: Olive

Characteristics

Olive is for people who are physically and emotionally exhausted.

AREA OF USE

Olive is used for the basic treatment of general weakness and impaired ability to perform, anemia, and heart insufficiency. Used to treat all pathological conditions related to exhaustion. In daily life, used to treat physical and/or spiritual exhaustion, generally after a great exertion or serious illness.

Causes and Symptoms of Olive Syndrome

This condition is characterized by a certain weakness and a low level of resilience. Harmoniously developed, the Olive type knows how to use her strengths wisely and avoids anything that will cause her to overexert herself. She knows her limits and organizes her life so that she will never exceed them. For example, she will choose an easy career, takes no exhausting trips, and regularly rests in the middle of the day. She is like a delicate plant that can flourish only under the most favorable circumstances and develops its own, still beauty. The Olive condition also corresponds to a natural biological phenomenon—the parasympathetic weakening and recuperation phase, which is accompanied by fatigue and is not indicative of an illness. It is a requisite for detoxification and regeneration.

When Olive syndrome is unfavorably developed, the latent weaknesses of the Olive type manifest themselves as an ever present fatigue and limit her in many ways. She carries herself tiredly through life, feels constantly exhausted, and requires excessive amounts of sleep. A medical cause could be weakness of the heart, anemia, or a shortage of vitamins or trace elements. When this condition—generally the result of a long illness or a severe strain—continues to worsen, it marks the beginning of the Olive syndrome, which can occur in anyone. We are at the end of our rope (often not just physically but emotionally as well), we cannot bring ourselves to go on, and we experience life as a painful burden. This means as well that the regenerative parasympathetic phase becomes a constant vegetative pathological state and cannot find its way back to full health and strength.

The Effects of Olive

Olive is the essence used to treat exhaustion. It has a general strengthening effect and can restore the psychic and physical functions to their normal levels. It has proved effective in treating weakened conditions of all kinds, especially of the heart.

Psychotherapeutic Notes

Olive syndrome is the result of chronic overexertion. Where the organism is normally able to bear heavy physical and emotional burdens, when the constitution is weakened (such as with the Olive syndrome), it takes only a small exertion to call forth the symptoms described here. A healthy organism can handle day-to-day stress with no problems. It mobilizes the body's reserves and moves into a state of generally heightened activity, to react as quickly and effectively as possible. In this "battle" phase (related to the sympathetic nervous system), the detoxifying and synthesizing functions are minimized and will return to normal levels when the problem is solved or the goal is reached, at which time the organism switches to the "relax" mode. Everyone is familiar with the weakness or weariness that sets in as soon as a period of stress is past. If the stressful phase was very strong or of long duration (such as a long period of exertion or a serious illness), the relaxation phase will also set in heavily or even pass over into the Olive condition.

This danger is especially present when the mobilized reserves are small, which is to say, with individuals whose ability to achieve or whose strength has been lessened by hereditary factors, illness, unfavorable life conditions, or, especially, an unhappy family life. Generational conflict also plays a significant role; in this context parents attempt to suppress the increasing competition they feel with their children—the mother with the daughter and the father with the son. From a biological and evolutionary point of view, children of the same sex as a parent pose a threat. The stronger the offspring becomes, the more of a threat he or she poses.

Normally, young people develop the strength for independent existence in this instinctual battle; they become independent or even drive out the parents from the parents' own territory. If they are not successful, they remain somewhat immature, undeveloped, and dependent on their parents. Among other things, this situation can result in disrupted sexuality, in a limp body or posture, in anxiety, in lack of physical and psychic development, or in a generally frail constitution. The Olive condition (and the Centaury and Larch conditions as well) can often persist in its subliminal nature or its characteristic weaknesses. If an Olive type finds herself in strange surroundings or if her parents die, however, she can sometimes develop into a strong, capable person. Mostly she remains in the shadows of her parents or teachers for her entire life. Only a course of psychotherapy that goes right to the core of her self-awareness can free her and set her on her way to an unimpeded process of becoming strong and growing up.

Anyone who has had firsthand experience with the Olive condition should learn to pay attention to the warning signs. Even the early signs of exhaustion should be taken seriously. If an Olive type learns to deal appropriately and carefully with her weaknesses, she will often outlast her stronger competition in the rat race. Aside from physical illness, the Olive type's weakness is often also the result of psychic overexertion from worries, fears, or negative expectations caused by a difficult, dissatisfying life or the constant denial of important needs. In such cases, the typical Olive type almost needs to undergo a thorough examination and reordering of her life, the object of which is to put an end to her constant troubles and self-denial.

We should think of an acutely weakened condition as a biological signal that marks a period of convalescence following a period of stress; by taking us out of circulation for a while, the organism is giving itself a needed rest so that the functions of synthesis and detoxification may resume. It is a mistake to expect an immediate return to full strength after a serious illness or an unusual mental or emotional trauma. Any therapy or treatment that acts to stimulate us is inappropriate and only inhibits the body's ability to carry on the essential acts of regeneration, so that we can never be fully rested. At best, we give ourselves up to the rhythms of nature (with the exception of life-threatening conditions), which will allow the organism to become active again only when the recovery is complete. We can learn a great deal by watching animals: when they are sick, they crawl away and hide until they are well again.

Common Combinations with Other Essences

Clematis (9/23): drowsiness, absentmindedness, hallucinations, or unconsciousness due to exhaustion

Elm (11/23): unconsciousness due to exhaustion

Gentian (12/23): exhausted and discouraged

Gorse (13/23): hopelessness caused by exhaustion

Honeysuckle (16/23): flight into the past brought about by exhaustion

Larch (19/23): self-doubt due to exhaustion

Mimulus (20/23): terrified and exhausted

Mustard (21/23): depression caused by exhaustion or exhaustion caused by depression

Pine (23/24): a guilt complex wearing one down

Red Chestnut (23/25): exhausting, debilitating worries

Star of Bethlehem (23/29): lack of mental resilience due to exhaustion

Walnut (23/33): easily influenced due to exhaustion

Water Violet (23/34): antisocial behavior due to exhaustion

Wild Rose (23/37): lack of drive due to exhaustion

24: Pine

Characteristics

Pine is for people who suffer from feelings of guilt and a bad conscience.

AREA OF USE

Pine is used for the basic treatment of guilt feelings, moralistic compulsions and drives, self-judgment, self-rejection, enslavement to authority, and pathological perfectionism. Used to treat all pathological conditions related to guilt. In daily life, used to treat unwarranted pangs of conscience and finickiness.

Causes and Symptoms of Pine Syndrome

This condition is characterized by a morally hued idealism and the tendency to place oneself in the service of a higher authority or by the fear of those stronger than oneself. Harmoniously developed, the Pine type is always oriented toward high moral values and ideals and guides his thoughts and actions accordingly. He always has the feeling that there is a higher (or divine) power or authority who is responsible for him. Once he realizes that something is right or obligates himself to something, he cannot be made to give up through promises or threats. He would rather suffer greatly than be deterred from his obligations or be led to betray those he serves. This can mean God, an institution, a community, an idea, or an individual—anything that seems worthy of his worship and respect. He is loyal, reliable, and incorruptible.

Unfavorably developed, the inborn, clear knowledge of conscious responsibility of the Pine type can turn into groundless or excessive feelings of guilt. This, in turn, can mean that the Pine type can lose his thoughtful self-awareness and his orientation to higher values and instead attempt to fulfill any moralistic demands that are placed on him. In fact, he will actively seek them out. Moreover, his desire for perfection and proper behavior can lead to an incessant, tormenting feeling of inadequacy. And so he suffers from excessive or groundless feelings of guilt, a bad conscience, or his need for perfection. He can never be content with his own achievements and often believes that he has not done his duty. This feeling of being in someone's debt is the reason that he feels guilty or sinful. Instead of repressing negative expectations, he is drawn to them. It seems as if he's addicted to blaming himself, and he loses his ability to be happy and to make others happy. Even if he is happy, he will eventually succeed in making himself miserable. He also has the uncanny ability to pass his own wretched guilt feelings on to those around him. Cultivating guilt is by no means a sign of high morals and virtue but a pathological and pathogenic phenomenon.

The Effects of Pine

Pine is the essence used to treat guilt feelings. It helps diminish a bad conscience, guilt complex, and compulsive perfectionism. It promotes self-affirmation, responsibility to ourselves, and mental independence. Pine should be used not just for current complaints but also as a treatment for the fundamental personality. It improves our ability to enjoy our lives naturally and without guilt and can often help treat morally related sexual problems as well.

Psychotherapeutic Notes

We cannot speak of guilt feelings without thoroughly examining the phenomenon of guilt, which represents one of the most common causes of disease among people raised in the Christian tradition. It is a given that whoever is born and raised in our culture knows what it is to feel guilt and is constantly confronted with unnatural demands that he can hardly hope to fulfill. We become guilty when we do not pay our debts, when we do not obey a law, or when we do not fulfill an obligation. In itself, this would be relatively harmless and only theoretical if it were not linked with painful consequences: the punishment! This makes guilt a terrifying phenomenon to be taken seriously and avoided.

The system of guilt and punishment is a very effective method for training and controlling people. It is relatively easy to make someone guilty and subject to punishment: one need only make a demand that the person can't (or won't) fulfill. In early childhood we acquire our first painful familiarity with this system. In being punished, we learn that there are limits that we may not exceed and demands that we must fulfill. Thus, we live in constant fear of being punished, which is always linked with our alleged guilt and becomes an integral part of our thoughts and feelings. These feelings are always active when we notice that we cannot be what everyone expects us to be.

This emotion, known as guilt, normally gives us the impression that a higher moral order (the conscience) is making us feel guilty. In truth, there are no higher morals involved, only the simple—and totally natural—fear of punishment. If there were no punishment, no one would have a guilty conscience. To survive, we must be "well brought up," follow the rules, and honor all the prohibitions that our overpowering surroundings impose on us. If we cannot meet these demands and expectations despite our best intentions (because they go against our grain or demand a great amount of self-deception), we develop feelings of guilt—as an expression of our fear of punishment—which become stronger the more sensitive we are and the more painful past punishments have been.

The Christian Church takes this system of guilt/punishment/fear to extremes and demands from us that we dedicate our lives to renunciation and self-denial, accept a dogma that runs counter to our natural sensibilities, and ignore our inborn needs to pursue and experience happiness, self-realization, and mental freedom. These demands are based on the irrational claim that Christ died on the cross for our endless and unredeemable sins, thereby "saving" us but putting us into an even greater debt to God and obliging us to spend our lives doing penance.

The Christian cannot help but feel that he is a continual failure and eternally guilty. He experiences a guilty conscience when things are going well and is always ready to deny himself happiness, or doesn't even expect it. In addition, he suffers from the constant fear of an all-knowing God who allegedly mercilessly punishes us for disregarding his rules. A typical Christian would never dare admit that this domineering, petty, and far from "loving" God conspicuously resembles those people who created this image of him. Furthermore, the skillful and manipulative linking of religious reverence and awe and natural fear of punishment prevents him from undergoing a thorough and clear-eyed examination of his alleged guilt. He might notice very quickly that these alleged rules and prohibitions in truth serve the interests of those who promulgate them.

Is it not always the powerful who preach to the weak, obedient flock, the "haves" who lecture the "have-nots" that they should not steal, the prudish and repressed puritan who condemns a natural sex life, the fanatic who insists on order, or the compulsive character who would eradicate the spontaneous, unplanned element in life? The Pine type is especially susceptible to such guilt because he is very easily influenced and in need of sympathy. Out of insecurity, he tries to make others happy by dancing to their drummer and ignoring his own, and it happens so often that he compulsively and enthusiastically accepts the behavioral norms imposed on him by others. He is sensitive and afraid of anyone who can assert herself and tends to subordinate himself to any power or authority. Here lies the source of his religiously tinged guilt feelings: he trembles at the thought of a divine punishment, but any concept of "God" is just an abstraction of all authority figures who have ever punished or suppressed him. His fear of them is so profound that even as an adult he doesn't dare question the role he assumed as early as childhood.

He must, however, understand this if he ever wants to be free of his guilt feelings. He must also grasp the following fact clearly: throughout history, "guilt" and "sin," despite the inhumane suppression and punishments they have inspired, have never been totally eliminated. This fact demonstrates that there is an elemental and essential factor involved. What is the irresistible power that makes us ignore a law or prohibition that is imposed upon us? It is our drive for self-realization and happiness (which is, in any case, totally subjective and cannot be governed or regulated by others). We cannot help but feel guilt if we are forbidden to do something that it is in our nature to do.

We could look at it the way the Christian religions often do; we could take it as a given that humans are by their very nature fallen, evil, sinful creatures and must always, therefore, be engaged in acts of penance. We can also look at it another way. Feelings of guilt and sin create pain and suffering and make us sick; they can be neither healthy nor natural, and they must be overcome, cured like an illness, if we want to live a free and happy life. Doesn't a happy life consist of joy, desire, and affirmation, and doesn't our natural instinct tell us to resist being tormented or engaging in unnecessary self-denial? Isn't denial a relative of death?

Accepting these simple and seemingly obvious insights is extremely important for the Pine type. Otherwise he cannot free himself from the vicious, life-negating, misery-inducing cycle of guilt/punishment/self-denial/morality. He should also realize that his alleged sins and transgressions are themselves integral components of life. In denying them and in striving for excessive perfection or trying to adjust his behavior to a morality imposed on him by others, he is fighting against himself and against life itself.

Some people, in order to avoid a bad conscience, try to fulfill scrupulously every expectation and demand that has been made of them. As long as we can keep up, our guilt (that is, our fear of punishment) remains mute, and we perceive this to be a "clear conscience"—but it pipes up again at the smallest slip. We are not the masters of our lives, we did not give ourselves the gift of life, and we cannot determine our own fate. We can only—consciously or unconsciously—pursue the course for which we are best suited with the tools with which we are born. We are not responsible for the way things are, and we don't behave badly intentionally. We act the best way we know how, given the particular circumstances.

Everything positive in our lives—happiness, love, health, beauty—comes about when we follow our inner voice, our longings, and our feelings; sadness, sorrow, and illness, on the other hand, are signs that we've strayed in thought or deed from our personal path. We must keep in mind that everything in this life, joy included, has many aspects and that the "higher" facets are also the most precious. When we strive for these higher values, and when we strive for the realization of our divine nature, it can certainly happen that we are asked to deny ourselves something. But we should not see it as a form of denial. When we give something up to receive true riches, we are not denying ourselves anything.

Common Combinations with Other Essences

....

Centaury (4/24): selflessness due to guilt feelings
Cerato (5/24): insecurity due to fear of a bad conscience
Crab Apple (10/24): moralistic compulsion for cleanliness
Mimulus (20/24): fear of guilt

Oak (22/24): unyielding perfectionism
Red Chestnut (24/25): worries caused by a bad conscience
Rock Water (24/27): compulsive perfectionism
Star of Bethlehem (24/29): unprocessed, guilt-related trauma
Walnut (24/33): weakness in defense against accusations
White Chestnut (24/35): compulsive thoughts with overtones
    of guilt

25: Red Chestnut

Characteristics

Red Chestnut is for people who worry very much about others and suffer greatly when others suffer.

AREA OF USE

Red Chestnut is used as the treatment for pathological worrying over others and neurotic sympathy. Used to treat all pathological conditions related to altruistic concerns. In daily life, used to treat oppressive sympathy or pathogenic worrying about others and excessive caring for others.

Causes and Symptoms of Red Chestnut Syndrome

This condition is characterized by an introverted but nonetheless altruistic personality characterized by sensitivity and sympathy. Harmoniously developed, the Red Chestnut type cares deeply about other people. Even though she herself never bothers others with her own needs or desires, she is glad to worry about the well-being of those around her. She sympathetically participates in their lives, is there for them when they need her, and gives them the comforting feeling that they are not alone in the world. In hard times, she doesn't waste her strength in useless worrying but helps effectively and without being asked, wherever and whenever she can. She makes sure, however, that those she helps do not grow too dependent on her or feel in any way obligated to her. She lets those she helps—especially her children—lead their own lives. She does not withdraw her affection if they do not meet her expectations. If she cannot help people—and she is clearly aware when she cannot—she is in the position to leave their fate up to them. She is wise enough to know that no one can really "fall from grace," and that nothing truly bad can happen. She believes that everything that happens serves a higher purpose.

Unfavorably developed—which is to say, when her faith in fate has been shaken—the Red Chestnut type adopts a pessimistic, fearful attitude and tends to expect the worst. These negative expectations have less to do with herself than with those near her; for no apparent reason she will fret excessively over them, all the while neglecting herself. One often has the impression that Red Chestnut types are addicted to worrying. In any case, they almost always find someone for whom they can feel sorry, even if nothing bad has happened—yet. Sometimes the Red Chestnut type can feel that there is something unhealthy in her behavior, but she can't help herself.

A typical example of this type is the mother who lives in constant, excessive, and unfounded worry and fear for her children. Indeed, such "worrisome selflessness" can have a function, and it fits well with our moralistic clichés. When it is excessive, however, it is useless and only causes unhappiness. It affects more than just the "victim," who feels unhappy (and is supremely bothered by the Red Chestnut type's incessant worrying); if you look closely, you can see that the Red Chestnut type herself has a troubled expression and suffers from inner tension, sleeplessness, and anxiety.

The Effects of Red Chestnut

Red Chestnut is the essence used to treat suffering and selfless worrying. It helps eliminate the habit of worrying about others while strengthening our confidence and restoring our trust in fate and a healthy level of egotism. Red Chestnut can treat any condition that is related to worrying, especially nervous conditions and circulatory and respiratory problems.

Psychotherapeutic Notes

The Red Chestnut type is sensitive and has an active imagination. When she experiences unhappiness, her sensitivity and imagination create her anxiety and fears, which are not directed at herself but toward other people. Behind every worry is a positive human element—the emotional investment in the fate of others and simultaneously the desire that things will work out for them. Under healthy, natural conditions, this means that we are concerned about someone else's welfare, while under unhealthy conditions, we worry and fret about them.

In the first case, we support the object of our concern in our actions and stand by him, as much as we are able, in times of need. And we remain aware of our own abilities and limits and protect ourselves from being infected with the problems of those we are trying to help. If this empathy should transform into an unhealthy form of sympathy, the suffering doubles, and the prospects of improvement are diminished. In order to help effectively, we must not be suffering or in need of help ourselves.

In the second case, we unconsciously project our own suffering and fears on the fate of someone else. This type of worrying is useless and senseless because it offers no prospects of improvement, no appropriate help, no end of suffering and unhappiness. It actually serves the purpose of providing an outlet for our own suffering and self-pity and allows us to avoid an embarrassing encounter with the lies that we tell ourselves to survive. We avoid having to ask ourselves why we're unhappy, what we need to change in our lives, or why we have such negative expectations of the future yet can give ourselves up to watching our own negativity (based on a totally speculative *potential* unhappiness) play itself out in someone else's life.

When we worry about someone else, we give expression to our own pessimism and also gain distance from it. Instead of paying attention to our own anxieties, we think that we are concerned with the well-being of other people. The clearly pathogenic anxiety and pessimism of the Red Chestnut type lead her to worry. Making a precise diagnosis of this condition is difficult because worrying about other people is often taken to be a sort of moral superiority or moral high ground. Who could possibly admit that one's seemingly selfless concern for the welfare of others is merely an expression of and a distraction from one's own fears?

The essential problem for the Red Chestnut type lies in her ignoring a basic truth of life: we cannot grasp the secret of our lives, and we are not in the position to judge our own fate. Our notions of "good" and "bad" are not sufficient because they are oriented toward superficial well-being and are merely expressions of our limited insight. This is just as true of our expectations of the future. How often have we experienced that what seemed to be a catastrophe turned out to be a blessing in disguise? We realize too seldom that there is a mysterious force, order, or wisdom at work, which obviously knows better than we what is good for us.

It is up to us whether we want to have positive expectations of the future or to fear the worst. While our expectations have no influence on the future, they can affect the present. Thus, we can determine, to a certain extent, whether we will be ruled by happiness or sadness. We cannot avoid every form of misery and unhappiness, but we can certainly avoid those that we create with our own pessimism and negativity.

The problem of the Red Chestnut type is not just a lack of trust in fate or in "God" but a dishonesty with herself. She recoils at the prospect of seeing her behavior at face value, of realizing that she is not living her life correctly, that she herself has created the fears with which she lives, that she has bothered and burdened her "victims" (especially children) and has intruded on their lives and perhaps even infected them with her unhealthy habits. The solution for her problems lies within herself. It won't help for her to convince herself, by careful consideration, that a particular worry is groundless; she must instead find a new way of behaving, which means trusting life, fate, or God. She should learn to see again that her life is an unbroken chain of positive, maturing learning experiences (positive because they help her grow), even when those experiences cause her unhappiness. She should let herself consciously examine her worries and expectations to recognize how groundless and laughable they are, and she should get used to telling herself that everything's going to be just fine.

Common Combinations with Other Essences

Agrimony (1/25): secret worries
Aspen (2/25): general, anxiety-induced worries
Centaury (4/25): worrying selflessness
Cherry Plum (6/25): rage-inducing worries
Chicory (8/25): total self-sacrifice
Impatiens (18/25): restless worrying
Mimulus (20/25): anxious, excessive concern for others
Mustard (21/25): depressive worrying
Olive (23/25): debilitating worries
Pine (24/25): worries caused by a bad conscience
Rock Rose (25/26): panic-inducing worries
Star of Bethlehem (25/29): excessive worries caused by
negative experiences
White Chestnut (25/35): fretful thoughts

26: Rock Rose

Characteristics

Rock Rose is the essence for emergencies, panic, and shock.

AREA OF USE

Rock Rose is used as the basic treatment for a tendency toward panic, psychic instability, and latent anxiety. Used to treat all pathological conditions related to psychic shock or panic. In daily life, used for emergencies, shocking experiences, fear, "blanking out" during exams, loss of presence of mind, and losing one's head.

Causes and Symptoms of Rock Rose Syndrome

This condition is characterized by emotional openness, an impressionable character, sensitivity, and great spontaneity. Harmoniously developed, the Rock Rose type is open to all impressions and reacts spontaneously. His emotions cannot be controlled by conditioning, habit, or negative experiences; they are not filtered, stifled, or faked but are expressed directly and naturally. He is not stubborn or inflexible and will not be thrown off balance by the unexpected; instead he reacts flexibly and without resistance to everything he sees and experiences, like a water plant swaying in the current. Like an innocent child, he has an open, unbiased, impartial spirit, and there is hardly anything that can surprise or frighten him. He has an inner security, natural resilience, and presence of mind.

Unfavorably developed, the sensitivity of the Rock Rose type can change to oversensitivity, his impressionable nature can cause him to be easily shaken or disturbed, and his spontaneity can lead to excessive, inappropriate reactions. Rock Rose syndrome stems from the inability to stand unusual experiences and manifests itself in panic or a breakdown. As a rule, people with the typical Rock Rose disposition end up this way. Under catastrophic conditions, these symptoms can appear in other types as well. We cannot remain calm and composed and keep our presence of mind at the sign of surprising or troublesome events; we lose our perspective, end up with an inner block, or behave unreasonably. This will happen in the case of accidents or sudden, violent conflicts with a hidden, bothersome problem with which we are confronted again and again. A typical example is when some-one is diagnosed with cancer. This diagnosis sends most people into a state of panic because they often mistakenly accept it as the equivalent of a death sentence, and they cannot get used to the idea that they might die at any time.

The Effects of Rock Rose

Rock Rose is first aid for panic. It restores our quiet, our composure, our presence of mind, our courage, and our clearheadedness. Rock Rose is help-ful in accidents or instances of sudden violence because it releases the blockages that these events can cause and restores the normal coordination of the mental and vegetative functions. It is an important ingredient in Rescue Remedy.

Psychotherapeutic Notes

The Rock Rose syndrome arises, as does any fear or anxiety, when an excess supply of psychic and physical defensive energy cannot be channeled appropriately, resulting in a sort of internal bottleneck. In addition, the nor-mal mental functions are thrown out of balance, and the result is that we panic or "lose our heads." Such conditions arise when we are faced with any kind of surprise or shock. From a biological point of view, a shock or sur-prise can signal a potential danger; the organism reacts by immediately mobilizing additional energy to flee or fight. Once the danger has been averted, the body returns to its normal state. If not, there is a buildup of excess defensive energy, and panic ensues. This situation comes about when we have overplanned our lives or feel too secure, but have left no room for anything unplanned or out of the ordinary. Sometimes our unprocessed negative experiences result in an anxiety-ridden oversensitivity with respect to certain life situations, and our body overreacts, as with an allergy.

There are two types or people who fall quite easily into a state of panic— the inflexible, rational person who controls and plans everything, who loses his perspective when he is confronted with an unexpected or inexplicable situation; and a sensitive person with a fragile constitution (the typical Rock Rose type!), who lives with deep-seated fears and quickly loses his cool when faced with unexpected, potentially threatening situations. Where the person of reason has too much need to control, the emotional person has too little. Essentially, both types suffer from an underlying fear that is kept in check only with great difficulty. These fears can be compared to allergies in that they can easily get out of control and themselves become a source of even more fear or panic. The rational self, which has not formed a flexible, realistic concept of life and has no room for the irrational or unexpected, has all it can do in trying to cope with everyday survival; eventually this type lose their heads and their reactions become unconscious and involuntary.

This happens especially in the case of accidents. The fundamental beliefs that shape their existence are shaken; an unexpected or intense event will disorient them and destroy their sense of perspective. They don't know anymore what they should do; shell-shocked, they stare at the remains of what used to be their perfect, infallible world: they become crippled or else react instinctively. If we find ourselves in this situation, we should try to get some rest, distance ourselves from the causes, and give the psyche a chance to restore its balance. Sometimes this approach can help neutralize the shock and replace it with a more positive perspective.

People in a pronounced Rock Rose condition need outside guidance, at least in the short term. They cannot deal with everyday problems and need the opportunity to withdraw into themselves and find a new starting point for their lives. In extreme cases, medication that can forcefully break through the pathological mental and emotional block is called for. As a rule, we should try to avoid such drastic situations, but we can use the little surprises and disappointments of everyday life to strengthen our flexibility, presence of mind, and sense of security. The basis for this is being open to experience and developing an acceptance of fate. If we have no expectations, we can't be disappointed; if we can accept and express our feelings, we can't be over-whelmed by them; and when we can face our fears, anxieties, and weaknesses, we cannot fall prey to them. When we can adopt a playful, open sense of life, we will never be overcome by it.

In order to reach this attitude, we must always make it clear to ourselves that, in the end, we cannot plan our lives and we cannot control or compre-hend all of its complexities. We have no power over our own fate, and we actually comprehend very little of the secrets of our existence. We can believe, however, that there is a guiding force (such as God) that creates and guides those mysteries that we don't comprehend as well as those things that daily fill us with wonder, gratitude, and awe.

Common Combinations with Other Essences

Agrimony (1/26): lack of feeling resulting from panic

Aspen (2/26): extreme anxiety-related panic

Cherry Plum (6/26): panic with the danger of losing the rational faculties

Clematis (9/26): tendency to lose consciousness with panic

Elm (11/26): panic accompanied by stress

Impatiens (18/26): driven behavior caused by panic

Mimulus (20/26): anxiety with a tendency toward panic

Scleranthus (26/28): unable to function when in a panic

Star of Bethlehem (26/29): psychic shock caused by panic

Sweet Chestnut (26/30): desperation caused by panic and fear

27: Rock Water (water from a rock spring with the power of the Sun)
Characteristics

Rock Water is for people who are too hard on themselves or have a tendency toward self-castigation.

AREA OF USE

Rock Water is used to treat ascetic, martyrlike behavior, excessive self-discipline and self-control, self-abuse with lack of joy, self-torment, compulsive fanaticism and dogmatism, and fear of emotions. Used to treat all pathological conditions related to obsessive/compulsive behavior or self-abuse. In daily life, used to treat excessive self-discipline, excessive need for planning and control, fanatical dieting, self-imposed self-denial, and strictness with oneself.

Causes and Symptoms of Rock Water Syndrome

This condition is introverted and is characterized by rationality, idealism, and a need for inner discipline. Harmoniously developed, the Rock Water type has enormous self-discipline and a highly developed sense of morals. She makes great, idealistically tinged demands of herself and sticks to them long after others have given up. She's reliable, but she never relies on herself. She can never be talked into something that she doesn't believe in. Although she never makes compromises with herself, she is forbearing and tolerant of others. She would never demand of anyone that they adopt her attitudes or fulfill her demands, because her philosophy is very personal and subjective and she accepts that each of us should follow his own path. She is, however, always aware of the responsibility that we all carry in that we should serve as examples for others; she strives unobtrusively to make herself a positive role model as a way of serving humanity. She is often seen as a symbol that even in today's corrupt, self-centered world there is room for pure ideals and a strong spirit. She gives those around her the courage to stay true to themselves.

Unfavorably developed, her life-affirming, understanding idealism can turn into dogmatic, alienated thinking, and she can lose her flexibility. Her inborn self-centeredness allows her to withdraw from her surroundings and suppress her natural feelings while masking them with an uncompromising rationality. The result is a dogmatic, introverted idealism that leads to an excessive sense of self-discipline. In this condition, the Rock Water type is unable to react flexibly and effectively to life's intensity, mutability, and contradictions. The stronger her feelings, the more rigorously she tries to suppress them; in doing so, she does not recoil from self-castigation or self-torment, as we know from certain "holy" people in their battle against sexual temptation. The typical Rock Water type strives to replace a less-than-perfect reality with an ideal and perfect inner world, and she tries to ward off life's uncomfortable unpredictability by sticking to a very rational and strictly held regime. She uses such methods as exact scheduling of her days, a strict diet or exercise regime, or religious or ideological dogmas. She is welcome wherever idealistic or morally oriented denial, self-denial, or martyrdom are practiced, such as in religious or ideological cults. Naturally, there are physical consequences to her behavior—tension and stress, which above all affect the musculature (in conditions such as rheumatism), the circulatory system (degeneration and calcification), the liver and gallbladder (infections, stones), and sexual dysfunction.

The Effects of Rock Water

Rock Water is the essence used to treat self-denial and self-rejection. It frees us from inflexible self-discipline, makes us more open to our own feelings, and promotes mental flexibility and a carefree, positive attitude. It also works against tension and hardening due to excessive self-control. Rock Water is a primal healing essence. This invisible essence from pure, pristine rock springs loaded with energy from the Sun is the elixir of life of the Bach essences because it removes self-destructive, life-negating tendencies and fosters a positive, constructive joy in life. It represents the life-affirming and sustaining principle of natural water.

Psychotherapeutic Notes

Because the Rock Water type cannot come to terms with the variety of life, she tries to grapple with it by painting everything in black and white;

because her feelings make her weak and susceptible to all kinds of influences and bring her into conflict with the strong need for a clear, regulated life, she suppresses these inclinations through her dogmatism. She treats herself harshly and rationally, like a stern father keeping his children in control, in order to keep her irrational impulses in check. And there is also a somewhat romantic element in her behavior, in that she has an inclination to have "noble" interests, such as ecology, natural medicine, spirituality, and religion. The Rock Water type's strict idealism, however noble its intentions, is nonetheless pathological and pathogenic because she tries to make the world fit into an arbitrary scheme. She tries with great force of will to realize her theoretical and often alienating ideas, but she is unable to live her life naturally, truthfully, and happily (which is to say, she is unable to live life as it really is; at times, she can be very depressed.

Rock Water behavior is very self-centered but still exerts a certain effect on other people, not just because of the Rock Water type's inability to compromise but also because of her inborn tendency toward self-negation, which is often taken as being superhuman. Life-negating misanthropes or self-tormenting ascetics are often mistaken for holy people. Actually, however, the true holy person is at peace with herself, modest, and content. She lives an unusual life, not out of some kind of unnatural inner compulsion or obsession but because she stays true to herself and realizes what lies within her and what she is suited for. Her mode of living is so exemplary and so rare that we can't help but marvel at it; because of the truth that it expresses, we call it holy. "Holy" in this case means "leading to salvation or redemption." While a true holy person would never want to be "holy" in this sense, the Rock Water type has this tendency.

The solution to this problem can be found in the very thing that created the Rock Water essence. The rock springs deep in the earth correspond to the deep recesses of the human subconscious; the water accumulates in clear rock pools, which correspond to rational thought and the process of becoming conscious. Finally, the water is energized with the power of the Sun, which corresponds to the eternal divine, godlike spirit. Even if we rely too heavily on our conscious selves, we can still be happy and healthy. We should take seriously our feelings, inspirations, and intuitions, which arise from the depths of our soul, and put them into a clear, meaningful order and charge them with inspiration.

If the Rock Water type dares to acknowledge her feelings, and if she can allow herself to take life as it comes to her, she can shed her fears and lead a free and natural life. Then she can begin to recognize any ultimate truths and validate her efforts. Reason can be manipulated and programmed, but the heart is incorruptible: it gives us the answer to our question according to the right and the good, which, in any case, does not lie in compulsive ideals, dogma, or rules. Its language is so simple that anyone can understand it; it is the direct, primitive, and often "immoral" joy of living against which the Rock Water type fights so intensely and vainly

Common Combinations with Other Essences

Aspen (2/27): anxiety-induced self-abuse

Beech (3/27): generosity with others and strictness with oneself

Cerato (5/27): mental dependence and self-abuse

Cherry Plum (6/27): psychic consequences of severe self-denial

Crab Apple (10/27): excessive cleanliness and discipline

Oak (22/27): self-tormenting desire to achieve

Pine (24/27): compulsive perfectionism

Vine (27/32): strict personality

Water Violet (27/34): fleeing from the world and self-castigation

Wild Oat (27/36): self-castigation as a replacement for a purpose in life

28: Scleranthus
Characteristics

Scleranthus is for people who have difficulties making decisions.

AREA OF USE

Scleranthus is used as the basic treatment for indecisiveness, inconsistency, instability, inner turmoil, erratic and unreliable behavior, lack of concentration, and illnesses with changeable symptoms. Used to treat all pathological conditions related to indecisiveness or mutability. In daily life, used to treat scatterbrained behavior, indecisiveness, absentmindedness, distracted behavior, moodiness, and lack of concentration.

Causes and Symptoms of Scleranthus Syndrome

This condition is characterized by an open, curious, and flexible mind. Harmoniously developed, the Scleranthus type is mentally flexible and has diverse interests. Because he can see both the positive and negative sides to everything, he can never act unjustifiably or out of a one-sided, closed-minded motivation. His ability to view the positive aspects of even the most gloomy events allows him to take everything in stride. He is not easily shaken or frightened. His uncomplicated, tolerant manner, his nonjudgmental understanding for everything that life throws at him, and his accepting, comprehensive worldview make him a popular and entertaining companion who serves as living proof that things are not so bad. He makes decisions easily, with his playful lightness and sense of security. He is more open and less apt to judge harshly and has more of a talent for seeing the "big picture" than most other people, and is not handicapped by preconceptions. He can adapt to changing circumstances and alter his priorities for action at any time. If necessary, he can reevaluate his decisions from one day to the next, without fretting about it for a long time.

Unfavorably developed, this mental eclecticism can lead to inner turmoil and a general inability to make decisions. This inclination can run so deeply that both conscious and unconscious actions and reactions can become muddled and confused and the instinctive sense of security that is so important in shaping our lives can take a backseat to indecisiveness.

Every action must be preceded by a clear decision, whether it is conscious or unconscious.

The unfavorably developed Scleranthus type is unable to make decisions quickly and sensibly. He finds himself constantly plagued by the tension between the many (often contradictory) aspects that he (almost against his will) discovers in everything, and he is tormented by the prospect of making a one-sided, biased decision. His diverse interests often compel him to undertake several projects at once, which he can only partially complete; this becomes another source of frustration. He should be aware that for him "less is more."

The Scleranthus type is easily distracted and finds it difficult to concentrate on one thought or act; new ideas are coming to him all the time. A venture begun will soon become boring to him; while he's working on one project, he's already thinking about the next one or even shifting his thoughts back and forth among several subjects. This jumble in his head can lead to an inability to think clearly, absentmindedness, muddleheadedness, flightiness, or problems with concentration.

The Scleranthus condition, marked by a mental block or inner chaos, also arises in normal people when they have to make decisions under pressure, for example, during examinations. When this happens, the wealth of knowledge either gets mashed into a muddled mess or the fear of failure prevents an orderly train of thought. The physical symptoms of Scleranthus syndrome are constantly changing symptoms or ailments that move about the body, fluctuating temperature, mood swings, vague symptoms, and relapses during convalescence.

The Effects of Scleranthus

Scleranthus is the essence used to treat indecisiveness. It brings about a certain mental clarity and consistency, is effective against erratic behavior and mental conflict, and improves the abilities for decision making and concentration. Scleranthus is often helpful for illnesses with incompatible or seemingly inappropriate symptoms.

Psychotherapeutic Notes

Making a decision means being content with that decision. Only when we are content to choose from myriad possibilities can we make a decision. The Scleranthus type, who has difficulty making decisions, needs to learn the conscious practice of contentment. This natural contentment does not consist of a willingness to stunt ourselves or ask for less than we feel we deserve, as in the case of moral contentment, but, quite the contrary, in consciously demanding the best and pushing the rest aside. (The "best" has less to do with material advantages than with anything that can be of value for the spirit.) Natural contentment is an element of coping with life in a conscious, healthy manner; moralistic contentment, on the other hand, is a false contentment, averse to life, because life never voluntarily denies itself what it needs. At most, it can be useful to survival in a society of people obsessed with possessions and power.

The Scleranthus type's indecisiveness can be overcome when he learns to consciously set priorities. This means making the most appropriate choices from a plethora of possibilities and, for the time being, putting everything else aside. He should be aware of where his psyche, with the help of his emotions and inspirations, will lead him. His survival instinct will serve him better and more clearly than his more rational, conditioned, learned responses. Some Scleranthus types try to overcome their indecisiveness by making totally arbitrary decisions, which they cannot truly stand behind. In doing this, they attack the problem only superficially and strengthen it internally, because they lack the motivation to learn discipline in shaping their lives. For Scleranthus types, there are only momentary solutions, not permanent ones. Because his life's path runs a zigzag course, he should try to keep his detours to a minimum, while continually living for the moment and adjusting his strategy for action to the ever changing conditions of life.

Common Combinations with Other Essences

Aspen (2/28): indecisiveness due to vague fears

Cerato (5/28): insecurity with difficulties in decision making

Chestnut Bud (7/28): learning difficulties due to distractedness

Clematis (9/28): indecisiveness due to daydreaming

Gentian (12/28): relapses during recovery from an illness

Impatiens (18/28): erratic and impatient

Mimulus (20/28): indecisiveness stemming from anxiety

Mustard (21/28): constant mood swings

Rock Rose (26/28): inability to act due to panic

Wild Oat (28/36): inner turmoil and life crisis

29: Star of Bethlehem

Characteristics

Star of Bethlehem is for people who do not have the strength to bear unhappy situations or devastating experiences.

AREA OF USE

Star of Bethlehem is used for basic treatment of unprocessed or unresolved psychic or physical trauma, seemingly unbearable life situations, inability to forget or let go, neuroses, and consequences of accidents. Used to treat all pathological conditions related to injuries or psychic trauma and shock. In daily life, used to treat unhappiness, grief, nightmares, psychic shock, excessive need for comfort, and injuries.

Causes and Symptoms of Star of Bethlehem Syndrome

This condition is characterized by a great sensitivity and a tendency to be easily influenced, a good memory, and a strong need for happiness and a perfect world that cannot be fulfilled owing to a lack of strength. Harmoniously developed, the Star of Bethlehem type is sensitive, open, and happy with her life and has a good instinct for avoiding anything that might hurt her. To this end, her unusually good memory is most useful, with the help of which she always remembers exactly if certain life conditions or behavioral patterns have pleasant or unpleasant results. This incessant caution regarding everything that can cause her sadness is unavoidable for her because her extreme sensitivity makes her suffer with any negative experiences. In addition to this outer protection, she also has an inner security that allows her to accept her fate. Because of her instinctive sensitivity, she has the ability to find an element that is right and good in everything that happens so that she doesn't suffer. She is the kind of person who calmly feels joy from her life by carefully putting all difficulties aside; in keeping a positive attitude, she can take the sting out of misery.

Unfavorably developed, which means under the influence of unbearable circumstances or a sudden, terrible experience, this sensitivity can turn into a heightened sensitivity that is the source of sorrow. The superior memory of the Star of Bethlehem type can cause her torment (this, by the way, can even occur in individuals who are psychically robust). The following symptoms illustrate Star of Bethlehem syndrome: inconsolable grief, nightmares, depressive moods, and fears or behavioral disorders related to unhappy circumstances or a traumatic event. Anyone in this condition has more or less lost the ability to have a positive attitude and the ability to focus on the future—she can think only about his misfortune. There are also people who cannot overcome a serious loss or a disappointment in love or whose lives have taken a sudden, radical turn for the worse owing to a catastrophe or who have experienced the shattering of an illusion on which their whole existence has depended or whose lives are simply miserable. They often give the impression that they have reached the low point and that their minds are fixated on the negative. It is evident to an observer that they have bottomed out.

The Effects of Star of Bethlehem

Star of Bethlehem is the great mind-altering essence if a deep and far-reaching process of awakening the consciousness is indicated. It is useful in overcoming psychic or physical trauma (or accidents) and can improve neurotic behavioral disorders. It helps us bear the burden of heavy life situations or work through terrible shocks. Nightmares are a special indication. We should always use Star of Bethlehem when we have the feeling that the process of recovery is being blocked for some unknown reason. It is one of the most important essences used in cancer treatment because cancer is often triggered by severe psychological trauma, and it cannot be brought into check without first healing the trauma (discovered by Dr. R. G. Hamer). The shock resulting from a cancer diagnosis is especially dangerous since, in their ignorance, most patients take it to be the same as a death sentence. Only the most stable individuals can overcome such a trauma, but the typical Star of Bethlehem type is shattered by such news and dies, in the end, not from the cancer itself but from the shock of receiving the diagnosis.

Psychotherapeutic Notes

Humans have a consciousness that separates us from all other living creatures and that follows a general principle of growth: substances or energy is consumed, changed according to need, and made to fit into the existing structure in an appropriate form. While the body metabolizes material in a complex process of selection, purification, and metamorphosis, the spirit assimilates psychic material—information, impressions, and knowledge—and puts it through a complicated metamorphosis. The result is the so-called expanding consciousness, which distinguishes us as conscious beings.

It is notable in this process of assimilation that not just what we take in (nutrition, information) but also the system that absorbs it undergoes a change. We really are what we eat. Just as food has an influence on the makeup of the body, the quality of the spiritual and mental material processed has an influence on a person's consciousness. The "nutrients" we receive are thus of prime importance to our mental and emotional growth. Raw, primitive, or intolerable influences affect us just as much as refined or humane ones. Depending on our upbringing, we can have a healthy, vital, naturally self-affirming spirit and be able to deal with life, or we can have an anxious, neurotic, and self-negating spirit.

Even the "digestibility" of what we absorb is important in this connection. If the food is too heavy, it drains the organism of strength or damages it; if it is too light, it will be easily consumed, but the organism cannot do much with it and does not derive much sustenance. The spirit needs appropriate stimuli that it can easily tolerate and process but that can also provide nourishment. If we are healthy, we look for tasks, themes, or problems that will serve to expand our knowledge or horizons. On the other hand, we can opt for lightweight, insubstantial fare that goes down easily but leaves us feeling empty and causes our mental faculties to atrophy.

Another factor plays a key role in mental and physical sustenance. If we hastily wolf down our food, if we don't chew thoroughly or don't take time to taste and enjoy our food, we don't derive any nutritional benefits. Accordingly, our consciousness also develops insufficiently, and we become frustrated and, finally, psychosomatically ill, if we will not pay attention positively and honestly to that which we need to feed our conscious selves.

The Star of Bethlehem syndrome is, to a certain extent, a spiritual digestive problem. Our "life's food" is too rich for the overly sensitive "psychic digestive tract" with which the pampered Star of Bethlehem type is equipped. She cannot get over the shock, the terror, the loss, the pain, the sorrow, the fateful blow; she can derive no psychic strength and cannot grow. She just sits, moaning and groaning in the corner, bemoaning her aching body and its failing functions. She can think only of the indigestible chunks fate has thrust down her throat.

In other words, anyone who finds herself with Star of Bethlehem syndrome has not experienced enough conflict in this life, has ignored the messages sent to teach her, and has neglected the abilities of her intellect and the quality of her spirit. She cannot digest the heavy fare that fate has served up for her, and this impedes her development. Unexpected events can take on a devastating character for her, and unhappy life circumstances are simply unbearable.

People with a sensitive and open demeanor and the good memory of the Star of Bethlehem type can defend themselves only with difficulty against harmful influences. They are like soft wax in which life effortlessly puts its stamp. Fate often leaves behind such clear marks in the psyche that if outside help is not available (in the form of therapy or a compensating positive experience), such people are always scarred by them. Star of Bethlehem types can naturally not recognize that such afflictions are actually signs that the spirit is trying to shake things up and find a new way of living; our psyche allows to rise to the surface only those things for which we are mentally and emotionally ready. The fact that a problem is cropping up in our lives means that we must face it; otherwise our spiritual development will be retarded.

If we are spiritually overwrought and blocked, we should try to free ourselves from this blockage so that no lasting neuroses or relationship problems remain. In general, these problems can be troubled family relationships, unhappy marriages, or humiliating or frustrating work situations. Help is relatively useless if we can't learn to come to terms with life and its surprises. We should always strive for honesty with ourselves and a clear-eyed attentiveness for the truth and be ready to look at fate in a positive light. The Star of Bethlehem type should try to consciously face everything that she finds disturbing or shocking. At least, she can practice on the little, relatively harmless shocks of everyday life.

Common Combinations with Other Essences

Agrimony (1/29): spiritual wounds behind a happy mask

Aspen (2/29): spiritual injury due to fear

Cerato (5/29): insecurity caused by a shocking experience

Cherry Plum (6/29): psychosis due to spiritual injury

Clematis (9/29): unconsciousness prompted by shocking experiences

Crab Apple (10/29): pathological loathing

Elm (11/29): breakdown caused by a spiritual shock

Gentian (12/29): weak will as the result of psychic trauma

Holly (15/29): aggression due to spiritual distress

Honeysuckle (16/29): unresolved loss

Larch (19/29): loss of self-confidence from spiritual trauma

Mimulus (20/29): anxiety due to psychic trauma

Mustard (21/29): depression caused by psychic trauma

Olive (23/29): lack of spiritual resistance due to exhaustion

Pine (24/29): unprocessed (unresolved) guilty trauma

Red Chestnut (25/29): excessive worries as the result of negative experiences

Rock Rose (26/29): psychic devastation and panic

Sweet Chestnut (29/30): despair caused by psychic devastation

Walnut (29/33): lack of resistance against (or caused by) psychic trauma

Water Violet (29/34): human contact problems stemming from spiritual trauma

White Chestnut (29/35): traumatic compulsive thoughts

Willow (29/38): bitterness caused by unprocessed or unresolved trauma

30: Sweet Chestnut
Characteristics

Sweet Chestnut is for people who are in total despair and stand on the verge of a breakdown.

AREA OF USE

Sweet Chestnut is used for the basic treatment of desperation, mental anguish, extreme depression, acute hopelessness, extreme spiritual suffering, and mental or physical breakdown. Used to treat all pathological conditions related to desperation. In daily life, Sweet Chestnut is seldom needed—only if we are at the end of our rope and don't know how to proceed.

Causes and Symptoms of Sweet Chestnut Syndrome

This condition is characterized by a great inner strength, self-responsibility, and the ability to suffer consciously. Harmoniously developed, the Sweet Chestnut type is independent, possesses an inner strength, and is up to meeting life's challenges. He doesn't avoid problems but sees them as a kind of personal test and an opportunity for mental and spiritual growth. He is sure to drain the bitter cup that life has offered him without falling to pieces. He is convinced that any life is essentially good and that even the pains and sorrows that life sends his way also serve to make him better. He knows that the spirit cannot be lost or defeated and that we are never faced with a test that is beyond our ability to pass (even though we may be pushed to our limits or lose our physical lives).

Unfavorably developed, the inner strength of the Sweet Chestnut type can turn into a pigheaded, arrogant inflexibility that puts him in a power struggle with his fate. Because this is a battle he cannot win, he becomes mired in a senseless and stubborn resistance to reality that takes him to the limits of his mental and emotional powers and leaves him desperate. It's as if he were in a trap from which there is no escape, and he feels that his next move—if he is even able to make it—will inevitably lead him to a breakdown or to his own destruction. He can't think anymore, can't feel anymore, can't act anymore, and waits like a mountain climber who—in the literal and figurative sense of the word—has gone too far and for whom there is no more forward or backward, only the final fall to the end, in which he sees a possible solution.

The Effects of Sweet Chestnut

Sweet Chestnut is the essence used against total desperation. It is a type of mental "softener" and enables us to release our resistance and our reservations in dealing with reality. It gives us an acceptable perspective to go on living and lets us find a way out of a seemingly hopeless situation. Once more optimistic, realistic, and more human, the Sweet Chestnut type can let go of his weaknesses and leave himself trustingly in the hands of fate. Sweet Chestnut can also be tried when the body is in an extreme state of reactive rigidity.

The basic theme of the Sweet Chestnut type is that of "conscious suffering." This does not mean inflicting on oneself a masochistic form of suffering or strengthening sorrows that already exist. It does mean, however, being clear with ourselves that we are suffering, why we are suffering, and that we are not entirely innocent. Most of us tend to shy away from this view because then we obligate ourselves to do something about our suffering, and this makes it impossible to act as if we are powerless to do anything. All of us, through either our behavior or our attitudes, contribute to our own misery. Suffering comes about essentially when we try to resist reality and want to have things other than the way they really are. If we understand conscious suffering, we can prevent extreme suffering by dealing attentively with our fate and our feelings, by correcting negative developments when they first arise, and by resolutely battling unhappiness.

Our life is like a line that travels in a zigzag path running between various life-determining poles. Our psyche wants to maintain its inner balance and reacts to every deviation from the personal ideal with a respective countermovement. It compels us, at the sign of frustrations, not just to correct life's constant little irregularities but also to mount an extreme counterreaction in the case of serious deviations.

Sweet Chestnut types are always faced with the dichotomy between strength and weakness and between fighting and giving up. They normally face their problems bravely and take them as personal tests; they fight earnestly against the difficulties and challenges of their fate. On occasion, they go too far and forget that fate, like a good-natured father with his child, only enters into the struggle playfully, in order to call forth the child's strengths and abilities. When the child (in this case the Sweet Chestnut type) tries too seriously or too stubbornly to oppose an unalterable reality, he learns who the master is, and his arrogant strength is transformed into extreme weakness and pushes him to the limits of sorrow.

Instinctively, we realize that we have brought about this situation ourselves. In truth, behind this behavior is a searching question: "Who are you, God? I challenge you to acknowledge me!" This question is an essential one for Sweet Chestnut types, who always have their lives in control because they have lost their elemental awareness that they are merely creatures and weak humans. In other words, the more inflexibly we behave and the more forcefully we refuse to accept that which fate offers us, the more deeply our soul compels us to the extreme limits in order to make us conscious of our own human pettiness and weaknesses. In the desperation of the Sweet Chestnut syndrome, we finally recognize the existence of "God"—and often so absolutely that we are not even capable of pleading or prayer. We are unable to take charge of our lives and are aware of our unconditional helplessness and absolute insignificance. The final solution lies in death or purification.

In principle, any of us could find ourselves in this situation; it occurs more commonly, however, in those with the symptoms described here. When this condition appears, reasonable words and advice do not help very much, because we are acting with an infantile helplessness. At best, the proper medication (Bach flowers and homeopathy) can bring about a rapid improvement under the right conditions; otherwise, we must—guardedly—wait until our psyche has found its way back to its normal condition.

We can avoid the Sweet Chestnut syndrome by paying attention to the warning signs, which our spirit offers us in the form of minor, frustrating losses or defeats. With its help, we can correct our inner behavior or external conditions. We can learn flexibility when we recognize that our plans are unrealistic; we can learn tractability when we cannot realize our desires; and we can learn to accept fate when things are not going well for us and to accept God when we have hit bottom.

Common Combinations with Other Essences

Cherry Plum (6/30): desperation due to emotional stress

Elm (11/30): desperation caused by overexertion

Gorse (13/30): absolutely hopeless desperation

Rock Rose (26/30): desperation due to panicky fear and anxiety

Star of Bethlehem (29/30): desperation due to a mental or emotional shock

31: Vervain
Characteristics

Vervain is for people who burden others with their convictions and missionary zeal.

AREA OF USE

Vervain is used for the basic treatment of missionary tendencies, intolerant idealism, a need to improve the world, fixed ideas, inflexible beliefs and convictions, fanaticism, and blindly zealous beliefs. Used to treat all pathological conditions related to excessive zeal or missionary tendencies that are pushy or insistent. In daily life, used to treat pushiness, excessive enthusiasm, one-sidedness, preconceptions, lack of a sense of proportion, stress, nervousness, and tension.

Causes and Symptoms of Vervain Syndrome

This condition is characterized by extroversion and consists of a humane sense of idealism, goal-oriented thinking, strength of will, and a need to dominate. Harmoniously developed, the Vervain type is an enthusiastic, can-do idealist who gladly places her talents and knowledge in the service of others. She has a view for what those around her need and is always ready to help them. Her selflessness is combined with an ambitious, active spirit and a strong will—thus she can achieve remarkable results where the well-being of others is concerned. Because she wishes for things to go well for those around her, it never occurs to her to impose her own opinions on them, to convert them to her way of thinking, or to place them in a kind of mental yoke. She is inspired to put her personal sense of mission into action. She feels "called" and sent to share her riches with those in need and to bring them what they need for body and soul, while taking care not to force upon them anything that will be harmful.

Unfavorably developed, her idealism can turn into intolerance, her readiness to help can change to a need to impose her will on others, and her natural superiority can become dominance, which turns the Vervain type into an intolerant do-gooder or a fanatical missionary. By nature oriented toward success and driven by a sense of mission, she can lose her feeling for the uniqueness and worth of other people; she cannot stop herself from barging uninvited into the lives of others or imposing on them what she feels is best for them. She interferes exactly because she has the best intentions, and many will rightly find her to be imposing, intolerant, or fanatical. Even when she is physically not robust, she can still mobilize an unusually great amount of strength to carry out her obsession with an idea or a mission. She is restless and undeterred, and she has a wonderful capacity for dedication and concentration when it comes to reaching her goals. She is helpless against life's diversity and mutability, however, and finds it difficult to direct her energies toward determining whether her ideas and intentions are realizable and sensible. Above all, she can become especially captivated by lofty moral values. When she loses the appropriate sense of proportion, she pursues a goal that she has set for herself like someone obsessed or tries to follow with missionary zeal what she takes to be the right path. This attitude creates an imbalance: there is more in the world than what the Vervain type thinks or feels is right. Reality has its own rules, and there are those who resist having someone else's form of "happiness" imposed upon them. Thus, all the energy she has gathered becomes directed at herself, and she becomes rushed, tense, sleepless, or stressed, without noticing how fanatical, pushy, or intolerant she has become.

The Effects of Vervain

Vervain is the essence used to treat stress-related, missionary overzealousness. It helps us respect the attitudes of others and allows us to let them live happily in their own manner. It broadens our horizons and brings about the realization that we do not have a monopoly on the truth. At the same time, it prevents zeal and enthusiasm from becoming ends in themselves and creating a source of stress. In appropriate cases, it works against nervous tension, insomnia, high blood pressure, or tension and can help initiate a healing relaxation phase in the case of overwork and overexertion or stress on the sympathetic nervous system.

Psychotherapeutic Notes

The problem of the Vervain type lies in her greatest virtue, her idealistic enthusiasm for helping, when it grows out of control and becomes superficial. In this case, our culture, which is predominately devoid of meaning, is responsible, for it does not allow us to be brought up to find ourselves and develop our own sense of the truth (truth not in the moral sense but in the sense of things *as they truly are*). Having failed in this regard, our society does not allow us to channel our energies in a meaningful manner. In any case, the Vervain type should become clear about the meaning of idealism and helping.

"Ideals" are essentially the creations of a dissatisfied psyche. When life does not offer us what we expect or desire, we often try to replace it with a better, made-up substitute—through a fantasy image in which we fill in only a one-sided version of what seems pleasant and good to us. All of the things we take to be negative or unhappy are left out. This fantasy is constituted of true and untrue elements, and if we take the end result for what it is (a theoretical model), it can enrich us psychologically, lend a little color to life, and nourish the tendencies that lead us on our life's path. We make a mistake if we follow and accept this false image uncritically, since only a part of it jibes with reality. In the depths of our being, we become even more discontent and enter into an even greater conflict with our less-than-perfect life, which we—despite our wishes—can lead only once.

While the ideals that we apply to ourselves do possess a certain amount of flexibility and our psyche tries to adapt to a certain degree to match reality, any ideal that we try to impose on others will lack this regulating element. Such ideas are largely theoretical because they arise predominately from our reason and often make us hard and intolerant. This is especially true (and often with disastrous effects) in education or politics, where such ideas can become dogmas. While the Vervain type acts with the best of intentions, her actions have harmful consequences for the "victims" (those she's trying to help). She's convinced that what is good for her is good for everyone else and judges the value and appropriateness of her actions in terms of whether they make her happy, not those that she's trying to help.

She overestimates the value of her own convictions, ideals, and goals because she mistakes them for reality; she underestimates the uniqueness and "otherness" of other people because she closes herself off to them; and she exaggerates her ability to do good deeds because her ideas and desires obscure her clear vision. Her limited view leads her to intolerance. She believes that helping consists of solving problems for other people, and she thinks that anything she wants must be desirable for others as well. Her great enthusiasm and active nature compel her to impose her advice and help on others. She never thinks that someone might need and be looking for something else, and it never occurs to her that help given too hastily and without forethought might be more harmful than helpful because it deprives the "helpless" of the chance to help themselves and thereby make themselves stronger.

In addition, she hurts herself because, carried away with her own strength and enthusiasm, she cannot read the multifarious internal and external signals that her busy, overworked body sends in the form of stress symptoms. It's important for her to be cool and composed, to gain a little distance (especially from herself) and concentrate on her positive aspects—her selfless enthusiasm and her pure motives. Once she does this, she can use her considerable powers of concentration and achievement sensibly and appropriately.

Common Combinations with Other Essences

Holly (15/31): the irritable do-gooder
Impatiens (18/31): stress and agitation
Oak (22/31): stress due to a compulsion for overwork
Vine (31/32): totally intolerant behavior
White Chestnut (31/35): fixed ideas

32: Vine

Characteristics

Vine is for self-confident, intolerant people who want others to march to their tune.

AREA OF USE

Vine is used for the basic treatment of obstinacy, intolerance, inflexible convictions, a need to dominate, dogmatism, and fanaticism. Used to treat all pathological conditions related to mental inflexibility or intolerant domination and a need to impose one's will. In daily life, used to treat pedantry, superiority (the know-it-all), dominating behavior, mental inflexibility, the perpetual teacher, and the domestic tyrant.

Causes and Symptoms of Vine Syndrome

This condition is extroverted and consists of self-confidence, very structured thinking, and a need to dominate others. Harmoniously developed, the Vine type is self-assured, has good judgment, and is up to tackling any problem. Because he always knows a solution, never feels desperate, and gladly places his knowledge at the service of others, he is an ideal and highly esteemed adviser. He has the ability to reduce problems to a few key factors, which goes a long way toward restraining desperation or insecurity. He also avoids trying to force his opinions on others because he knows his own limits. In whatever position he finds himself—teacher or head of a family, philosopher or statesman, priest or soldier—those around him inevitably yield to him and appoint him to a leadership position, which he assumes skillfully and convincingly. His self-assured convictions, his finely tuned sense of responsibility, and his clear and orderly mind are blessings in emergencies and catastrophes; he never loses his head and always knows how things must turn out.

Unfavorably developed, his clear opinion can turn into an obstinate dogmatism, his love of order can change to intolerance, and his readiness to help can become a need to dominate. In this situation, the Vine type takes himself to be exemplary or without fault and tries with great intolerance to force his own opinions on others. Sometimes his abilities to act in a goal-oriented, uncompromising manner turn into a small-minded thoughtlessness, making life difficult for those around him—whether he is a pedantic boss or small-minded teacher, a fanatical slave driver or a leader without compassion, a pigheaded policeman or an intolerant ideologue, or a petty, compulsive, domestic tyrant. Anything he cannot have, others should not be able to have either. Because he has a great need for clearly defined relationships, he always makes sure to keep "order" or "do the right thing." Disorder, lack of clarity, or chaos make him profoundly insecure and lead to obstinate, blind thinking. In their less blatant forms, the Vine tendencies can also manifest as excessive love of order, small-mindedness, a need to impose one's will on others, an inability to accept other points of view, narrow-mindedness, mental inflexibility, dogmatism, intolerant self-righteousness, or compulsive thinking.

The Effects of Vine

Vine is the essence used to treat intolerance. It promotes mental flexibility and the ability to learn and acquire new knowledge, and it breaks down pettiness and fanatical obstinacy. It frees us from the compulsion of blind convictions or dogmatic thoughts, makes us more tolerant, open-minded, kinder, and happier. It loosens up excessive discipline, releases tension, and works against all illnesses related to an insufficient inner flexibility and tractability, such as calcification (hardening of the arteries) or high blood pressure.

Psychotherapeutic Notes

Humanity can be divided into many categories, among them leaders and followers. While those who will be led always have a sense of powerlessness or helplessness and feel that they are merely small cogs in a very big machine, those who lead are filled with a sense of personal responsibility and believe that their lives, or even the well-being of humankind, depend upon their actions. Vine types belong to this category. They cannot live their lives passively, cannot simply sit back and allow themselves to be guided; they must always have their hands on the wheel and attempt to shape the world to fit their way of thinking. The passive and active approaches to life are equal, complementary opposites. What would become of a leader without his followers, and vice versa? How can an active impulse be put into play without a corresponding passive act of giving way, or an act of devotion without a corresponding act of receiving? We all carry such contradictory impulses and attributes within us; today we must be active and tomorrow passive, here we must take and there we must receive, and on and on in a constant flux, according to the circumstances.

In order to be physically and spiritually healthy, we must realize our potentials and inclinations as fully as we are able. This means that we must be true to our natures. A sensitive, shy person should not be a robust daredevil, and an active, thick-skinned, practical person will never become a sensitive aesthete. The same applies to social behavior: anyone who does not feel called to serve his fellow human beings should preferably follow more egotistical, "taking" pursuits, while anyone who is born to be a warrior should take care not to be a caretaker. All such predispositions have their justifications (precisely because they exist) and can exist only in the presence of their complements. It is this interplay that ensures the existence of our world.

The problem of the Vine type is not the predisposition in itself, but the extent to which and the manner in which it manifests. As long as he comes into conflict neither with himself nor with his environment, he behaves properly. His strength of will, his clear thinking, and his tendency to impose his will, give commands, or lead can be true blessings, especially in emergencies or times of need; he helps keep order and gets done those things that need to be done. There are situations in which the good of the community depends upon concentration, the unwillingness to compromise, and the strength of will of its leader. In daily life—in the family, in relationships, in management, in politics, and in intellectual life—the stabilizing influence and leadership qualities of the Vine type are useful.

When the self-confident leadership qualities get the upper hand, however, they can squelch the Vine type's ability to compromise and cause him to become intolerant of and ignore the needs of others or to act arbitrarily and without justification; the condition becomes pathological and pathogenic. Sensible and even necessary in chaotic situations, such behavior in daily life is unhealthy and, when it becomes a habit, makes the Vine type unable to live flexibly and sensibly. When he becomes conscious of his strengths, he can prevent them from becoming weaknesses that will cause unhappiness that can destroy his own life and the lives of others, leading him to social isolation.

The physical symptoms accompanying such a condition—high blood pressure, degeneration of the joints, liver dysfunction, calcification—are all warning signs. His mission is clear—to be an upstanding, incorruptible, self-critical master teacher or leader who can simplify problems and make them solvable, convey his convictions and act as a negotiator, and find new ways so that he may show others. He can do all of this only if he is asked and if he is needed.

Common Combinations with Other Essences

Beech (3/32): total intolerance
Crab Apple (10/32): petty fanaticism for cleanliness
Holly (15/32): rage caused by opposition or errors
Oak (22/32): dogmatic compulsion to achieve
Rock Water (27/32): strict personality
Vervain (31/32): absolutely intolerant behavior
White Chestnut (32/35): compulsive dogmatism
Willow (32/38): embittered domestic tyrant

33: Walnut

Characteristics

Walnut is for people who are too easily influenced or who need more stability in a personal crisis.

AREA OF USE

Walnut is used as the treatment for weak personality, lack of self-assertiveness, sensitivity to outside influences, personal crises, lack of self-confidence, excessive need to conform, changes in life, dependence, puberty, menopause, teething (or losing the first teeth), death, and birth. Used to treat all pathological conditions related to physical or emotional defenses or a lack of inner stability. In daily life, used to combat being too easily influenced, frailness, a trusting innocence, and bad habits.

Causes and Symptoms of Walnut Syndrome

This condition is characterized by great mental and emotional openness and influenceability. Harmoniously developed, the Walnut type is open with everyone. She is a pleasant, innocently trusting, and guileless companion who neither judges nor mistrusts. Her mind and spirit are uninhibited and free from preconceived opinions. The rational and irrational, the wonderful and the banal, dream and reality penetrate her so profoundly that she has a rich, comprehensive inner view of existence. Where others see with blinders, she sees an entire panorama. She lives in her mind like the great philosopher who expressed the quintessence of his life of reflection with the words "I know that I know nothing!" She knows that behind the external, banal appearances there is endless complexity and that what most of us take to be irrefutable facts are only fleeting impressions from fixed points of view and can be refuted or annulled by other points of view—in short, the Walnut type knows that human consciousness is denied absolute knowledge, that everything is relative, and that in all things there are thousands of possibilities. With this instinctive view of life, she goes on her sometimes puzzling way, following only her inspirations, interests, and feelings. Like the child in the fairy tale, she reaches her personal goal safely; there are no life crises filled with self-doubt and errors. She has an inner compass, and if it seems that she may be too easily influenced, too gullible, and too inconsistent, it is only a sign that the observer is too deeply entrenched in preconceptions and has no sense of the unusual and the wonderful.

Unfavorably developed, this unbiased attitude can give way to an excessive tendency to be influenced. The Walnut type's openness toward mental and emotional impressions often leads her to become insecure or can divert her from her original path. With authority figures especially, Walnut types often cannot assert themselves and find themselves in situations that they did not want to get into, such as a frustrating career, an unhappy partnership, or an unsuitable living situation. Because their spirit is suffering, it reacts with frustration or depression or takes the form of an illness—especially of the skin, lymph, or hormone system—which is a sign that something is not right.

The Effects of Walnut

Walnut is the essence for defensive strength and inner stability. It gives us a thicker skin to withstand outside influences, especially when we want to start out on a new life path. It minimizes naive and gullible behavior and excessive trustfulness when it is not called for; it strengthens the personality and allows for the development and realization of our own life concept. Natural processes of development are directed against any opposition (such as psychic and moralistic conditioning). We acquire the ability to give up old habits; to act decisively against the pressures of a hostile, unsympathetic environment; to free ourselves from dependence; or just generally to become ourselves. Walnut does not simply protect against negative influences—such as infections—but also helps in times of important life changes, such as teething or losing the first teeth, puberty, menopause, birth, or illness, and it helps us survive them relatively unscarred. It is almost always needed for its stabilizing influence (in concert with Agrimony) when we want to get rid of neurotic, defensive behavior.

Psychotherapeutic Notes

Life means expansion, growth, and self-realization. The driving force in our lives is the need for unimpeded expression of our natural abilities and potential. This naturally leads to conflict—eat or be eaten. As conscious humans, we can avoid many conflicts through our highly developed insight, and from sympathy for our fellow humans, we can limit the murderous fight for survival to only the necessary battles and reign in our "scavenger instinct." We are nonetheless ruled by our fundamental biological structure, and we are part of the natural struggle.

There are, of course, differences from one individual to the next. While one person strives toward mental and spiritual values, another tries to succeed on the physical/material level. In the struggle for survival and self-realization, the most important elements of a personality are protected, and, when necessary, the less meaningful ones are sacrificed. For the sake of sheer existence, one tosses her beautiful ideals overboard, while another sacrifices life and limb for her morals and convictions. (This must not be taken as a moral judgment, since each of us finds self-realization in our own manner and with our own justification.)

In this struggle, the Walnut type can easily get the short end of the stick; because she is easily influenced and because of her naive, innocent trust, her lack of boundaries provokes her "enemies" to attack. She is compelled, influenced, persuaded, put off her own goals, misused, made to pursue goals that are not her own, made insecure, and manipulated—in short, she does everything except what is important for her life.

This cannot last long, however, since the spirit—the real person—must express itself and pursue its own goals. To this end, it creates various warning signs, depending on the extent of self-alienation: aggression, frustration, depression, psychoses, neuroses, behavioral problems, or physical illnesses. Life changes (during which the organism develops special new qualities), such as losing the first teeth, puberty, menopause, birth, or death are critical junctures and indications of the Walnut syndrome. The more freedom that is given to our inner rhythms, the more freedom we have to express our unique qualities, and we can follow our life's path more seriously and with more determination. Once this is done without internal or external resistance, things will go better for us, and we can be healthier and more humane.

The Walnut type should control her easy, trusting nature and give in only when it makes sense to do so. She should consciously examine her independence and, as much as possible, try to follow her own path. Staying true to oneself is often difficult; betraying oneself without a compelling reason can be hell.

Common Combinations with Other Essences

Agrimony (1/33): total self-alienation

Centaury (4/33): dependent and easily influenced

Cerato (5/33): insecurity caused by being easily influenced

Gentian (12/33): despair precipitated by a life change

Larch (19/33): a lack of self-confidence causing one to be easily influenced

Mimulus (20/33): timidity leading one to be too easily influenced

Olive (23/33): exhaustion prompting one to be easily influenced

Pine (24/33): weak defense against accusations

Star of Bethlehem (29/33): lack of resistance against or caused by psychic trauma

Wild Oat (33/36): lacking a life goal

34: Water Violet
Characteristics

Water Violet is for loners who have problems with human contact.

AREA OF USE
Water Violet is used for the treatment of problems with human contact, fear of attachment, reserved behavior, shyness, being a "loner," arrogance, contempt, coldness of emotions, disapproval of others, and pride. Used to treat all pathological conditions related to human contact problems. In daily life, used to treat shyness, reserved behavior, being unapproachable, and being a loner.

Causes and Symptoms of Water Violet Syndrome

This condition is characterized by introverted behavior, mental independence, and a strong need for freedom. Harmoniously developed, the Water Violet type is self-sufficient and independent and expresses his individuality. Freedom and independence are the pillars of his existence. To keep these, he avoids anyone who wants to obligate him in any form whatsoever, and he spends time only with those who understand him; given his unique views, this happens very rarely. In any case, he does not want other people to become involved in his affairs or help him solve his problems, because he wants to remain independent and because there are very few people who understand his ideas. His inborn extravagance—an unusual appearance, a singular manner of thinking, uncommon preferences, special abilities, or a unique background—ensures that he generally goes his own way to protect his individuality. He gives the impression that he needs very little outside stimulus, and this attitude allows him even more rest for himself. He is a pleasant companion because he bothers no one with demands, is very tolerant, and allows everyone to do as they please.

Unfavorably developed, his disposition loses its carefree, happy tone and transforms itself into the Water Violet syndrome: the inborn, supercilious independence can lead to human contact problems or to a cold pride, and his unusual characteristics can make him an eccentric outsider. This sensitive independence can transform the Water Violet type into an unhappy misanthrope or a shy person, filled with complexes. The desire to be alone drives him into a painful loneliness and makes it impossible for him to accept human companionship or gifts or advice. He reduces his contact with other people more and more, either by an active withdrawal or by a passive retreat into himself, thus alienating him from the rest of society. This retreat can have a truly irritating effect on even the most good-natured of his friends. The Water Chestnut type feels that an unsympathetic and uncomprehending environment has forced him to be the way he is. We often find Water Violet syndrome at work in outsiders, rootless people, recluses, or with people who are cool and keep their distance. We often have the impression that they don't want to be the way they are, but circumstances forced the role of the outsider upon them and offered them a chance for survival. We also find this situation at work in shy, "loner" children who misunderstand themselves and feel compelled to act in a way that is not natural to them, choosing to seek their salvation by retreating into themselves.

The Effects of Water Violet

Water Violet is the essence used to treat problems with human contact. It makes us more sociable, more open, and friendlier to other people, and it works against loneliness. It is particularly helpful (especially in children) when negative circumstances or a developing illness make us shy away from people and become antisocial. It is also indicated in cases of unnatural pride, arrogance, or excessive reserve, since these are often neurotic defense mechanisms.

Psychotherapeutic Notes

An interest in other people and the need to exchange thoughts and feelings with them are fundamental characteristics of the human spirit and essential for our psychic health. Contact with other people enriches us by exposing us to new ideas and information and stimulating our emotions; above all, it serves our developing consciousness. Our companions are reflections of ourselves: they react to our behavior—like an echo—and all the qualities we see in them are counterparts of our own.

The need for communication varies from one person to the next. While an extrovert needs human contact as much as he needs air, an introvert might need only a limited amount. While the extrovert merely stores his impressions, the introvert's go straight to the depths of his psyche, where they are distilled. The more attention and energy he must devote to this process, the less he is able to take in new impressions, and his psyche essentially shuts itself down to them. He becomes less social and wants only to be alone, much as an animal that has just eaten will seek out a quiet place to "digest."

The Water Violet type is introverted by nature and needs this downtime more than most. When he is bombarded with too many impressions or influences, he begins to withdraw, as a protective mechanism. Under very difficult circumstances, such as a severe shock, an injury, or a major disappointment, this withdrawal can take on pathological proportions and lead to extremely cold and isolated behavior. He can no longer distinguish between those influences that are useful and those that are harmful, and, for this reason, he limits the amount of contact he allows himself to have much more than he would like and more than is actually good for him. He avoids everyone, becomes taciturn, sullen, lonesome, and unhappy.

Sometimes this happens at the onset of an illness. Monosyllabic responses, withdrawn behavior, and a need to be alone are all signs that there is an internal problem that must be worked through, not in a dialogue with others but in a dialogue with oneself. Illness is a kind of healing reaction that expels all sorts of toxins from the body and attempts to restore order. Treatment for the Water Violet type includes quiet and rest, a calm understanding, and a constant willingness to communicate. He must reach a balance between introversion and extroversion and be able to have as much contact with other people as he needs. Anything more than that he must learn to bear lightly.

Common Combinations with Other Essences

Agrimony (1/34): interpersonal problems due to a lack of openness

Aspen (2/34): human contact difficulties caused by vague fears

Beech (3/34): excessively tolerant, yet unapproachable

Chestnut Bud (7/34): closed-mindedness

Holly (15/34): the irritable misanthrope

Larch (19/34): problems with human contact related to an
inferiority complex

Mustard (21/34): severe depression and interpersonal
problems

Oak (22/34): ambition leading to loneliness

Olive (23/34): antisocial due to exhaustion

Rock Water (27/34): flight from the world and self-castigation

Star of Bethlehem (29/34): human contact problems due to a
mental and emotional trauma

Willow (34/38): bitterness stemming from restricted freedom

35: White Chestnut

Characteristics

White Chestnut is for people who are tyrannized by certain unpleasant thoughts or ideas.

AREA OF USE

White Chestnut is used for the basic treatment of compulsive thoughts, fixations, and mental and emotional overstimulation. Used to treat all pathological conditions related to compulsive thoughts or fixations. In daily life, used to treat sleep disorders, jumbled thoughts, difficulties with concentration, "wired" behavior, and headaches due to excessive mental and emotional stress.

Causes and Symptoms of White Chestnut Syndrome

This condition is characterized by mental alertness, great sensitivity, and intensive thought processes. Harmoniously developed, the White Chestnut type has an agile mind and a powerful imagination. Everything she undertakes, she engages in with great intensity, concentration, and imagination—to the extent that everything else not related to the subject at hand just disappears. She is very effective at mental work and can jump easily from one subject to another and turn her attention to whatever idea, problem, or question is occupying her.

Unfavorably developed, the intensive mental processes of the White Chestnut type can result in uncontrollable, obsessive thoughts; certain thoughts or ideas can just take over. (This can happen to anyone who has been through a devastating experience.) Generally, these thoughts take on a decidedly unpleasant character, in the form of worries, fears, or problems. Sometimes a positive thought will push its way so prominently to the foreground that she can't think of anything else. Her thoughts become stuck like a broken record; her reason becomes a prisoner of fixations or obsessions that keep spinning around in her head without any rhyme or reason. A song, a phrase, or a word will repeat itself over and over without interruption, and she is powerless to do anything about it. She takes to brooding, can't relax, can't shut off her obsessions, and can't form any new thoughts. This condition is often accompanied by headaches or sleep disorders.

The Effects of White Chestnut

White Chestnut is the essence for mental clarity. It frees us from tormenting ideas and helps us break out of vicious mental cycles, inhibits obsessive thoughts, and supports positive suppressive behavior. It encourages our ability to concentrate, helps us order our thoughts, and aids us in solving problems or storing them away in our subconscious. It can improve headaches or sleep disorders caused by obsessive thoughts.

Psychotherapeutic Notes

We all know what good it does us to express our anger or our pain, say by screaming or howling; it allows our internal emotional energies an outlet and frees up emotional blockage. We all know someone who is temperamental and uninhibited, and we've seen how they release their intense emotions immediately, which makes them feel much better and more relaxed. When we try to hold back our problems, worries, pains, fears, or aggressions, it's like chewing on something bitter or rotten; when we swallow, it makes us sick and unhappy.

This happens especially with introverts. Everything affects them deeply, and their experiences are processed and changed into another form—either as a new realization or awareness or as something more negative—and then integrated into the personality. This is also the case with the White Chestnut type, but she has another problem: everything affects her with great intensity and profundity, and her thoughts become so emotionally charged and full of conflict that she can't get them out of her head. It's like chewing on a bone for hours without deriving any nutrients from it. She is plagued by thoughts that she doesn't want to acknowledge; worries, fears, and needs that she doesn't want to give up; problems that she doesn't want to solve for reasons she doesn't want to admit. Her consciousness is often so dominated by negative ideas or intense desires that she can no longer think rationally.

Normally, such overbearing thoughts are suppressed by the psyche, which examines countless thoughts, impressions, and bits of information and determines whether they contribute to our physical or spiritual growth. Anything that is not deemed appropriate for immediate use is stored away in the subconscious and will be recalled when it's needed. This process ensures that we don't suffer from an overload of information or from thoughts or impressions that might be too difficult to distill. This material can be recalled when we are ready to accept it and take it in, and it can be incorporated into another phase of personal growth. At that point, it is time to face this material and integrate it in a meaningful way into our lives, for example, by expanding our worldview, modifying a personal assumption, or making a practical change in how we live.

Most of us find ourselves plagued by this aspect of the White Chestnut condition at one time or another. When we see the symptoms, we should try to clarify our emotions, face our problems, and make sure our outer lives are appropriate to meet our internal needs. When a problem becomes so serious that it causes us to suffer, suppression is no longer a viable strategy; it must be confronted and worked through. We should ask why a particular thought keeps running through our heads and look for a new answer to the fundamental question that is plaguing us. Too often, we try to avoid these questions. We should not be afraid of taboos that are no longer meaningful.

This search alone will often lead to breaking up the vicious cycle of tormenting thoughts. Sometimes, as a drastic measure, we can only try to replace these thoughts with their more positive opposites, in an attempt to reprogram ourselves; the conscious mind can then distance itself from these unsolvable problems and questions, and the psyche can work on finding an intuitive, subconscious solution.

Common Combinations with Other Essences

Aspen (2/35): mental block caused by nebulous fears

Cherry Plum (6/35): mental obsession

Chestnut Bud (7/35): compulsive thoughts leading to distraction

Chicory (8/35): obsessive love

Clematis (9/35): obsessive daydreaming and planning

Crab Apple (10/35): tormented by dirt and filth

Heather (14/35): obsessive vanity

Holly (15/35): aggressive, obsessive thoughts

Honeysuckle (16/35): obsessive memories

Impatiens (18/35): mentally "driven"

Mimulus (20/35): obsessive anxieties

Oak (22/35): obsessed with success

Pine (24/35): obsessed with guilt

Red Chestnut (25/35): worried thoughts

Star of Bethlehem (29/35): obsessed with traumatic thoughts

Vervain (31/35): obsessive dogmatism

Willow (35/38): bitter, obsessive thoughts

36: Wild Oat
Characteristics

Wild Oat is for people who want to do something sensible and meaningful but don't know how to go about it.

AREA OF USE

Wild Oat is used as the basic treatment for a feeling of pointlessness, lack of clarity, lack of goals, self-alienation, crises related to new beginnings, life crises, and depression caused by lack of purpose in life. Used to treat all pathological conditions related to frustration and a lack of purpose. In daily life, used to treat discontent and frustration with our daily lives, indecisiveness, and a lack of clarity.

Causes and Symptoms of Wild Oat Syndrome

This condition is characterized by openness and enthusiasm and a strong need for a meaning and purpose in life. Harmoniously developed, the Wild Oat type understands how to give meaning and purpose to his life. He doesn't waste his time or energy on trivialities but follows his inner voice with determination and does what is important to him. His goals can be materialistic or spiritual in nature, superficial or deep, but they always speak to his wants and needs and are tailor-made for him alone. From his orientation and his theoretical needs and possibilities, on the one hand, to his more practical life situation, on the other, he achieves great peace of mind, which allows him to be objectively successful. The harmoniously developed Wild Oat type always knows what he wants, goes after it without hesitation, and does what makes him happy. He is successful and knows how to make the best of things—not because he goes after life with blind ambition but because he lives his life with dedication, concentration, and confidence. He is often interested in philosophy, religion, or the arts and, at the very least, has a natural sense of the more profound questions of life.

Unfavorably developed, his tendency to seek meaning in life can become so strong that he constantly searches for it but never finds it. He loses his clarity and his reliable instinct, which otherwise guide him so well. He will begin a project and, soon after, decide that it's not right for him. Then he'll start something new and decide that that's not right for him either. Alternatively, he will plan a project but never get around to actually carrying it out. He longs desperately for a meaningful life or a satisfying occupation. He doesn't want to compromise but is so unclear that he can never reach a goal. He is so incapable of finding a calling or the right path that it makes him depressed and unhappy.

This could happen to anyone. Sometimes we see this condition in young people who are just beginning to assert their independence and are filled with expectations and enthusiasm but don't know exactly where to begin. It also happens quite often when we are faced with a crisis of life, work, or a relationship in which we feel that we must change something, but we don't know what or how. We make a few halfhearted attempts to change; we do something foolish—change our job or our partner—and, in the end, we feel that we've left ourselves hanging, frustrated, and depressed.

The Effects of Wild Oat

Wild Oat is the essence for clarity and self-realization. Taken over a longer period (months!), it restores our inner order and imperceptibly opens our eyes to the ongoing process of recognizing our spiritual needs. It brings us clarity and decisiveness, lets us find our calling, helps us choose a career or a partner, helps us make a new beginning in life, and fights depression or any illnesses related to discontent or a lack of inner clarity. It can also be used when we lack a goal or purpose in life.

Psychotherapeutic Notes

The need to find a meaning in everything is a typically human trait and an expression of our consciousness. Whether we're nihilists, materialists, esotericists, religious people, philosophers, rationalists, dreamers, idealists, ideologues, or free spirits, we all need to find meaning, be it positive or negative, in what we experience and what we do with our lives. We seek this meaning by developing great philosophical ideas, religious visions, or intuitive works of art or in catastrophes, laws of nature, or even physical laws or any kind of connection in which we can seek to bring order and meaning to our lives.

This search for meaning plays a definitive role in our personal lives as well, which is a kind of ongoing work of art that gives evidence of our inner maturity. Depending on our age, certain aspects become more prominent. In childhood and youth, we try to achieve an external ordering of the world and society, whereas in our later years, this becomes a striving for self-awareness and developing our relationship to the transcendent side of the world. Normally, this development takes place in small steps and is given direction by all of our feelings, intuitions, and inspirations. These elements, and not our rational faculties, are what guide us through life, because they more fully reflect the complexity of our nature. When we ignore these less rational impulses, we run the risk of one day being faced with a violent reaction in the depths of our soul; we begin to question everything we believe, and we lose our orientation. Everything that seemed to hold water loses its value. A less forceful version of this process happens in young people because they sense never-ending frustration and see that they cannot make a connection with their lives.

It is important for Wild Oat types to rediscover (or to learn for the first time) what is right for them. They must learn to take their impressions, intuitions, and feelings seriously and to pay attention to the signs that life sends them every day. Frustration and happiness will show them the way. They must get to know themselves better so that they can make a new beginning consciously and seriously. In this process, meaningless taboos will be jettisoned, no longer valid morals will be tossed aside, and personal compulsions and obsessions will be overcome. Sometimes this process can take years. They will be encouraged once they feel they are on the right track, and they will have the needed determination to overcome their frequent lean periods. We can be reborn, perhaps with a new career, a new partner, new surroundings—or, in any case, with new behavior that harmoniously combines the subjective and objective, internal and external elements of life.

Common Combinations with Other Essences

Agrimony (1/36): lack of self-awareness

Cerato (5/36): insecurity due to a lack of goals

Chestnut Bud (7/36): lacking life goals because of inattentiveness

Larch (19/36): no purpose in life stemming from a lack of self-confidence

Mustard (21/36): depression resulting from a feeling of meaninglessness

Rock Water (27/36): self-castigation as a replacement for a purpose in life

Scleranthus (28/36): internally broken and suffering a life crisis

Walnut (33/36): lacking a purpose in life

Wild Rose (36/37): lack of drive due to a lack of purpose

37: Wild Rose

Characteristics

Wild Rose is for people who are resigned and who can't bring themselves to be active.

AREA OF USE

Wild Rose is used as the basic treatment for apathy, lack of drive, resignation, pathological resignation, convalescence, or illnesses that sap the energy. Used to treat all pathological conditions related to a lack of drive, resignation, or a lack of willpower. In daily life, used to treat lack of interest and enthusiasm.

Causes and Symptoms of Wild Rose Syndrome

This condition is characterized by adaptability, dedication, and a certain awareness of fate. Harmoniously developed, the Wild Rose type is able to adapt to constantly changing situations without losing sight of the positive side. He has no problem with his destiny because he gives himself up fearlessly and without resistance to the greater powers that determine everything in this life. As a realist in the best sense, he never tries to make reality (that which has happened) into something different but instead has an innocent, positive attitude and takes everything as it comes. His lack of prejudice and refusal to take things for granted makes it difficult for him to encounter any situation that will make him unhappy. Like a sapling that sways with the wind, he allows himself to be taken here and there by the whims of fate, dreamily, playfully, and willingly. He never looks at reality with preconceptions or stubborn ideas; he can see things with an inner freedom and innocence that allow him to make the best of anything he encounters.

Unfavorably developed, his passive, accepting nature can get the better of him. He allows himself to go through life without will or drive, and he has no interest in his life; he develops a kind of resignation that has a hint of a departure from life. He is no longer able to clearly assess his situation, to take reasonable countermeasures when required, or to ask for help. The Wild Rose syndrome does not usually consist of extreme resignation but of a lessened enthusiasm and a tendency just to let things run as they are. One has the impression that the Wild Rose type uses only a fraction of his potential and does not develop himself fully. He is not able to accomplish as much as he should and needs to stop and rest often, which leads to a limited life. If he should start a project, he comes immediately to a halt, like a vehicle stuck in the sand. His potential remains unfulfilled, he just hangs around aimlessly, and, even when things are not going well for him, he can't pick himself up to do anything about it. He'll do nothing to change an unhealthy living situation, he'll stay with a lousy marriage, and he'll take any wretched situation as it comes. If his behavior were a conscious and aware answer to an unavoidable circumstance, it would make sense as a kind of survival tactic. In this case, however, it is a sign of a pathological lack of interest and vitality and an extensive loss of creativity.

The Effects of Wild Rose

Wild Rose is the essence for enthusiasm and interest in life. It fosters an attention to life and makes us more interested and invested and more open and enthusiastic. It minimizes indifference, mental passivity, and resignation. If these symptoms appear in connection with an illness, they could accompany a decisive deterioration, and Wild Rose is indicated. It is generally helpful during any phase of convalescence and should be used as an adjunct to medical treatment in any case of anemia, vitamin or mineral deficiency, or other organic condition.

Psychotherapeutic Notes

Resignation should by no means be confused with an acceptance of fate. This distinction becomes especially clear when we examine the Wild Rose syndrome. Acceptance of fate means trusting ourselves to the hands of fate because we recognize a greater positive order, power, or being (God) at work. With this attitude, we can learn to accept reality and strive to make the best of it. We still try to fulfill our desires the best we are able, but we also know enough to give up when we recognize we're in over our heads. We can change our plans without any regrets.

Resignation, on the other hand, means rejecting fate. Where acceptance of fate is distinguished by positive expectations, resignation means troubling ourselves with only those things that we encounter directly and living our lives without resistance, without investing our selves, and without active participation; life just passes us by. Resignation is still a pathological phenomenon even when it is not extreme. It can affect our physical functions, in the form of bad posture, a weak spine, poor circulation, or a reduced sexual drive. Typical Wild Rose types share similarities with Centaury, Larch, and Olive types, and they are usually the product of mistreatment in early childhood by dominating, egocentric parents or teachers. This sort of upbringing downplays the tendency to compete and causes the child to lead a sort of shadow life, undemanding, "sweet," and unobtrusive. He becomes used to suppressing his wishes for happiness and self-realization and learns to accept obediently whatever he is allowed. This profound loss of his natural initiative and enthusiasm dominates his character later in life as well and makes him into a person who is unable to "follow through."

People who are resigned become ill much more easily than more life-affirming types. Conversely, a serious illness can cause us to be resigned and lose our will to live and our will to become healthy again. This is always a bad sign. As already discussed in the section (see Mustard), there are several distinct phases in an illness: the aggressive phase, in which we fight actively and vitally against an encroaching illness; the frustration phase, in which our aggression abates; the depressive phase, in which our aggression is blocked and our behavior becomes more self-defeating; and resignation, the final phase before death, which means that we are broken—we've given up the fight and are ready for the end.

The Wild Rose syndrome is not easily overcome. In any case, it's important to determine whether an organic illness (heart, kidneys, hormone system) or some deficiency (vitamins, trace elements) might play a role and institute the appropriate treatment. Sometimes resignation is a consequence of a severe but passing psychic trauma. In this case, we need only wait (while using the appropriate Bach Flower essence) in quiet until the psyche rebounds like a blade of grass that has been trod upon. Long-term loss of enthusiasm or initiative is more difficult to combat, and it can have far-reaching effects on a person's overall behavior. The Wild Rose type usually finds it challenging to pull himself up by his bootstraps (this would indicate the recovery phase of an illness), and he often needs help. This help must include supporting him while he becomes healthy again.

Giving him words of encouragement is not enough. Even when we can persuade him to act, after a short time he will lose interest, and his troubles will be back.

Wild Rose types do not have a natural, innate, positive attitude. Their tendency, in difficult times, to let things run their course indicates a (pathological) inclination to leave everything up to fate. Wild Rose types need to find a better, more personal, and more conscious relationship to whatever gives meaning to their lives, but they can't come to this point because they've been cut short in their quest for self-realization. Finding meaning in life means having a goal. Having a goal allows us to channel our strength and to become more active. Finding meaning in life means living with our senses open and discovering whatever makes us happy and whatever our hearts need. Psychotherapy can be useful for the Wild Rose type by making him aware of how his self-realization is being stifled and which desires and longings he is sacrificing. When he finally has the courage to reward himself with what he needs and to take what he deserves, and when he is finally able to let himself be happy, the life-affirming spirit within him will awaken.

Common Combinations with Other Essences

Centaury (4/37): resignation due to a weak personality

Chestnut Bud (7/37): distracted and resigned

Clematis (9/37): resignation and a longing for death

Gentian (12/37): resigned and weak willed

Gorse (13/37): total resignation

Honeysuckle (16/37): wistful resignation

Hornbeam (17/37): lack of drive caused by stress and overwork

Larch (19/37): lack of drive due to a lack of self-confidence

Mustard (21/37): depressive resignation

Olive (23/37): lack of drive due to exhaustion

Star of Bethlehem (29/37): resignation resulting from mental and emotional trauma

Wild Oat (36/37): lack of drive stemming from a sense of meaninglessness and futility

38: Willow

Characteristics

Willow is for people who are disappointed, bitter, or offended.

AREA OF USE

Willow is used for the basic treatment of bitterness, resentment, a need for revenge, an inability to reconcile, and being at odds with fate. Used to treat all pathological conditions related to disappointment or bitterness. In daily life, used to treat disappointment or feeling offended or slighted.

Causes and Symptoms of Willow Syndrome

This condition is characterized by a pronounced sense of justice and an intensive need for love and happiness. Harmoniously developed, the Willow type can come to terms with the ever changing circumstances of her life and can take the good with the bad. She can accept her defeats, losses, and difficulties just as she can enjoy the happier aspects of her life. This is a valuable ability, and it is seldom found. In the case of the Willow type, it stems from her finely tuned, incorruptible sense of justice, which is not preoccupied with external factors but with the truth. It is a justice that seeks what is right, a justice that does not seek personal advantage but is the expression of an unknowable divine order. It is clear to her that things simply are the way they are and that everything is right and just whether or not she likes or understands it. From this "higher" sense of justice, she learns to accept what life, fate, or God have arranged. She reacts coolly and thoughtfully to situations that make others angry and bitter. Life for her is not a dangerous struggle for existence but a glorious adventure that she faces with a wide-eyed innocence and openness, a fascinating journey to unknown dimensions in which conflict, defeats, and losses all serve as signs to mark the way.

She has a clear, strong yearning for happiness. These feeling are very genuine and very real; she has no sweet delusions or expectations, and this spares her from becoming bitter. In her life-affirming attitudes and behavior, the Willow type is living proof that there is a higher, divine justice that speaks for all of us, including those who are petty or corrupt. When we accept this justice, we can never think that we're being treated unfairly, and we're spared a lot of suffering.

Unfavorably developed, the inborn sense of justice can turn into a sense of self-righteousness that in itself can lead only to injustice. This is what gives the unfavorably developed Willow type the feeling that she has been treated unfairly, which causes her to become bitter and resentful and to want revenge. When she reacts in this way, she shows that she hasn't learned from the lessons or advice that life has given her. These lessons simply don't fit into her self-righteous worldview. She refuses to examine thoroughly whether her expectations and wishes are truly just, and she feels hurt, offended, bitter, or disappointed; she sulks, feels resentment, and wants to get even. Her unhappiness is contagious. Indeed, it often seems that she derives a certain amount of pleasure in drawing others into her negativity and bitterness. She is a miserable companion and becomes a burden on herself and others. When she finally sees that she is not always in the right or that everything is not as bad as she thought, she will calm down. As a rule, she doesn't learn her lesson, and it is only a matter of time until she suffers the next insult.

The Effects of Willow

Willow is the essence for conciliation and forgiveness. It counters the tendency to feel that we've been treated unjustly and the need for revenge; it makes us more conciliatory, understanding, and content. It's useful for children who get their way through sulking or tantrums, and it is especially suitable for people who cannot accept their fate and who become sick as a result. As long as they maintain this attitude, they'll never recover.

Psychotherapeutic Notes

When dealing with someone who is bitter or sullen, we must first ask whether the behavior is genuine; many people, especially children, will pretend to be hurt in order to have their way. The more successful they are, the more strongly they develop as emotional tyrants who take advantage of the sensitivity, sympathy, or guilt feelings of their parents or companions. This kind of emotional blackmail should not be tolerated, because it does no good for anyone involved. The Willow type will learn to act sullen and hurt every time life puts an obstacle in her way. Life, however, does not allow itself to be blackmailed; it gives us the options only of meeting its challenges or dying, of sinking or swimming. We should all learn (especially children) the fundamental lesson that we need to be realistic in our expectations and satisfied with what we are given.

In training us for life, parents or teachers must make these lessons clear. They must be sure that their word is respected and that the child learns that she can't have everything she wants, that there are limits. When a child learns these fundamental lessons, she'll be able to deal with life's many disappointments. We must be careful not to let ourselves be blackmailed by "strategic" sullenness and sulking but allow our blackmailer to simmer in her own juices for a while until she understands that she can't always have her way and readjusts her behavior accordingly.

A genuine Willow condition is something entirely different and has a destructive potential. The otherwise positive attitudes and behavior of the Willow type and her pronounced need for happiness turn into their opposites when her expectations can't be fulfilled. She is truly disappointed and embittered, injured and hurt; she becomes sullen and withdraws from the world and from other people or she feels that life has treated her unfairly. Her positive, life-affirming energy becomes an equally intense negativity. She becomes aggressive to everything that stands in her way—in extreme cases against the world or against fate itself—or, if she is more introverted, directs her negative energy against herself in the form of a bitter and disappointed renunciation of the world.

In the genuine Willow condition, we should assume that the Willow type—at least subjectively—is justified in her views and, if the condition is serious, make sure to help; excessive unyieldingness can run the risk of ongoing psychic damage (especially with children, who can be deeply disappointed or injured through incidents that seem meaningless to an observer). In such cases, it is pointless to exert more pressure; you will only be adding fuel to a raging fire. Better to leave disappointed or embittered people in quiet and try to point out to them (in a nonthreatening manner) that their behavior is leading them to a dead end. They are trying to fight against an intractable reality, and they stand to lose the most.

People who tend to suffer from disappointment, hurt, and bitterness need to make a fundamental change in their attitude. They need to realize that they are only hurting themselves with their denials, accusations, and "facts"; life is not concerned with their opinions. They also need to develop a more realistic view that includes the true facts and that takes into account that humans are merely feeble creatures dependent on their creator.

As long as the Willow type is convinced that someone is taking a personal and intentional interest in her misfortune, she takes it very personally, and it goes straight to her heart. When it is made clear to her, however, that everything that happens is part of a larger scheme and that everything and everyone—including the Willow type—serves as a tool for an unknowable fate, she'll be able to take her misfortune in stride and look at it as just another fateful event. It would also be helpful to get her to make the same demands on herself that she makes on others, since this would allow her to see matters in a gentler, more forgiving light (by the way, it often transpires that even the things that disappoint her have a way of turning out for the best). Life is a process of development and maturity with a secret goal toward which all that we experience plays a part—this includes unpleasant and negative experiences. It's like a fruit with a prickly skin that hides a delicious core. Overcoming the Willow condition means getting past the prickly part and finding the sweet fruit.

Common Combinations with Other Essences

Chicory (8/38): bitterness due to rejection or ungratefulness
Holly (15/38): bitterness combined with rage or hate
Honeysuckle (16/38): bitterness due to a loss
Mustard (21/38): depression caused by bitterness
Oak (22/38): relentless desire for revenge
Star of Bethlehem (29/38): bitterness caused by an
     unprocessed or unresolved trauma
Vine (32/38): embittered, domestic tyrant
Water Violet (34/48): bitterness due to restricted freedom
White Chestnut (35/38): bitter obsessive/compulsive thoughts

TWO

THE NEW COMBINATIONS

Rescue Remedy

The essence for an emergency, Rescue Remedy is the most well-known and most often used combination of essences. It was first mixed and used by Dr. Bach himself. Since then, it has been employed in countless critical situations, and it has often worked wonders. Rescue Remedy consists of the following essences:

6: Cherry Plum
9: Clematis
18: Impatiens
26: Rock Rose
29: Star of Bethlehem

This mixture belongs in every household, travel first-aid kit, and car. It should always be taken in any kind of emergency—for example, in all types of accidents, collapse, anger or panic, threat of suicide, heart attack, stroke, burns, and injuries. It calms, stabilizes, and heals. The normal dosage is three drops on the tongue at short intervals (approximately ten minutes); repeat until there is improvement, and then take after longer intervals. If oral ingestion is not possible, just put some drops on the lips or rub in to the forehead.

1/2 Agrimony/Aspen

Suppression due to fears or fears due to suppression

Agrimony/Aspen is for people who try to ignore and suppress their problems until they become unclear, overwhelming, and unpredictable. This results in a vicious cycle in which the fears provoke suppression and suppression gives rise to fears, causing a fear of fear itself. This combination can make us braver and more open and internally free and be helpful in consciously overcoming problems that cause fears and anxieties. Possible complementary essences: *Mimulus, Red Chestnut, Rock Rose, Star of Bethlehem, Walnut.*

1/3 Agrimony/Beech

Artificial, false tolerance

Agrimony/Beech is for people who hide their fear of conflict and their dislikes and aversions behind a mask of tolerance and tend to gloss over even those things that rub them the wrong way. This combination can be helpful in acknowledging and coming to terms with our likes and dislikes while still being friendly and tolerant. Possible complementary essences: *Heather, Larch.*

1/4 Agrimony/Centaury

Pathological good-naturedness

Agrimony/Centaury is for people who allow themselves to be used without resistance or who behave too obligingly because they have a fear of conflict. They hide their fear behind a mask of affable naïveté. This combination can make us more able to face conflict and help restore a healthy sense of ego. It gives us more courage to speak our minds and to think of our own needs and concerns. Possible complementary essences: *Aspen, Cerato, Gentian, Larch, Mimulus, Star of Bethlehem, Walnut.*

1/6 Agrimony/Cherry Plum

Suppression creating a danger of excessive psychological pressure

Agrimony/Cherry Plum is for people who are under excessive psychological pressure because they suppress strong emotions or drives and try to keep them hidden. There is the danger that at the next minor strain they will go over the edge or go crazy. This combination can help us be more positive and open in conflicts and express our feelings and emotions more openly, which in turn helps to reduce the pressure. Possible complementary essences: *Rock Rose, Sweet Chestnut, White Chestnut.*

1/7 Agrimony/Chestnut Bud

Learning difficulties or immaturity caused by shirking

Agrimony/Chestnut Bud is for people who cannot acknowledge unpleasantness and who avoid difficulties. They remain immature, inexperienced, and cowardly. This combination can make us more engaged and less afraid so that we can confront the duties or problems that face us and we can thereby learn from them. It is often used to treat lazy, indolent children. Possible complementary essences: *Clematis, Gentian, Honeysuckle, Hornbeam, Larch.*

1/19 Agrimony/Larch

Excessive or suppressed inferiority complex

Agrimony/Larch is for people who suffer from an inferiority complex; the more insecure and despondent they are internally, the more carefree and supercilious they become externally. This combination can make us more self-confident and natural, allowing us to admit to our weaknesses without feeling inferior. Possible complementary essence: *Heather.*

1/20 Agrimony/Mimulus

Repressed or secret fears

Agrimony/Mimulus is for people who are very timid but hide their timidity behind a carefree, courageous demeanor. This combination helps us admit to our fears and consciously work on overcoming them. Possible complementary essences: *Aspen, Larch, Red Chestnut, Rock Rose, Star of Bethlehem.*

1/25 Agrimony/Red Chestnut

Secret worries

Agrimony/Red Chestnut is for people who constantly worry about others but don't want to show it. They try to appear carefree and optimistic, but secretly worry, trying to hide their pessimistic fears, so that they can never truly relax or be happy. This combination minimizes these exaggerated worries and allows us to discuss them freely and reach clarity. Possible complementary essences: *Aspen, Chicory, Mimulus, Star of Bethlehem.*

1/26 Agrimony/Rock Rose

Stiffening due to panic

Agrimony/Rock Rose is for people who feel under pressure of a panic situation. They cannot sufficiently release the emotion and have a psychic inflexibility or painful irritation in the muscles, tendons, joints, or spine. This combination can lift the blockade. Possible complementary essences: *Aspen, Crab Apple, Oak, Rock Water, Star of Bethlehem.*

1/29 Agrimony/Star of Bethlehem

Emotional wounds behind a happy mask

Agrimony/Star of Bethlehem is for people who hide unhappiness or a psychic injury behind a carefree facade of optimism. This combination gives us more courage to express our feelings and makes us able to consciously face our problems, for example, in conversation with others. The resulting lifting of our burden helps us lay the groundwork for peacefully coming to terms with life. Possible complementary essences: *Larch, Mimulus, Water Violet, Willow.*

1/33 Agrimony/Walnut

Total self-alienation

Agrimony/Walnut is for people who are alienated from themselves and cannot live as they should, because they let themselves be influenced so strongly and they don't dare to be honest with themselves. Although they appear happy and content, inside they are sad. This combination can help us rediscover ourselves and begin life anew. It motivates us to deal seriously with our problems and helps us develop our own personality, independent of the expectations of those around us. It is an essential accompaniment to psychotherapy because it prevents the fears that often appear when old behaviors are being broken down and new ones are being formed. Possible complementary essences: *Centaury, Cerato, Heather, Star of Bethlehem, Wild Oat.*

1/34 Agrimony/Water Violet

Human contact problems based on a lack of openness

Agrimony/Water Violet is for people who find it difficult to have contact with others because they are trying to hide something, such as a problem, a fear, or a weakness. Although they know instinctively that they would be better off if they could trust someone and open up to them, they are unable to overcome the gulf that separates them from others and remain disconnected, lonely, and unhappy. This combination helps us become more open, more content with human contact, more trusting—and thereby more able to overcome our tormenting isolation. Possible complementary essences: *Larch, Star of Bethlehem.*

1/36 Agrimony/Wild Oat

Lack of self-awareness

Agrimony/Wild Oat is for people who, owing to constant repression, don't know themselves anymore or perhaps never did know themselves. They avoid all confrontations and are afraid to face the truth about themselves. They don't know how to bring about improvement in their lives or how to find meaning in their lives. This combination is useful at the beginning of any kind of personality development. It helps us reach self-awareness and is always indicated when we don't know which essence we should take first. Possible complementary essences: *Cerato, Scleranthus, Walnut.*

2/6 Aspen/Cherry Plum

Sudden feeling of fear and danger of a total breakdown

Aspen/Cherry Plum is for people who feel fear and panic, suddenly and for no recognizable reason, and are on the verge of breaking down or going crazy. Used to treat conditions of psychotic fear caused by emotional trauma. This combination can ease dangerous, fear-induced emotional blockages, preventing psychoses, and prepare us to find a solution by stimulating our awareness. Possible complementary essences: *Mimulus, Rock Rose, Star of Bethlehem.*

2/20 Aspen/Mimulus

Absolute timidity

Aspen/Mimulus is for people who suffer from all sorts of clear and unclear fears and anxieties. In part they arise from clearly defined sources and in part from deep ungrounded fears. This combination can alleviate strong, generalized fears and give us more courage to examine ideas or situations that make us afraid. Possible complementary essences: *Agrimony, Chestnut Bud, Rock Rose, Star of Bethlehem.*

2/21 Aspen/Mustard

Anxious depression

Aspen/Mustard is for people who are constantly stricken with anxiety and fear-inducing ideas. They see everything in black and are afraid of all kinds of misfortune. Often these symptoms appear in concert with a heart or liver illness. This combination can alleviate our fears and make us more mentally and emotionally stable and optimistic. Possible complementary essences: *Gentian, Gorse, Honeysuckle, Hornbeam, Olive, Rock Rose, Star of Bethlehem, Wild Rose.*

2/25 Aspen/Red Chestnut

General, anxiety-induced worries

Aspen/Red Chestnut is for people who worry excessively about others. They are plagued by the terrible fear that some kind of misfortune will strike those close to them. This combination can drive away our fear and allow us to see reality more clearly and to realize that for the most part, things are not as bad as they seem. Possible complementary essences: *Chicory, Mimulus, White Chestnut.*

2/26 Aspen/Rock Rose

Absolute panic

Aspen/Rock Rose is for people who are suddenly stricken with panic and fear. This combination can help us clear our heads when we are stricken with horror or panic—regardless of the cause. Possible complementary essences: *Cherry Plum, Mustard, Sweet Chestnut, White Chestnut.*

2/27 Aspen/Rock Water

Fear-induced self-abuse

Aspen/Rock Water is for people who impose on themselves a strong sense of self-discipline in order to neutralize their fears and anxieties. They keep, for example, a strict order, a strict diet, or a strictly regimented form of behavior because they want to make themselves "watertight" from any sub-conscious, often unnamable fears and anxieties or dangers. The discipline leaves them with a feeling of security. In reality, however, they exchange one form of insecurity for another. As soon as they deviate from their strict rules, they are overcome with terror. This combination can temper our tendencies for compulsive behavior and also ease general fears so that we may live a more natural, carefree life. Possible complementary essences: *Agrimony, Crab Apple, Mimulus, Pine, Vine.*

2/28 Aspen/Scleranthus

Indecisiveness due to vague fears and anxieties

Aspen/Scleranthus is for people whose minds are so occupied with general-ized fears and anxieties that they are unable to think clearly and make decisions. They do not know what they should do because they expect negative consequences from any possible decision. This combination can mitigate our fears and make the mind and spirit clearer so that we regain the ability to act. Possible complementary essences: *Cerato, Mimulus, Rock Rose, Star of Bethlehem, Wild Oat.*

2/29 Aspen/Star of Bethlehem

Mental and emotional vulnerability due to anxious, timid behavior; fear caused by psychic trauma

Aspen/Star of Bethlehem is for people who, because of a general timidity, are easily shaken by unexpected or troubling events or who have lost their faith in life after a terrifying experience. This combination can make us more courageous and able to deal with life and to process fear-related psychic traumas. Possible complementary essences: *Gentian, Honeysuckle, Mimulus, Rock Rose, Walnut.*

2/34 Aspen/Water Violet

Human contact problems caused by generalized, vague fears

Aspen/Water Violet is for people who lose contact with their surroundings because of inexplicable or generalized fears and anxieties, which above all can happen in old age as the consequence of a mental breakdown. This combination can strengthen our trust in other people and awaken the desire for human contact. It helps against loneliness caused by mistrust. Possible complementary essences: *Mimulus, Mustard, Star of Bethlehem, Wild Rose.*

2/35 Aspen/White Chestnut

Mental block caused by vague, undefined fears

Aspen/White Chestnut is for people who are so obsessed with the idea that "something bad" will happen to them that they are barely able to think rationally. This combination can lessen our fears and help us think more realistically and clearly. Possible complementary essences: *Cerato, Cherry Plum, Mimulus, Red Chestnut, Star of Bethlehem.*

3/14 Beech/Heather

Opportunistic tolerance

Beech/Heather is for people who force themselves to be tolerant and generous to make themselves popular. The effect, however, is actually artificial or forced. This combination helps us recognize our own natural preferences and dislikes and, if necessary, deal with being unpopular. Possible complementary essences: *Agrimony, Chicory, Larch, Walnut.*

3/15 Beech/Holly

Allergic shock reaction

Beech/Holly is for people who have strong or excessive allergic reactions to substances or life situations. This combination can lessen reactions or reduce the propensity to have them. Possible complementary essences: *Clematis, Crab Apple, Elm, Rock Rose, Vine.*

3/19 Beech/Larch

Tolerance due to a lack of self-confidence

Beech/Larch is for people who, because of a lack of self-confidence, do not dare to practice justifiable and appropriate criticism and instead try to understand and be tolerant of everything. This combination can strengthen our self-confidence and our ability to face unpleasant truths. Possible complementary essences: *Agrimony, Heather, Mimulus, Walnut.*

3/20 Beech/Mimulus

Tolerance due to timidity

Beech/Mimulus is for people who, due to a fear of eventual consequences, do not dare to criticize appropriately and instead try to understand and tolerate everything. This combination can minimize the fear and anxiety of the consequences of personal and natural aversions and give us the courage to have unpleasant opinions. Possible complementary essences: *Agrimony, Heather, Larch, Walnut.*

3/24 Beech/Pine

Tolerance on moralistic grounds

Beech/Pine is for people who feel they are failing when they cannot see everything in a positive light and try desperately to show generosity and tolerance. This combination promotes responsibility and frees us from the compulsion to be better and more tolerant than we really are. Possible complementary essences: *Agrimony, Crab Apple, Rock Water, Walnut.*

3/27 Beech/Rock Water

Generosity with others and strictness with oneself

Beech/Rock Water is for people who are decidedly generous and tolerant with others but strict and petty with themselves. One has the feeling that something is not right with their behavior. This combination helps us treat ourselves naturally, truthfully, and more objectively. Generosity and incorruptibility come together in a balanced relationship. Possible complementary essences: *Crab Apple, Larch, Wild Oat.*

3/32 Beech/Vine

Total intolerance

Beech/Vine is for people who are intolerant in their emotions, thoughts, and actions. They always find themselves on the defensive (which often manifests itself in allergies, among other things) and constantly try to shape their surroundings according to their needs. They criticize or avoid anything new or unusual. Even if they make a conscious effort to be accepting, it's no more than lip service; they'll soon be back to their old ways of criticizing or wanting to have their hands in everything. They are never truly happy, and they are a burden to those around them. This condition is often accompanied by liver ailments. This combination can make us more open, more generous, and more tolerant. Possible complementary essences: *Crab Apple, Holly, Oak, Pine, Vervain.*

3/34 Beech/Water Violet

Overly tolerant yet unapproachable

Beech/Water Violet is for people who think of themselves as tolerant and understanding in order to avoid deeper contact and to keep others at a distance. This combination helps us shape our relationship to our surroundings more naturally, encourages us to express our critical opinions, and lets us accept personal relationships. Possible complementary essences: *Agrimony, Heather, Mimulus.*

4/5 Centaury/Cerato

Dependence due to a weak personality

Centaury/Cerato is for people who have never learned to act independently and who need to have someone else prescribe for them how they should behave and what they should do. They are even-tempered, let themselves be used, and do not have their own opinions. This combination can develop our personality, making us stronger, braver, and more independent. It is often used for overly dependent children. Possible complementary essences: *Crab Apple, Larch, Pine, Walnut, Wild Oat.*

4/8 Centaury/Chicory

Selfish self-sacrifice

Centaury/Chicory is for people who gladly sacrifice themselves, but their motivation is a mix of selflessness and selfishness. Their tendency to latch on to others through worrying or playing the victim is both strengthened and weakened by their natural devotion. It becomes difficult for the "victims" of their good deeds to free themselves from this relationship. This combination can limit the dependent, exploitative nature of relationships. Possible complementary essences: *Pine, Red Chestnut, Walnut, Wild Oat.*

4/12 Centaury/Gentian

Weak will and weak personality

Centaury/Gentian is for people who have so little self-assertiveness or will to see things through that they are easily manipulated, used, and discouraged. They are often depressed because they can never have what they really want. This combination can strengthen our personality and will so that we can resist being manipulated and pressured and not let potential failures muddle our judgment. Possible complementary essences: *Cerato, Clematis, Honeysuckle, Hornbeam, Larch, Star of Bethlehem, Wild Rose.*

4/13 Centaury/Gorse

Compliance due to hopelessness

Centaury/Gorse is for people who have given up hope on their own life, who deny themselves and put themselves in the service of other people or let themselves be used by others. Taken over a longer time period, this combination can change our pessimism and motivate us to think again of ourselves. Possible complementary essences: *Gentian, Star of Bethlehem, Wild Rose.*

4/17 Centaury/Hornbeam

Feelings of stress and overwork due to dependence

Centaury/Hornbeam is for people who do not feel up to life's challenges, as the result of undeveloped independence. They are not as successful as they would like to be, especially where work is concerned. This combination can strengthen our personality, our enthusiasm, and our willingness to undertake new things. Possible complementary essences: *Aspen, Gentian, Larch, Olive.*

4/19 Centaury/Larch

Readiness to help caused by an inferiority complex

Centaury/Larch is for dependent people with an inferiority complex who do not risk leading their own lives and act in an overly helpful, friendly manner. This combination can make us more independent and self-aware so that we begin to think of our own interests. Possible complementary essences: *Cerato, Gentian, Hornbeam, Mimulus, Walnut.*

4/20 Centaury/Mimulus

Fearful submissiveness

Centaury/Mimulus is for people who let themselves be used out of fear of others. Their noticeably affable demeanor has a decidedly obsequious tone. This combination can make us braver and more self-aware so that we begin to assert our own rights and do not allow ourselves to be used anymore. It is especially useful for children and can help spinal complaints, which are connected to servile behavior. Possible complementary essences: *Cerato, Hornbeam, Larch, Star of Bethlehem, Walnut.*

4/24 Centaury/Pine

Self-sacrifice caused by feelings of guilt

Centaury/Pine is for people who deny themselves owing to feelings of guilt. Their inborn selflessness will become pathologically strengthened through the opinion that they do not have a right to be happy or to have their own life. This combination can allow us to look after our own well-being without suffering a guilty conscience. Possible complementary essences: *Cerato, Larch, Rock Water, Star of Bethlehem, Walnut.*

4/25 Centaury/Red Chestnut

Worried selflessness

Centaury/Red Chestnut is for people who are overly selfless and constantly worried. This combination can make us naturally free of worries and allows us a healthy amount of egotism, while giving us the ability to leave others to their own fate. Possible complementary essences: *Aspen, Chicory, Mimulus, Pine, Star of Bethlehem, Walnut.*

4/33 Centaury/Walnut

Dependent and easily influenced

Centaury/Walnut is for people who let themselves be too easily influenced by others and can't lead their own lives. This combination can make us more independent and strong willed, allowing us to think more of ourselves and do what we truly want. Possible complementary essences: *Cerato, Heather, Larch, Pine, Wild Oat.*

4/37 Centaury/Wild Rose

Resignation due to a weak personality

Centaury/Wild Rose is for people who allow themselves to be used and to serve others and who put forth no objections. They have resigned themselves and tend to let themselves be pushed around by others instead of trying to improve their own situation. This combination strengthens the personality and awakens in us a new interest in life so that we can finally begin to think of ourselves and our future. Possible complementary essences: *Gentian, Larch, Olive, Star of Bethlehem, Walnut.*

5/7 Cerato/Chestnut Bud

Perplexity due to carelessness

Cerato/Chestnut Bud is for people who do not know how they should act because they are not attentive and do not learn enough from their experiences. Although they constantly receive advice, they make the same mistakes again and again. Used to help mentally lazy children who constantly ask questions without thinking. This combination can awaken our interest in our experiences so that we can better mentally process events and become independent and able to make decisions. Possible complementary essences: *Clematis, Hornbeam, Larch, Scleranthus, Wild Oat.*

5/19 Cerato/Larch

Insecurity due to feelings of inferiority

Cerato/Larch is for people who do not dare act spontaneously because they feel themselves to be incapable or inferior. At every opportunity, they ask what they should be doing or how they should behave. This combination can make us more self-aware and independent. It helps us act without asking for advice or validation. Possible complementary essences: *Agrimony, Centaury, Gentian, Mimulus, Walnut, Wild Oat.*

5/20 Cerato/Mimulus

Timidity and insecurity

Cerato/Mimulus is for people who fear excessively that they are acting wrongly and constantly ask for the opinions of others. This combination can alleviate our fear of making mistakes and helps us act intuitively, freely, and according to our own judgment. Possible complementary essences: *Centaury, Gentian, Larch, Walnut, Wild Oat.*

5/24 Cerato/Pine

Insecurity due to fear of a bad conscience

Cerato/Pine is for people who fear being guilty and do not dare to act as they really want; they constantly ask for advice to be sure that they're doing the right thing. This combination can free us from our groundless feelings of guilt and make us responsible for ourselves and more secure. Possible complementary essences: *Centaury, Crab Apple, Larch, Mimulus, Red Chestnut, Walnut, Wild Oat.*

5/27 Cerato/Rock Water

Mental dependence and self-abuse

Cerato/Rock Water is for people who do not trust their own instincts and often follow strictly some teaching, religion, or dogma, even though it may be against their own interests. This combination can make us unaffected, natural, and self-assured. Possible complementary essences: *Crab Apple, Larch, Pine, Walnut, Wild Oat.*

5/28 Cerato/Scleranthus

Insecurity and indecisiveness

Cerato/Scleranthus is for people who have no idea what they should do because they don't trust their own opinions and find it difficult to make a decision. This combination helps promote our abilities to make decisions independently. Possible complementary essences: *Chestnut Bud, Gentian, Larch, Walnut, Wild Oat.*

5/29 Cerato/Star of Bethlehem

Insecurity caused by a traumatic experience

Cerato/Star of Bethlehem is for people who have become so insecure from a particular experience or event that they have lost the ability to act independently and self-confidently. Still under the influence of a shock, they are so desperate to assure themselves that they'll ask anyone for advice. This combination helps us overcome psychic trauma and be ourselves again. Possible complementary essences: *Aspen, Centaury, Gentian, Larch, Mimulus, Walnut, Wild Oat.*

5/33 Cerato/Walnut

Insecurity due to being easily influenced

Cerato/Walnut is for people who are easily influenced and are again and again put off their goals by bad advice. This combination can make us more secure and self-confident and helps us follow our own path without straying. Possible complementary essences: *Centaury, Gentian, Larch, Pine, Scleranthus, Wild Oat.*

5/36 Cerato/Wild Oat

Lack of life plans leading to insecurity

Cerato/Wild Oat is for people who are lacking a goal in life to orient themselves and their actions. Internally insecure, they are in constant search of an adviser or leader. Because they cannot judge whether these leaders are right for them, they often find themselves on the wrong path. This combination helps us reach a point of clarity on the important aspects of our lives and take action. Possible complementary essences: *Centaury, Gentian, Mustard, Scleranthus, Walnut.*

6/11 Cherry Plum/Elm

At the limits of psychic and physical endurance

Cherry Plum/Elm is for people who have demanded too much of themselves physically and psychically and can lose their physical and rational faculties. This combination can prevent a potential collapse by easing self-induced pressure and allows us to reward ourselves with happiness and rest. Possible complementary essences: *Agrimony, Oak, Pine, Rock Rose, Rock Water, Sweet Chestnut.*

6/15 Cherry Plum/Holly

Uncontrollable fits of rage

Cherry Plum/Holly is for people who suffer under very strong emotional pressure and are susceptible to fits of aggression and rage. This combination is for exceptional situations. It should be taken when we feel that we're about to burst from anger and rage. It can reduce tension and protect us from the worst. Possible complementary essences: *Impatiens, White Chestnut, Willow.*

6/18 Cherry Plum/Impatiens

Prepsychotic restlessness

Cherry Plum/Impatiens is for people who react to severe emotional pressure by being restless or by excessive, inappropriate actions. It's as if they might go over the edge if they were to have to stand still for just a moment. This combination can make us calmer and more relaxed. Possible complementary essences: *Agrimony, Elm, Holly, Scleranthus, Vervain, White Chestnut.*

6/20 Cherry Plum/Mimulus

Severe internal conflict due to fear

Cherry Plum/Mimulus is for people who are in danger of cracking under pressure, owing to particular fears that they cannot consciously express or work through. This combination is for emergency situations. It can reduce internal, anxious pressure and must be taken frequently. Possible complementary essences: *Aspen, Impatiens, Rock Rose, Sweet Chestnut, White Chestnut.*

6/22 Cherry Plum/Oak

On the verge of an emotional breakdown
due to stress and overwork

Cherry Plum/Oak is for people who demand more of themselves than they can actually achieve and are thus under such internal pressure that they are in danger of a breakdown. Instinctively, they begin to sacrifice their own happiness in order to fulfill their own overambitious plans and feel the irresistible urge to throw everything overboard that represents order and reason. This combination can reduce inner tension by minimizing self-imposed pressures and helping us see them as unnecessary and destructive. Possible complementary essences: *Elm, Holly, Rock Water, Sweet Chestnut, Vervain.*

6/25 Cherry Plum/Red Chestnut

Raging worries

Cherry Plum/Red Chestnut is for people who worry about someone so much that they are on the edge of a breakdown. Perhaps they've tried too hard and for too long to suppress their fears or perhaps other anxieties combine with their worries to create a psychic pressure cooker. This combination can lessen the internal pressures caused by our worrying. It makes us more optimistic and able to consciously face our own fears. Possible complementary essences: *Aspen, Chicory, Impatiens, Mimulus, Rock Rose, Sweet Chestnut, White Chestnut.*

6/26 Cherry Plum/Rock Rose

Panic, with the danger of losing one's reason

Cherry Plum/Rock Rose is for situations in which sudden, panicky fear puts us in danger of going over the edge. We cannot think straight or listen to reason. This combination can minimize the acute danger by bringing us more distance, quiet, and clarity. Possible complementary essences: *Aspen, Clematis, Impatiens, Mimulus, Sweet Chestnut.*

6/27 Cherry Plum/Rock Water

Psychosis as the result of an excessive self-imposed pressure

Cherry Plum/Rock Water is for people who have put themselves under too much pressure; an unexpected psychic trauma puts them in danger of losing self-control. This combination can calm and relax us as it helps us deal more flexibly with our emotions and psychic needs. Possible complementary essences: *Crab Apple, Impatiens, Oak, Pine, Vine.*

6/29 Cherry Plum/Star of Bethlehem

Psychosis caused by a mental or spiritual injury

Cherry Plum/Star of Bethlehem is for people whose psyche has been so shaken from some shocking event that they are on the verge of a breakdown or are generally so unstable and sensitive that even a minor shock will send them over the edge. This combination can make us psychically more stable by tempering our oversensitivity or lessening the trauma. Possible complementary essences: *Aspen, Holly, Impatiens, Mimulus, Walnut, Willow.*

6/30 Cherry Plum/Sweet Chestnut

Desperation due to emotional stress

Cherry Plum/Sweet Chestnut is for people who have lost sight of the "big picture" as the result of emotional stress and feel lost and desperate. This combination is for exceptional situations. It can reduce the inner pressure and return our hope of somehow making life clear again. Possible complementary essences: *Aspen, Elm, Gorse, Star of Bethlehem.*

6/35 Cherry Plum/White Chestnut

Mental obsession

Cherry Plum/White Chestnut is for people who are so obsessed with a particular thought that they can go insane. This combination can limit mental and emotional obsessions and relax us so that we can face our problems rationally. Possible complementary essences: *Holly, Impatiens, Pine, Oak, Rock Water, Star of Bethlehem, Vervain, Willow.*

7/9 Chestnut Bud/Clematis

Carelessness and daydreaming

Chestnut Bud/Clematis is for people who make mistakes again and again because they depend too much on their daydreams and illusions. For dreamy children with learning disabilities. This combination can make us more attentive, more interested, and more circumspect. Possible complementary essences: *Gentian, Honeysuckle, Larch, Wild Rose.*

7/12 Chestnut Bud/Gentian

Lack of attentiveness leading to a relapse

Chestnut Bud/Gentian is for people who do not pay enough attention to their experiences. This laxity will often lead to setbacks at work, which, in turn, causes them to be frustrated and give up prematurely. It can also lead to a standstill or relapse in the healing process. If we have a tendency to neglect our own needs, this combination can help us get back on our feet after an illness. It is also useful with children who lose their thirst for learning because they constantly make mistakes. Possible complementary essences: *Clematis, Holly, Hornbeam, Impatiens, Olive, Scleranthus, Star of Bethlehem, Wild Rose.*

7/16 Chestnut Bud/Honeysuckle

Inattentiveness due to nostalgic daydreaming

Chestnut Bud/Honeysuckle is for people who often make mistakes because their thoughts are stuck in the past. This combination helps us let go of the past and apply ourselves constructively to the present. It is good for children who have learning difficulties due to homesickness. Possible complementary essences: *Centaury, Clematis, Gentian, Mustard, Wild Rose.*

7/28 Chestnut Bud/Scleranthus

Learning difficulties caused by attention deficit

Chestnut Bud/Scleranthus is for people who are poor learners because they are too easily distracted. This combination helps us stay on track and concentrate on that which needs to be learned. Possible complementary essences: *Cerato, Clematis, Gentian, Honeysuckle, Impatiens, Wild Oat.*

7/34 Chestnut Bud/Water Violet

Closed-mindedness

Chestnut Bud/Water Violet is for people who close themselves off to every new experience. Intellectual conflicts, new knowledge, and stimulating or unaccustomed human contact are all unpleasant. This combination can make us more receptive, more mentally flexible, more interested and enthusiastic, and more open to human contact. It is especially suitable for withdrawn children who lack enthusiasm. Possible complementary essences: *Clematis, Honeysuckle, Larch, Mimulus, Star of Bethlehem, Wild Rose.*

7/35 Chestnut Bud/White Chestnut

Distraction due to obsessive thoughts

Chestnut Bud/White Chestnut is for people who are so dominated by certain thoughts that they cannot get their minds off them or learn something new. This combination can free our thoughts from pointless obsessions and help our memory. Possible complementary essences: *Clematis, Crab Apple, Honeysuckle, Pine, Rock Water, Star of Bethlehem, Vervain, Vine.*

7/36 Chestnut Bud/Wild Oat
Lack of goals due to inattentiveness

Chestnut Bud/Wild Oat is for people who do not learn from their experiences and therefore have no useful life concept or goals. This combination (which must often be taken for months) helps us recognize our purpose in life. Possible complementary essences: *Centaury, Cerato, Clematis, Gentian, Honeysuckle, Larch, Scleranthus, Walnut.*

7/37 Chestnut Bud/Wild Rose
Inattentive and resigned

Chestnut Bud/Wild Rose is for people who continually make mistakes because they have no interest in life. Used to treat generally unenthusiastic children who lack initiative and who have learning difficulties. This combination can make us more attentive, more circumspect, and more enthusiastic. Possible complementary essences: *Clematis, Honeysuckle, Hornbeam, Mustard, Olive, Star of Bethlehem.*

8/14 Chicory/Heather
Overpowering need to be loved and admired

Chicory/Heather is for people who crave attention and admiration. They care about other people, but they also toot their own horn at every chance. Their need to be loved and admired is so strong that they are deeply hurt if someone doesn't notice them. This combination can make us more discreet, more natural, and more independent of others. Vain children who crave love need it often. Possible complementary essences: *Agrimony, Cerato, Holly, Larch, Mimulus, Star of Bethlehem, Walnut, Willow.*

8/15 Chicory/Holly

Love-hate

Chicory/Holly is for people whose disappointed love turns to hate. They are unfriendly and hateful or aggressive because they do not get the attention they desire. This combination is often used for family or relationship problems, for example, if a partnership is about to break up or a child wants to be rid of his or her parents. It can prevent a serious disappointment and promote calm understanding. Possible complementary essences: *Red Chestnut, Star of Bethlehem, Willow.*

8/16 Chicory/Honeysuckle

Sadness due to a lost love

Chicory/Honeysuckle is for people who cannot get over the loss of a close relationship, such as the love of a person or an animal. Their thoughts are stuck in the past, when the world still made sense to them, and they feel deeply hurt. This combination helps us overcome the sadness that comes from not being able to let go. Once we are free, we can turn our attention again to the present. It is good for children who are torn away from their accustomed surroundings. Possible complementary essences: *Holly, Star of Bethlehem, Wild Rose, Willow.*

8/20 Chicory/Mimulus

Anxious clinging

Chicory/Mimulus is for people who cling to someone out of fear or for people (especially children) who constantly live in the fear of losing the person whom they most love and trust. This combination can make us more secure, confident, and independent. Possible complementary essences: *Aspen, Centaury, Larch, Red Chestnut, Star of Bethlehem.*

8/21 Chicory/Mustard

Depression caused by unrequited love

Chicory/Mustard is for people who are always stricken with sadness or depression because their love is not returned. This combination can make us more content and realistic in our life's desires. Possible complementary essences: *Gentian, Heather, Honeysuckle, Star of Bethlehem, Willow, Wild Oat.*

8/22 Chicory/Oak

Stubborn, insistent attention or love

Chicory/Oak is for people who cannot get over their obsession with helping someone, even though the assistance or attention is not welcome. This combination helps us keep the right distance when we find ourselves in a futile or unhappy relationship. Possible complementary essences: *Holly, Honeysuckle, Vervain, Willow.*

8/25 Chicory/Red Chestnut

Total self-sacrifice

Chicory/Red Chestnut is for people who tend to sacrifice themselves for other people out of an unusual combination of egotism and selflessness. This combination of essences helps us put more distance between ourselves and those we love and allows us to think more about ourselves. Possible complementary essences: *Aspen, Impatiens, Mimulus, Walnut, White Chestnut.*

8/35 Chicory/White Chestnut

Obsessive thoughts of love

Chicory/White Chestnut is for people who can think only of catching their beloved's attention or of how they'll never get over it if they don't succeed. This combination can bring us around to other thoughts again and normalize our perspective where love is concerned. Possible complementary essences: *Honeysuckle, Oak, Star of Bethlehem, Willow.*

8/38 Chicory/Willow

Bitterness caused by rejection or ingratitude

Chicory/Willow is for people who are embittered because someone they cared about very much has ignored them or treated them ungraciously. This combination can prevent or ease bitterness and resentment when they are reactions to unrequited love or ingratitude. Possible complementary essences: *Heather, Holly, Larch, Star of Bethlehem, Water Violet.*

9/12 Clematis/Gentian

Weak will and daydreaming

Clematis/Gentian is for people who give up too quickly at the sign of failure or difficulties and begin to take refuge in dreams or illusions. Used to treat dreamy, weak-willed children. This combination can make us more strong willed and realistic and enable us to better master our lives. Possible complementary essences: *Centaury, Honeysuckle, Hornbeam, Larch, Wild Rose.*

9/16 Clematis/Honeysuckle

Total daydreaming

Clematis/Honeysuckle is for people who are not realistic enough. At one moment they cling to pleasant memories, and the next they dream of better times; they have little interest in the present. They can't concentrate well on their work and are often unhappy with their lives. This combination can help us concentrate and make us more realistic and able to cope with life. It reduces pathological tendencies to flee from reality. Possible complementary essences: *Gentian, Larch, Star of Bethlehem, White Chestnut, Wild Rose.*

9/23 Clematis/Olive

Sleepiness, absentmindedness, hallucinations, or unconsciousness due to exhaustion

Clematis/Olive is for people who are so exhausted that they have a hard time concentrating. Their thoughts tend to roam or are vague and unclear. They often fall asleep or fall into a state of daydreaming at inappropriate times. In more serious cases, they can end up unconscious or longing for death. This combination can restore us to strength and clarity. It is especially useful for serious mental or emotional exertion, such as examinations or debilitating illnesses that drain the strength. Possible complementary essences: *Gentian, Gorse, Star of Bethlehem, Wild Rose.*

9/26 Clematis/Rock Rose

Tendency toward fainting in panic situations

Clematis/Rock Rose is for people who lose consciousness or presence of mind in a panic situation. This combination is an ingredient of Rescue Remedy. It helps us keep our presence of mind in emergencies and can also be taken as a preventive if we tend to become unconscious when faced with unusual psychic stress. It can be given with Agrimony in cases of epilepsy. Possible complementary essences: *Aspen, Cherry Plum, Elm, Gentian, Star of Bethlehem, Sweet Chestnut.*

9/28 Clematis/Scleranthus

Indecisiveness due to daydreaming

Clematis/Scleranthus is for people who have difficulties making decisions because speculation and illusions have taken away their clear view of reality. Generally, they wait for matters to take care of themselves. This combination can make us more realistic and decisive. Possible complementary essences: *Cerato, Gentian, Wild Oat.*

9/29 Clematis/Star of Bethlehem

Unconsciousness in traumatic situations

Clematis/Star of Bethlehem is for people who tend to pass out when faced with a shocking or unhappy situation. This combination generally restores our presence of mind and makes us mentally and emotionally more resistant. In accidents it can help us avoid unconsciousness. It is a component of Rescue Remedy. Possible complementary essences: *Aspen, Elm, Olive, Rock Rose, Walnut, Wild Rose.*

9/35 Clematis/White Chestnut

Obsessive dreams of the future

Clematis/White Chestnut is for eccentric daydreamers and people whose minds are always filled with future plans and dreams. They cannot think of anything else, live only in their fantasies and dreams, and are also unable to deal with the present. This combination can bring us back to reason. Possible complementary essences: *Chestnut Bud, Honeysuckle, Wild Oat.*

9/37 Clematis/Wild Rose

Drowsiness, lack of initiative or resignation, and a longing for death

Clematis/Wild Rose is for people who cannot think clearly and cannot bring themselves to act. They simply have no drive and often feel in a funk. In the case of a serious illness, this can often lead to resignation and a longing for death. This combination can reawaken the mind and spirit and make us more interested and engaged. Possible complementary essences: *Gentian, Honeysuckle, Olive, Star of Bethlehem.*

10/19 Crab Apple/Larch

Feelings of impurity and self-loathing

Crab Apple/Larch is for people who feel physically and spiritually unclean and inferior. There are two tendencies here: first, they have feelings of inferiority because they think of themselves as unclean, and second, their low self-esteem causes them to place excessive and pathological demands on themselves. This combination enables us to feel more at home in our own skin and pay more attention to our own needs. Possible complementary essences: *Centaury, Cerato, Pine, Star of Bethlehem, Walnut.*

10/20 Crab Apple/Mimulus

Excessive fear of filth

Crab Apple/Mimulus is for people who have an intense, groundless fear of filth, contagion, or toxins. They are sterile and artificial and can no longer be content with a "normal" life. Often, fear of contagion or uncleanliness can have a detrimental effect on their sexuality. This combination can make us more casual in questions of cleanliness, help us overcome our loathing, and give us the courage to indulge our guilty pleasures when called for. Possible complementary essences: *Agrimony, Aspen, Cerato, Larch, Pine, Star of Bethlehem, Walnut, Wild Oat.*

10/24 Crab Apple/Pine
Morally motivated obsession with cleanliness

Crab Apple/Pine is for people who strive toward absolute internal and external cleanliness on moral as well as hygienic grounds. They feel guilty when they can't be clean and orderly. This combination can mitigate our moral obsessions and make us able to be happy with life, even when it falls outside the norms of cleanliness, order, and morality. Possible complementary essences: *Cerato, Larch, Mimulus, Rock Water, Star of Bethlehem, Walnut.*

10/27 Crab Apple/Rock Water
Excessively clean and disciplined

Crab Apple/Rock Water is for people who drive themselves to excessive order, cleanliness, and discipline. This impulse makes them unpleasant, tense companions. This combination can make us more natural, unaffected, and tolerant in matters of cleanliness. Possible complementary essences: *Mimulus, Oak, Pine, Vine, Wild Oat.*

10/29 Crab Apple/Star of Bethlehem
Pathological loathing

Crab Apple/Star of Bethlehem is for people who react with excessive defensiveness or pathological disgust to dirt or filth as the result of a traumatic experience. This combination can normalize our relationship to "filth." Possible complementary essences: *Agrimony, Aspen, Mimulus, Rock Rose.*

10/32 Crab Apple/Vine

Petty fanaticism for cleanliness

Crab Apple/Vine is for people who have a strong need for cleanliness and order, not only for themselves but also for their environment. Their obsessions can make them petty, intolerant, and tyrannical. This combination can loosen our inflexible attitudes about order, morality, and cleanliness. Possible complementary essences: *Aspen, Mimulus, Pine, Rock Water, Star of Bethlehem, Vervain, White Chestnut.*

10/35 Crab Apple/White Chestnut

Tormenting feelings of being filthy

Crab Apple/White Chestnut is for people who are obsessed with the idea of being impure or poisoned and can no longer think clearly. These compulsive ideas can concern the physical (filth, toxins, contagion) or the spiritual (immorality, sins). This combination can free us from our obsessive attitudes so that we can feel at home in our own skin. Possible complementary essences: *Aspen, Mimulus, Pine, Rock Water, Vine.*

11/12 Elm/Gentian

Discouraged, overworked, and overwhelmed

Elm/Gentian is for people who suddenly do not feel up to a burden or responsibility and want to give up, even though they may have the strength to continue. Also for people who are normally very healthy and who suddenly become ill and can't recover. This combination helps us endure in extreme psychic or physical situations and, when we feel at the end of our rope, helps us go on. It can liberate our healing abilities in the case of serious, sudden illnesses. Possible complementary essences: *Gorse, Larch, Mimulus, Star of Bethlehem, Walnut.*

11/13 Elm/Gorse

Sudden hopelessness caused by overexertion

Elm/Gorse is for people who suddenly lose faith in their ability to succeed, under the pressure of a great burden or responsibility. They become mired in a kind of internal crippling and are no longer capable of hope. This combination is not often needed; used at the right moment, however, it can help us avoid a catastrophe. It can restore in us the hope that there is a solution for everything and return to us our lost optimism as well. Possible combinations: *Gentian, Star of Bethlehem, Sweet Chestnut, Wild Rose.*

11/17 Elm/Hornbeam

Acute performance anxiety

Elm/Hornbeam is for people who are on the verge of collapsing when life seems too difficult or when they are under a special strain. The origins of this condition are more psychic than physical. This combination can have a stabilizing effect in acute crises brought about by "performance anxiety" and can help alleviate fear of failure of all types. It is used for special traumas of all kinds, especially for pessimistic people. Possible complementary essences: *Gentian, Larch, Mimulus, Olive, Vervain.*

11/19 Elm/Larch

Sudden loss of self-confidence

Elm/Larch is for people with weak self-confidence who suddenly lose all courage in the face of a special mission or responsibility and are on the verge of a breakdown. This combination can restore our strength and self-confidence so that we may go on. Possible complementary essences: *Gentian, Hornbeam, Mimulus, Olive, Rock Rose, Star of Bethlehem.*

11/20 Elm/Mimulus

Sudden fear of failure

Elm/Mimulus is for people who are suddenly stricken with a fear of not being able to complete a task or not being able to fulfill a responsibility. Normally they are competent and love to take on a lot for themselves; all of a sudden, however, they become despondent and fearful. This combination can restore our accustomed courage and fill us with a new confidence in our ability to achieve. Possible complementary essences: *Aspen, Gentian, Hornbeam, Larch, Rock Rose, Star of Bethlehem.*

11/22 Elm/Oak

Overly demanding as the result of a compulsion to achieve

Elm/Oak is for people who always make extreme demands on themselves and find it difficult to lower their goals or give up when their goals are too unrealistic. Their ambitious, uncompromising behavior often pushes them to the edge of a breakdown, destroys their happiness, and, in the long term, undermines their health. This combination can temper our obsession with achievement and responsibility and help us better assess our abilities, which, in turn, will improve our performance. Possible complementary essences: *Rock Water, Vine.*

11/23 Elm/Olive

Severe physical, mental, and emotional exhaustion

Elm/Olive is for people who are pushed to the edge of their abilities and who feel mentally and physically drained. This combination can mobilize our reserves of physical and psychic strength. Possible complementary essences: *Gentian, Gorse, Hornbeam, Larch, Star of Bethlehem.*

11/26 Elm/Rock Rose

Panic due to stress

Elm/Rock Rose is for people who quickly fall into a state of panic when they are stressed. This combination can bring us the needed cold-bloodedness and efficiency in times of stress and keep us from losing our heads. Possible complementary essences: *Aspen, Cherry Plum, Impatiens, Mimulus, Star of Bethlehem.*

11/29 Elm/Star of Bethlehem

Collapse as the result of psychological trauma

Elm/Star of Bethlehem is for people who break down (or are on the verge of breaking down) when faced with a traumatic experience. This combination can restore our strength, our inner distance, and our mental clarity, in order to deal with several traumatic situations. Possible complementary essences: *Gorse, Rock Rose, Sweet Chestnut.*

11/30 Elm/Sweet Chestnut

Desperation due to overexertion

Elm/Sweet Chestnut is for people who are thrown into absolute desperation from a sudden feeling of overexertion and overwork. Normally, they can muster great reserves of strength in such situations, but in this case, the situation simply seems overwhelming. They don't know any longer how to proceed and are ready to throw in the towel. This combination can help us overcome the depths. It is not often used, but when it is, it should be taken frequently. Possible complementary essences: *Gentian, Hornbeam, Larch, Oak, Star of Bethlehem.*

12/13 Gentian/Gorse

Weak will and hopelessness

Gentian/Gorse is for people who are discouraged and pessimistic after a long history of failures. They undertake nothing with true conviction and decisiveness and give up at the first sign of difficulties. This combination can make us more optimistic, enthusiastic, and proactive. It is especially useful for debilitating, serious illnesses when a positive trend stops, and it can ensure small advances in the recovery process. Possible complementary essences: *Hornbeam, Olive, Star of Bethlehem, Wild Rose.*

12/16 Gentian/Honeysuckle

Excessive nostalgia and pining for the past

Gentian/Honeysuckle is for people who live more in the past than in the present and therefore are not up to the challenges of their lives. They are no longer interested in success and give up very easily. This is found in children who suffer from homesickness or with people who have lost their connection to life after a serious loss. This combination helps us forget the past and face the challenges of life. Possible complementary essences: *Clematis, Hornbeam, Mustard, Olive, Star of Bethlehem, Wild Rose.*

12/17 Gentian/Hornbeam

Pessimistic and weak willed

Gentian/Hornbeam is for people who always feel overworked and stressed, and who are essentially geared toward failure and readily give up in the face of difficulties. This combination can make us more proactive and strong willed. Possible complementary essences: *Centaury, Larch, Mimulus, Star of Bethlehem, Wild Rose.*

12/19 Gentian/Larch

Weak willed, with a lack of self-confidence

Gentian/Larch is for people who are programmed to fail because they trust nothing and throw in the towel at the first sign of difficulties. This is especially true of children who are too sensitive for the human rat race. This combination can give us more self-confidence and drive. Possible complementary essences: *Centaury, Heather, Mimulus, Star of Bethlehem, Wild Rose.*

12/20 Gentian/Mimulus

Tractable and timid

Gentian/Mimulus is for people who always shrink from problems, owing to their timidity. They break off appointments, abandon plans, or give up their rights because they are afraid that insisting on what's due them could have negative consequences. This combination can make us more brave and strong willed. Possible complementary essences: *Aspen, Centaury, Hornbeam, Larch, Star of Bethlehem, Walnut.*

12/21 Gentian/Mustard

Bad moods or depression

Gentian/Mustard is for people who are constantly in bad moods or suffer depression, sometimes with and sometimes without good reason. This combination helps against depressive moods of all kinds. It can stabilize mood and generally make us more optimistic. Possible complementary essences: *Centaury, Chicory, Hornbeam, Larch, Olive, Star of Bethlehem, Wild Oat.*

12/23 Gentian/Olive

Exhausted and discouraged

Gentian/Olive is for people who cannot take care of their obligations and affairs properly owing to serious exhaustion; they give up at the first sign of difficulties and, worn out, withdraw into themselves. This combination can mobilize reserves of strength and make us more strong willed and proactive. Possible complementary essences: *Centaury, Clematis, Honeysuckle, Hornbeam, Mustard, Star of Bethlehem, Wild Rose.*

12/28 Gentian/Scleranthus

Relapse during the recovery phase

Gentian/Scleranthus is for people who suffer setbacks or disruptions during a process of recovery, a recurring setback in an illness that we thought was defeated. One has the impression that the organism itself has not been totally convinced that it should become healthy again. This combination promotes consistency in the healing and recovery process and minimizes the danger of a relapse. It is especially appropriate in psychically unstable people who more or less unconsciously have not (or at least not sufficiently) reached the resolution of their illness because the motivation to become healthy again is still not strong enough. Possible complementary essences: *Cerato, Chestnut Bud, Walnut, Wild Rose.*

12/29 Gentian/Star of Bethlehem

Weak will caused by psychic trauma

Gentian/Star of Bethlehem is for people whose will is diminished by a terrifying experience or emotionally difficult circumstances. They shrink away in terror from every problem because they still suffer from a lingering shock, and it seems as if they will never recover. This combination can make us able to face life again by healing mental and emotional wounds and strengthening the will. Possible complementary essences: *Centaury, Hornbeam, Larch, Olive, Wild Rose.*

12/33 Gentian/Walnut

Despair accompanying life changes

Gentian/Walnut is for people who face losing their optimism and endurance during phases of important personal development. The problem arises when shaping the form of a new life comes to a standstill. This combination can give us the strength and resolve to follow our own path so that neither setbacks nor other people can deter us from realizing our goals. Possible complementary essences: *Centaury, Hornbeam, Larch, Mimulus, Olive, Scleranthus, Wild Oat.*

12/37 Gentian/Wild Rose

Resignation and weak will

Gentian/Wild Rose is for people for whom it takes a great effort to gather themselves together to undertake a project and who give up at the first sign of difficulty. Nothing interests them, and they let themselves drift; when they finally make a halfhearted effort to get on their feet again, they sabotage themselves by giving up immediately. This combination helps us find our way back to an active life by promoting an enthusiastic and energetic nature. Possible complementary essences: *Centaury, Hornbeam, Larch, Olive, Star of Bethlehem.*

13/21 Gorse/Mustard

Depression caused by hopelessness

Gorse/Mustard is for people who sink into depression again and again because they suffer from a deep-seated hopelessness that permeates their entire being. Although they lead a halfway normal life in their "good" phases, internally they are resigned and unhappy. This combination can limit the frequency and intensity of bouts with depression and make us, on the whole, more optimistic. It should be taken over an extended period of time. Possible complementary essences: *Centaury, Gentian, Hornbeam, Olive, Star of Bethlehem.*

13/23 Gorse/Olive

Hopelessness caused by exhaustion

Gorse/Olive is for people who have no more strength to go on living after long or intense suffering. The body has used up its reserves, and the spirit has lost all hope. They simply wait (consciously or unconsciously) for the end. This combination can strengthen the body and also awaken positive mental strength; in doing so, it can help bring about a general change for the better and, at the very least, make life worth living. It should be taken in cases of advancing cancer. Possible complementary essences: *Centaury, Clematis, Elm, Gentian, Hornbeam, Larch, Mustard, Star of Bethlehem, Sweet Chestnut, Wild Rose.*

13/29 Gorse/Star of Bethlehem

Hopelessness caused by severe trauma

Gorse/Star of Bethlehem is for people who have been deeply affected, psychically or physically, by a terrifying experience or accident to the extent that they have lost all hope of an improvement. Filled with a profound sense of pessimism, they can no longer imagine themselves being happy or healthy. Taken over the long term, this combination can heal our wounds and awaken new hope. Possible complementary essences: *Centaury, Clematis, Gentian, Hornbeam, Larch, Mustard, Olive, Wild Rose.*

13/30 Gorse/Sweet Chestnut

Absolute, hopeless desperation

Gorse/Sweet Chestnut is for people who are so desperate that they see no way out and no hope of better times. Something inside them seems to be broken. This combination is needed only in rare emergency situations; it makes the hopelessly desperate more responsive and helps them direct their energies toward life. This creates the groundwork for a new beginning. It must be taken often and tried in various potencies. Possible complementary essences: *Larch, Mustard, Wild Rose, Willow.*

13/37 Gorse/Wild Rose

Total resignation

Gorse/Wild Rose is for people who have lost all hope and all interest in life. They behave totally passively because everything seems meaningless and empty. When someone tries to help, they let it pass right by, taking no notice. This combination can reawaken our interest in life and help promote positive expectations. It must be taken over a long period of time, and after a time it should be combined with other essences appropriate to the personality. Possible complementary essences: *Centaury, Gentian, Hornbeam, Larch, Mustard, Olive, Star of Bethlehem.*

14/16 Heather/Honeysuckle

Vain youth

Heather/Honeysuckle is for people whose vanity will not allow them to grow old. They are afraid to lose recognition and acceptance because they are no longer as beautiful, strong, or capable as they were. For this reason, they try to stop the clock, so to speak, and remain as they always were. This combination helps us accept aging with more composure. Possible complementary essences: *Larch, Mustard, Star of Bethlehem, Walnut, Wild Oat.*

14/19 Heather/Larch

Boasting and showing off due to an inferiority complex

Heather/Larch is for people who have a lack of self-confidence and feel inferior; they often compensate by being overbearing and boasting of their talents and accomplishments in an imperious manner. This combination is often used and can help us become more self-confident and discreet; we don't need to show off to become more pleasant and generally more valued by others. Possible complementary essences: *Agrimony, Vervain, Walnut.*

14/20 Heather/Mimulus

Pushiness caused by a fear of loneliness

Heather/Mimulus is for people who are afraid of being rejected and lonely and who constantly draw attention to themselves by showing off in a chattering and talkative manner, which is exactly why no one will have anything to do with them. This combination can help us become more independent of others and enable us to be alone. Possible complementary essences: *Agrimony, Aspen, Cerato, Larch, Mustard, Walnut.*

14/21 Heather/Mustard

Depression caused by rejection and loneliness

Heather/Mustard is for people who are constantly depressed because they get no attention or companionship, which they need. This combination helps us be more independent of others and allows us to see life more positively. Possible complementary essences: *Cerato, Larch, Walnut, Willow.*

14/29 Heather/Star of Bethlehem

Psychic trauma due to humiliation

Heather/Star of Bethlehem is for people who are traumatized by their weakness, which is a need for recognition and affection. Perhaps someone has ridiculed them, or perhaps they have been closed out of society. In any case, they can't get over it, and they become sick. This combination helps us overcome trauma and the need for the recognition and approval of others. Possible complementary essences: *Cerato, Chicory, Mustard, Walnut.*

14/35 Heather/White Chestnut

Compulsive vanity

Heather/White Chestnut is for people who can think only of fulfilling their wish to be recognized and admired and are constantly preoccupied with how they can show themselves in a favorable light to those around them or with the fear of not being successful at it. This combination can temper our egotism and allows us to think of something besides ourselves. Possible complementary essences: *Agrimony, Cherry Plum, Impatiens, Mimulus, Walnut.*

15/18 Holly/Impatiens

Impatient and irritable

Holly/Impatiens is for people who are irritable or aggressive because things do not go as quickly or as smoothly as their usual impatience can tolerate. Waiting or being held up for anything is pure poison to them. This combination is suitable for treating an existing condition as well as the general constitution. It can diminish restlessness and aggression. Naturally, it won't make a fast-thinking and -acting person into a thoughtful and slow person, but it can, in most cases, significantly minimize the frequency and intensity of outbursts and prevent the worst manifestations of acute cases. Possible complementary essences: *Oak, Scleranthus, Vervain, Wild Oat.*

15/20 Holly/Mimulus

Anxious irritability

Holly/Mimulus is for people who become nervous and irritable out of fear or anxiety. They tend to react aggressively when faced with problems or when they find themselves in a state of anxious tension. This aggression provides a certain relief. This combination can make us calmer and more stable by alleviating our anxiety and irritability. Possible complementary essences: *Aspen, Impatiens, Rock Rose, Scleranthus.*

15/29 Holly/Star of Bethlehem

Aggression caused by mental and emotional stress

Holly/Star of Bethlehem is for people who react too aggressively to mental or emotional distress. This combination can soften a situation and help us confront it constructively. Possible complementary essences: *Aspen, Mimulus, Rock Rose.*

15/31 Holly/Vervain

Irritable do-gooder

Holly/Vervain is for people with missionary tendencies who become enraged if they encounter any resistance. They want the best for others, but their strong, easily irritable temperament is often difficult to restrain. This combination can make us more affable and also dampen our drive to manipulate the lives of others. Possible complementary essences: *Beech, Chicory, Oak, Vine*

15/32 Holly/Vine

Rage due to opposition or errors

Holly/Vine is for people who become angry when someone tries to oppose them or behaves in a manner other than what they think is proper—for example, a closed-minded boss or a petty domestic tyrant. They often suffer from gall-related problems. This combination can make us more affable, easygoing, generous, and tolerant. It allows us to let others live their own lives and gives us the ability to laugh at ourselves. Possible complementary essences: *Beech, Chicory, Impatiens, Vervain.*

15/34 Holly/Water Violet

Irritable misanthrope

Holly/Water Violet is for people who cannot bear any human contact. They become enraged when spoken to and only want to be left in peace. Their need for introspection and self-exploration has been overdeveloped by a lack of prolonged contact with others or reduced by a prolonged illness. This combination can balance our temperament and make us more willing to have contact with others. It is good for acute conditions and for making us more easygoing. It often helps prevent the outbreak of an encroaching illness if, for no apparent reason, we suddenly become irritable and do not wish to have any contact with other people. Possible complementary essences: *Elm, Star of Bethlehem, Walnut.*

15/35 Holly/White Chestnut

Aggressive, obsessive thoughts

Holly/White Chestnut is for people who become so enraged or irritated that they are incapable of rational thought. They hurt themselves more than anyone else because they can no longer think properly and cannot find a solution to their fundamental problem. This combination has a twofold stabilizing effect: it lowers the level of irritability and clears the mind. Possible complementary essences: *Chicory, Impatiens, Oak, Rock Water.*

15/38 Holly/Willow

Bitterness combined with anger or hate

Holly/Willow is for people who cannot overcome disappointment and react aggressively. They cannot simply release their anger and then forget about it but instead develop resentment or bitterness, which is then expressed in appropriate or inappropriate situations in the form of abusive behavior or bad, irritable moods. They often have liver conditions. This combination can make us more conciliatory and able to enjoy life. It helps us to forget (if not forgive) any real or alleged injustices. Possible complementary essences: *Chicory, Star of Bethlehem, Vine.*

16/17 Honeysuckle/Hornbeam

Flight into the past due to feelings of stress and overwork

Honeysuckle/Hornbeam is for people who do not feel up to the challenges of daily life and take refuge in the past. They compensate the lack of desire that reality instills in them with memories of the "good old days" and believe that things would be much easier if only they were the way they used to be. This leads them to not being able to gather themselves together to do what must be done. This combination can make us more realistic and more able to achieve what we need to achieve. Memories fade, and life seems easier to handle. Possible complementary essences: *Centaury, Clematis, Gentian, Larch, Mustard, Star of Bethlehem, Wild Rose.*

16/19 Honeysuckle/Larch

Retreat into the past due to a lack of self-confidence

Honeysuckle/Larch is for people who flee into the past as the result of shyness or a lack of self-confidence and pacify themselves with memories of better, more prosperous times instead of facing the challenges that life presents them in the present. This combination restores our self-confidence and interest in life. Possible complementary essences: *Clematis, Gentian, Hornbeam, Mustard, Star of Bethlehem, Wild Rose.*

16/20 Honeysuckle/Mimulus

Flight into the past caused by timidity

Honeysuckle/Mimulus is for people who retreat into pleasant memories because they are afraid of the present challenges and problems they must face. They bury their heads in the sand. This combination can make us more courageous and willing to undertake new endeavors. It is often used for children. Possible complementary essences: *Aspen, Larch, Mustard, Star of Bethlehem, Wild Rose.*

16/21 Honeysuckle/Mustard

Depression due to loss

Honeysuckle/Mustard is for people who have no joy in life owing to a serious loss; they become depressed from time to time and fall into painful memories. This combination helps us overcome our losses and find happiness again in our lives. Possible complementary essences: *Centaury, Gentian, Star of Bethlehem, Wild Rose.*

16/23 Honeysuckle/Olive

Flight into the past caused by exhaustion

Honeysuckle/Olive is for people who are too weary to take control of their own reality and instead give themselves up to memories of (allegedly) simpler and happier times. This combination can restore our lost strength and free us from the undertow of pleasant memories so that we can again turn our attention to life in the present. Possible complementary essences: *Centaury, Gentian, Hornbeam, Larch, Mustard, Star of Bethlehem, Wild Rose.*

16/29 Honeysuckle/Star of Bethlehem

Insurmountable loss

Honeysuckle/Star of Bethlehem is for people who have been so shaken by a serious loss that they can no longer come to terms with life. Because they cannot overcome the shock, they lose touch with the present. This combination helps us overcome painful feelings and memories and accept what has happened. Possible complementary essences: *Clematis, Mustard, Wild Rose, Willow.*

16/35 Honeysuckle/White Chestnut
Persistent memories

Honeysuckle/White Chestnut is for people who cannot rid themselves of certain memories (usually those of better times). They are incapable of thinking of anything else and have little interest in the present or future. This combination can make us think clearly so that we can deal directly with reality. Possible complementary essences: *Chicory, Rock Rose, Star of Bethlehem, Willow.*

16/37 Honeysuckle/Wild Rose
Melancholic resignation

Honeysuckle/Wild Rose is for people who go through life without interest and with a feeling of resignation because they have lost something close to their heart and cannot replace it in the present. This combination can allow our memories to fade and can rekindle our enthusiasm. Possible complementary essences: *Gentian, Gorse, Larch, Mustard, Star of Bethlehem.*

16/38 Honeysuckle/Willow
Bitterness caused by a loss

Honeysuckle/Willow is for people who are at odds with their fate or harbor resentment as the result of a loss. This combination can make us more conciliatory and positive; it helps us find closure with the past and accept our fate. Possible complementary essences: *Chicory, Holly, Star of Bethlehem.*

17/19 Hornbeam/Larch
Feelings of stress and overwork due to a lack of self-confidence

Hornbeam/Larch is for people who underestimate their capabilities and overestimate their problems because they constantly feel overworked and under pressure. This combination can make us more self-confident and able to work up to our abilities. It eases the feeling of being under excessive stress. Possible complementary essences: *Centaury, Gentian, Elm, Mimulus, Mustard, Olive, Star of Bethlehem.*

17/20 Hornbeam/Mimulus

Fear of failure

Hornbeam/Mimulus is for anxious people who always see problems, even though objectively these problems don't exist or at least not to the extent they believe. As the saying goes, they make a mountain out of a molehill. This combination can make us braver, more realistic, and more optimistic. Possible complementary essences: *Aspen, Cerato, Elm, Gentian, Larch, Mustard, Star of Bethlehem.*

17/37 Hornbeam/Wild Rose

Lack of drive due to a feeling of overexertion

Hornbeam/Wild Rose is for people who just let themselves muddle through the day because they believe that everything is too difficult for them. In the morning they think about all that they must accomplish during the day, and they feel overwhelmed and lose their enthusiasm. They can't get motivated to do anything and end up just hanging around. This combination can reawaken our interest in life and our desire to accomplish. Possible complementary essences: *Gentian, Larch, Mustard, Olive, Star of Bethlehem, Wild Oat.*

18/29 Impatiens/Mimulus

Anxious restlessness

Impatiens/Mimulus is for people who become nervous and restless from fear. This combination can make us calmer and more relaxed. Possible complementary essences: *Aspen, Red Chestnut, Rock Rose.*

18/25 Impatiens/Red Chestnut

Worried restlessness

Impatiens/Red Chestnut is for people who become restless and nervous by worrying about others (for example, in the case of an operation or a dangerous undertaking). This combination can allow us to be calmer and more confident. It is often needed for worried parents. Possible complementary essences: *Aspen, Chicory, Mimulus, Star of Bethlehem, Walnut.*

18/26 Impatiens/Rock Rose

Panicky, driven behavior

Impatiens/Rock Rose is for people who find themselves in a state of panic and cannot think or act calmly and thoughtfully. This can also occur when we are under pressure of a deadline (for example, a difficult job, a test, or an important appointment) and makes us prone to costly mistakes. This combination can avoid panic and alleviate our nervousness. It must be taken frequently. Possible complementary essences: *Cherry Plum, Elm, Larch, Mimulus, Star of Bethlehem, Vervain.*

18/28 Impatiens/Scleranthus

Erratic and impatient

Impatiens/Scleranthus is for very restless, impatient, and erratic people. One day, they will be busy with one thing, and the next they will be concentrating just as intensely on something completely different. This combination can make us more calm and circumspect, allowing us to make clear decisions and follow them through to completion. Possible complementary essences: *Cerato, Vervain, Wild Oat.*

18/31 Impatiens/Vervain

Stress and haste

Impatiens/Vervain is for people who go at everything full bore. Even at the slightest impediment or setback, they feel themselves under stress and become impatient and nervous. Also for situations in which one approaches a goal restlessly and in haste. This combination helps us pursue our plans, desires, and goals more patiently, prudently, and flexibly. It is often used to alleviate job-related stress or the stress caused by an anticipated appointment or event. Possible complementary essences: *Elm, Holly, Oak, Vine.*

18/35 Impatiens/White Chestnut

Mental overactivity

Impatiens/White Chestnut is for people who tend to put their ideas into action much too impatiently. They are often obsessed with certain ideas or desires, and nothing can go fast enough for them until these ideas are realized. They are often nervous, careless, hectic, or pushy and lose the big picture where life is concerned. Possible complementary essences: *Cherry Plum, Holly, Oak, Vine, Vervain.*

19/20 Larch/Mimulus

Anxiety due to a lack of self-confidence

Larch/Mimulus is for people who are afraid at every possible opportunity because they have no confidence in their abilities. This combination can make us more sure of ourselves and brave. Possible complementary essences: *Aspen, Centaury, Cerato, Gentian, Mustard, Star of Bethlehem, Walnut.*

19/23 Larch/Olive

Self-doubt due to exhaustion

Larch/Olive is for people who are so exhausted that they no longer believe in themselves or for people who quickly become exhausted due to a lack of self-confidence. This combination can help make us more capable of achieving our goals and gives us more self-assurance. Possible complementary essences: *Centaury, Elm, Gentian, Hornbeam, Mustard, Star of Bethlehem, Wild Rose.*

19/24 Larch/Pine

Feelings of moral inferiority

Larch/Pine is for people who, because of moral reservations or guilt feelings, doubt their own worth or tend to blame themselves out of a feeling of inferiority. This combination can reduce our guilt feelings and boost our feelings of self-worth. Possible complementary essences: *Centaury, Crab Apple, Mustard, Star of Bethlehem.*

19/27 Larch/Rock Water

Feelings of inferiority due to idealistic demands on oneself

Larch/Rock Water is for people who place great demands on themselves but feel themselves to be inferior because they cannot fulfill their own demands or who expect too much of themselves. They secretly believe that they are failures. They cannot recognize that ideals never correspond with reality. This combination can allow us to achieve reconciliation so that we never impose excessive discipline on ourselves. It allows us to reach a positive feeling of self-worth. Possible complementary essences: *Crab Apple, Pine, Vine, Walnut.*

19/29 Larch/Star of Bethlehem

Loss of self-confidence due to mental or emotional trauma

Larch/Star of Bethlehem is for people who have lost their self-assurance as the result of an experience they have not been able to get over (generally it is a defeat or a disgrace). Somewhat shy by nature, they dare not undertake anything else. This combination can strengthen our self-esteem and help us see such traumatic experiences with new eyes. Possible complementary essences: *Aspen, Centaury, Crab Apple, Gentian, Pine, Rock Water, Walnut.*

19/33 Larch/Walnut

Easily influenced owing to a lack of self-confidence

Larch/Walnut is for people who have too little confidence in themselves and are therefore too easily influenced by others. This leads them to not be able to put their plans into action or to be led to do things they actually do not want to do. This combination can give us more support; we develop confidence in our own abilities and can resist any influences that threaten to lead us astray from our path. Possible complementary essences: *Agrimony, Mimulus, Mustard, Star of Bethlehem.*

19/36 Larch/Wild Oat
No life goals due to a lack of self-confidence

Larch/Wild Oat is for people who are not in the position to shape their lives meaningfully and to their satisfaction because they lack confidence in themselves. This combination can make us more sure of ourselves and able to have contact with others. It is especially suitable for schoolchildren or businesspeople. Possible complementary essences: *Aspen, Centaury, Gentian, Hornbeam, Mustard, Star of Bethlehem, Walnut.*

19/37 Larch/Wild Rose
Lack of drive and self-confidence

Larch/Wild Rose is for people who have lost their interest in the struggle for survival because they do not believe in their own success. They let many opportunities pass them by or cede their rights and claims to others without a fight. This combination can make us more self-assured and give us more interest in actively participating in life. Possible complementary essences: *Aspen, Gentian, Hornbeam, Mimulus, Mustard, Olive, Star of Bethlehem, Wild Oat.*

20/23 Mimulus/Olive
Anxious and exhausted

Mimulus/Olive is for people in whom fear and exhaustion increase symbiotically; a great or long-lasting fear has sapped their strength, while the exhaustion undermines their courage. This combination can give us more courage through more strength and more strength through more courage. Possible complementary essences: *Aspen, Gentian, Hornbeam, Larch, Mustard, Star of Bethlehem.*

20/24 Mimulus/Pine

Fear of guilt

Mimulus/Pine is for people who do not dare to live as they would like from fear or feelings of guilt. This combination is important in that it helps us replace morality or values imposed upon us by others with our own. It can minimize our tendencies for self-judgment and give us the courage to be accountable to ourselves. Possible complementary essences: *Centaury, Cerato, Gentian, Larch, Mustard, Star of Bethlehem, Walnut.*

20/25 Mimulus/Red Chestnut

Anxious and excessive worry

Mimulus/Red Chestnut is for people who are in continual fear that something terrible is about to happen to their loved ones. This combination can allow us to let those to whom we are close go their own way. It is used often by parents. Possible complementary essences: *Aspen, Chicory, Impatiens, Mustard, Star of Bethlehem, Vine.*

20/26 Mimulus/Rock Rose

Anxiety with tendencies toward panic

Mimulus/Rock Rose is for people who are generally afraid and tend to react with panic when they are in a situation that causes them anxiety. This combination can make us more calm or generally acts to mitigate the fears that cause us to panic. Possible complementary essences: *Aspen, Elm, Larch, Star of Bethlehem, Walnut.*

20/28 Mimulus/Scleranthus

Indecisiveness caused by fear

Mimulus/Scleranthus is for people who have so much fear of a particular situation that they no longer know what they should do. They are emotional cripples and simply cannot make a decision. This combination can help us circumvent a block and can also be taken as a preventive measure. It eases our fears and simultaneously clears our view, so that we can make the right decision. Possible complementary essences: *Aspen, Cherry Plum, Gentian, Larch, Rock Rose, Star of Bethlehem, Walnut, Wild Oat.*

20/29 Mimulus/Star of Bethlehem
Anxiety due to psychic trauma

Mimulus/Star of Bethlehem is for people who have undergone a terrible experience and, as a result, have become abnormally afraid. The fear either is related to certain circumstances or determines the nature of a person's overall conduct. This combination can heal our inner wounds and restore our normal confidence and courage. Possible complementary essences: *Aspen, Centaury, Hornbeam, Larch, Mustard, Walnut.*

20/33 Mimulus/Walnut
Easily influenced owing to anxiety

Mimulus/Walnut is for people who feel that they must start out in a new direction in life, but fear of the consequences makes them put it off again and again. This combination is important for sensitive, easily influenced people who find themselves confronted with a change in life circumstances. It can give us the courage to follow our own path and to be deterred neither by the opinions of others nor by threats and blackmail. Possible complementary essences: *Centaury, Cerato, Gentian, Larch, Mustard, Wild Oat.*

20/35 Mimulus/White Chestnut
Anxious obsessive thoughts

Mimulus/White Chestnut is for people whose fears make them unable to think clearly. This combination can suppress our fears and help us think through the problems causing our fears and solve them; it can also allow us to occupy ourselves with other matters. It is usually needed only on a temporary basis but should be taken frequently. Possible complementary essences: *Agrimony, Aspen, Cerato, Cherry Plum, Larch, Rock Rose, Star of Bethlehem.*

21/23 Mustard/Olive

Depression due to exhaustion or exhaustion due to depression

Mustard/Olive is for people who become so exhausted from a serious strain or a long illness that they can find no more joy in life. This combination can restore our strength and our positive attitude. It can halt a dangerous development, especially in the case of an illness, or, if taken in a timely manner, prevent an illness. Possible complementary essences: *Centaury, Clematis, Gentian, Hornbeam, Larch, Star of Bethlehem, Wild Rose.*

21/24 Mustard/Pine

Depression caused by feelings of guilt

Mustard/Pine is for people who are repeatedly overtaken by a depressive mood because of displaced guilt feelings. They do not face their problems consciously and can tend to be dominated by them. This has a continuous, pernicious influence on their moods and prevents them from being happy. They are afflicted with depression that seems to come from nowhere. This combination can make us happier with our lives by assuaging guilt feelings and minimizing the tendency to be melancholic. Possible complementary essences: *Centaury, Crab Apple, Larch, Rock Water, Walnut, Wild Oat.*

21/25 Mustard/Red Chestnut

Anxious depression

Mustard/Red Chestnut is for people who worry about others too often and too much and find themselves with feelings of despondency that increase over time. The basic depression fosters the tendency toward an anxious pessimism. This essence can make us happier and less worried. Possible complementary essences: *Aspen, Centaury, Gentian, Star of Bethlehem.*

21/28 Mustard/Scleranthus

Frequent mood swings

Mustard/Scleranthus is for people who suffer from unpredictable mood swings and become melancholic for no apparent reason. This combination helps us consciously guide our moods. It can bring us balance and make us generally happier. Possible complementary essences: *Cerato, Impatiens, Larch, Wild Oat.*

21/29 Mustard/Star of Bethlehem

Depression due to psychic trauma

Mustard/Star of Bethlehem is for people who are frequently depressed as the result of a terrible experience or dreadful circumstances. This combination can help us see our difficulties in a more positive light, make our psyche aware of other possibilities, put us at peace, and generally improve our mood. Possible complementary essences: *Aspen, Clematis, Gentian, Honeysuckle, Larch, Pine, Red Chestnut, Wild Rose.*

21/34 Mustard/Water Violet

Serious, depressive human contact difficulties

Mustard/Water Violet is for people who, from time to time and seemingly without reason, are overcome with melancholy and withdraw from the world. This combination can make us happier and encourages a desire to be in contact with others again. It should be used over a long period of time. Possible complementary essences: *Agrimony, Clematis, Larch, Star of Bethlehem, Willow.*

21/36 Mustard/Wild Oat

Depression due to a feeling of pointlessness

Mustard/Wild Oat is for people who can find no real meaning in their lives and are frequently depressed. This combination can improve our mood and make it seem that life makes sense. Possible complementary essences: *Centaury, Cerato, Clematis, Gentian, Larch, Scleranthus, Star of Bethlehem.*

21/37 Mustard/Wild Rose

Depressed resignation

Mustard/Wild Rose is for people who have lost their interest in life owing to a fundamental feeling of depression. They have been unaware for some time of how they came to be this way. This combination can weaken our negative attitudes and reawaken our interest in life. Possible complementary essences: *Centaury, Cerato, Clematis, Gentian, Larch, Scleranthus, Star of Bethlehem.*

21/38 Mustard/Willow

Depression caused by bitterness

Mustard/Willow is for people who are deeply embittered because of an imagined injustice or a serious disappointment. This depression can manifest itself not in an extroverted hate but rather in an introverted rejection of life. This combination helps us see life in a more positive, conciliatory light. Possible complementary essences: *Chicory, Clematis, Gentian, Larch, Star of Bethlehem.*

22/24 Oak/Pine

Uncompromising perfectionism

Oak/Pine is for people who have a strong sense of obligation combined with great ambition, which drives them to perfectionism. They often lose a sense of perspective of their abilities, which results in pathogenic stress. This combination can free us from our compulsions so that we can allow ourselves a slip now and then and not have our happiness fall prey to our ambition. Possible complementary essences: *Crab Apple, Larch, Rock Water, Vervain, Vine, Water Violet.*

22/27 Oak/Rock Water

Self-tormenting compulsion to achieve

Oak/Rock Water is for decidedly disciplined people who put themselves under excessive strain and stress. This combination can help us limit the demands we place on ourselves and allow us to take it easy on ourselves. Possible complementary essences: *Crab Apple, Impatiens, Pine, Vine.*

22/31 Oak/Vervain

Stress due to a drive to accomplish

Oak/Vervain is for people whose relentless will and great enthusiasm combine to create uncontrollable stress. This combination can make us more circumspect, more flexible, and more yielding so that we may better control and dole out our strength. Possible complementary essences: *Chicory, Holly, Impatiens, Red Chestnut, Rock Water, Vine.*

22/32 Oak/Vine

Dogmatic compulsion to achieve

Oak/Vine is for people who are compelled to put their convictions into practice at any price. They are convinced of the rightness of their (often petty and dogmatic) opinions, and this makes them humorless, grumpy, and tense. This combination can make us more tolerant, more conciliatory, and more sociable so that we can accept other opinions, examine our own, and let things run their course. Possible complementary essences: *Chicory, Holly, Impatiens, Red Chestnut, Rock Water, Vervain.*

22/34 Oak/Water Violet

Loneliness due to ambition

Oak/Water Violet is for people who live only for their goals and ambitions and need no human contact. They feel that if they were to share themselves or spend their time in society, they would be wasting their time and energy and be distracted from their true purpose in life. They become lonely, one-dimensional, and grimly determined. This combination can make us more flexible and yielding, more sociable, and more able to have contact with others. Possible complementary essences: *Elm, Holly, Impatiens, Rock Water.*

22/35 Oak/White Chestnut

Obsessed with success

Oak/White Chestnut is for people who have no place in their thoughts for anything other than goals and plans and thus find themselves in a constant state of mental and physical stress. This combination can make us mentally flexible and allow us to think of other things besides our plans. Possible complementary essences: *Chicory, Red Chestnut, Rock Water, Vervain, Vine.*

22/38 Oak/Willow

Relentless lust for revenge

Oak/Willow is for people who are consumed with a lust for revenge because they have been treated unfairly or feel offended. Even if they want things to be otherwise, they cannot forgive and forget. This combination can make us more conciliatory and cooperative. Possible complementary essences: *Chicory, Star of Bethlehem, Vine.*

23/24 Olive/Pine

Debilitating guilt complex

Olive/Pine is for people who suffer so much from guilt feelings that they have no more strength for a normal life. This combination can give us a better conscience and more energy. Possible complementary essences: *Centaury, Crab Apple, Gentian, Larch, Mustard, Star of Bethlehem, Walnut.*

23/25 Olive/Red Chestnut

Debilitating worries

Olive/Red Chestnut is for people who are at the end of their strength because they have worried too much about someone. This combination can make us stronger and help minimize our worries. Possible complementary essences: *Aspen, Hornbeam, Mimulus, Mustard, Star of Bethlehem, Walnut, White Chestnut.*

23/29 Olive/Star of Bethlehem

**Lack of mental and emotional resistance
due to exhaustion**

Olive/Star of Bethlehem is for people who are so weak that they cannot cope with any sort of psychological strain or are exhausted as the result of serious psychological duress. This combination can restore our resilience. Possible complementary essences: *Aspen, Centaury, Gentian, Gorse, Hornbeam, Larch, Mimulus, Wild Rose.*

23/33 Olive/Walnut

Easily influenced as the result of exhaustion

Olive/Walnut is for people who are so exhausted that they cannot resist being influenced by others and find themselves in circumstances they did not wish for themselves. This combination can give us the independence and strength to shape our own lives. It is also useful for renewing our strength during difficult negotiations. Possible complementary essences: *Centaury, Cerato, Gentian, Hornbeam, Larch, Mimulus, Wild Rose.*

23/34 Olive/Water Violet

Antisocial due to exhaustion

Olive/Water Violet is for people who are too exhausted to have any contact with other people or to find happiness in the company of others. They withdraw in order to recuperate in peace and quiet. This combination can make us stronger and more willing to have contact with others. It is often useful in treating serious illnesses. Possible complementary essences: *Gentian, Larch, Mustard, Star of Bethlehem, Walnut, Wild Rose.*

23/37 Olive/Wild Rose

Lack of drive due to exhaustion

Olive/Wild Rose is for people whose strength has been drained to the extent that they can only vegetate and be resigned and uninterested. This combination (which should be taken in tandem with any essence used to treat the cause of the exhaustion) can strengthen us and renew our need to be active. Possible complementary essences: *Gentian, Hornbeam, Mustard, Star of Bethlehem.*

24/25 Pine/Red Chestnut

Worries due to a bad conscience

Pine/Red Chestnut is for people who worry about another owing to their own feelings of guilt. They feel responsible for others and ignore themselves. This combination helps us maintain a good conscience and allows us to care about our own well-being. Possible complementary essences: Aspen, Chicory, Crab Apple, Mimulus, Mustard, Star of Bethlehem, Walnut.

24/27 Pine/Rock Water

Compulsive perfectionism

Pine/Rock Water is for people who have a guilty conscience when they are not perfect and put themselves under strict discipline. They become tense and unhappy. This combination can lessen our tendency to judge and torment ourselves and enable us to accept our shortcomings more easily. Possible complementary essences: *Crab Apple, Larch, Star of Bethlehem, Vine, Walnut.*

24/29 Pine/Star of Bethlehem

Unprocessed, unresolved guilty trauma

Pine/Star of Bethlehem is for people who cannot overcome the strong feelings related to a shocking experience. This combination is useful in promoting the psychotherapeutic processing of a guilt-inducing trauma. It can free our conscience and restore our inner order. Possible complementary essences: *Centaury, Crab Apple, Larch, Mustard, Rock Water, Walnut.*

24/33 Pine/Walnut

Not being able to stand up for oneself against accusations

Pine/Walnut is for people who let themselves develop a guilty conscience too easily from the reproach of others. This combination can give us more self-confidence and the strength not to become insecure when we are faced with barbed accusations. Possible complementary essences: *Centaury, Cerato, Crab Apple, Gentian, Larch, Mustard, Rock Water, Star of Bethlehem.*

24/35 Pine/White Chestnut

Obsessed with guilt

Pine/White Chestnut is for people who cannot free themselves from their guilty conscience. The idea of their real or imagined guilt blocks all other thoughts and robs them of their inner peace and clarity. This combination can free us from tormenting guilty thoughts and allow us to think normally again. Possible complementary essences: *Centaury, Cherry Plum, Crab Apple, Elm, Larch, Mustard, Oak, Star of Bethlehem, Walnut.*

25/26 Red Chestnut/Rock Rose

Panicky worries

Red Chestnut/Rock Rose is for people who find themselves in (or on the verge of) a panic and in danger of losing their heads through excessive worrying about someone else. This combination can make us worry-free and more relaxed. Possible complementary essences: *Aspen, Cherry Plum, Chicory, Impatiens, Mimulus, Star of Bethlehem, Walnut.*

25/29 Red Chestnut/Star of Bethlehem

Excessive worries due to negative experiences

Red Chestnut/Star of Bethlehem is for people who have undergone a terrible experience and fear that something similar will happen to someone close to them. This combination can help heal trauma and drive away our worries. Possible complementary essences: *Aspen, Cherry Plum, Chicory, Gentian, Mimulus, Mustard, Rock Rose, White Chestnut.*

25/35 Red Chestnut/White Chestnut

Troubled thoughts

Red Chestnut/White Chestnut is for people who can think only of the worries of others. They always have ideas in their heads that make them afraid, and these fears plague their dreams. This combination restores our optimism. Possible complementary essences: *Aspen, Honeysuckle, Impatiens, Mimulus, Rock Rose.*

26/28 Rock Rose/Scleranthus

Frozen in panic

Rock Rose/Scleranthus is for people who are in such a state of panic that they are blocked to the extent that they cannot act. This combination helps us make clear decisions in emergency situations. People who tend to be nervous can take it as a preventive measure to have more presence of mind. Possible complementary essences: *Aspen, Cerato, Impatiens, Larch, Mimulus, Wild Oat.*

26/29 Rock Rose/Star of Bethlehem

Psychic trauma with panic

Rock Rose/Star of Bethlehem is for people who are thrown into a state of panic due to a terrifying experience. This combination is an ingredient of Rescue Remedy. It can make us more relaxed and restore our presence of mind. Possible complementary essences: *Aspen, Cherry Plum, Clematis, Gentian, Impatiens, Larch, Mimulus, Walnut.*

26/30 Rock Rose/Sweet Chestnut

Desperation caused by panic and fear

Rock Rose/Sweet Chestnut is for people who are overwhelmed by a severe panicky fear to the extent that their psyche is blocked and they fall into an inescapable state of desperation. They are not in a position to think or feel clearly and cannot see a way out. This combination is used only in case of extreme emergencies. It can release us from impediments and help us find a sense of perspective to go on living. Possible complementary essences: *Aspen, Elm, Wild Oat.*

27/32 Rock Water/Vine
A rigid personality

Rock Water/Vine is for people who are dogmatic with others and with themselves. It is difficult for them to make exceptions; they impose a strict form of discipline and expect everyone to live up to their rules and expectations. This combination can make us more generous, more lenient, and more flexible. Possible complementary essences: *Crab Apple, Holly, Mimulus, Oak, Pine, Star of Bethlehem, Willow.*

27/34 Rock Water/Water Violet
Flight from the world and self-castigation

Rock Water/Water Violet is for people with an excessive tendency toward discipline and solitude. They believe that if they place strict demands on themselves and reward themselves very little—which includes denying themselves human contact—their value as human beings will increase. They become lonely and unable to enjoy life. This combination encourages us to seek out the company of others and makes us happier and more relaxed. Possible complementary essences: *Crab Apple, Oak, Pine, Vine.*

27/36 Rock Water/Wild Oat
Self-castigation as a replacement for a meaning in life

Rock Water/Wild Oat is for people who try to counter their frustration over the meaninglessness of life with self-discipline. They are strict with themselves and falsely hope that this will give their life more worth or help them find a calling. This combination can lessen our obsession with asceticism and help us find meaning in life. It must be taken over a long period of time. Possible complementary essences: *Crab Apple, Pine, Vine, Walnut.*

28/36 Scleranthus/Wild Oat

Inner turmoil and life crisis

Scleranthus/Wild Oat is for people who are totally up in the air. They neither know how their lives should continue, nor can they make clear and simple everyday decisions. It is tormenting for them because they want to proceed in some way. This combination helps us find a meaningful goal in life and take the proper steps toward reaching it. It is often used for young people who must decide on a specific life path and don't know where to begin. It is also given to people in the midst of a midlife crisis, who feel that they should begin a new life but find themselves unable to get rid of their old habits. Possible complementary essences: *Cerato, Gentian, Larch, Mimulus, Star of Bethlehem, Walnut.*

29/30 Star of Bethlehem/Sweet Chestnut

Desperation due to psychological distress

Star of Bethlehem/Sweet Chestnut is for people who have been thrown so far off track by a distressing experience that life has lost its meaning and they do not know how to proceed. This combination can resolve our inner numbness and make us able to positively absorb a fatal blow. It is suitable for extreme emergencies. Possible complementary essences: *Aspen, Oak, Rock Rose, Walnut.*

29/33 Star of Bethlehem/Walnut

Lack of resistance due to an unresolved trauma

Star of Bethlehem/Walnut is for people who do not have sufficient defenses as the result of a great mental or psychological strain. This combination can help us in two ways—through a strengthening of the psychological defenses and through alleviating psychological strain. It is useful if someone is thrown off track by a traumatic experience and wants to make a new beginning. Possible complementary essences: *Centaury, Cerato, Gentian, Hornbeam, Larch, Olive, Wild Oat.*

29/34 Star of Bethlehem/Water Violet

Problems with human contact due to a psychological trauma

Star of Bethlehem/Water Violet is for people who have experienced something so terrible or unhappy that they desire no further contact with anyone. They shy away from people like an abused dog and give others a wide berth, which makes them very lonely. This combination helps us resolve such negative experiences and makes us more able and willing to seek out the company of others. Possible complementary essences: *Aspen, Gentian, Larch, Mimulus, Walnut, Willow.*

29/35 Star of Bethlehem/White Chestnut

Traumatic obsessive thoughts

Star of Bethlehem/White Chestnut is for people who ceaselessly think of a shocking experience or an unhappy situation. They are obsessed by these thoughts but can make no sense of them. This combination can gain us more distance from our problems, allowing us either to solve them or put them aside. Possible complementary essences: *Aspen, Crab Apple, Impatiens, Mimulus, Oak, Pine, Vine.*

29/37 Star of Bethlehem/Wild Rose

Resignation caused by a psychic trauma

Star of Bethlehem/Wild Rose is for people who have been so shaken by a terrible experience that they have lost all interest in life. They feel like "damaged goods," have lost their purpose, and keep to themselves. This combination can heal our inner wounds and lead us back to the living. It must be taken over a long period of time. Possible complementary essences: *Centaury, Gentian, Honeysuckle, Larch, Wild Oat.*

29/38 Star of Bethlehem/Willow

Bitterness due to unresolved trauma

Star of Bethlehem/Willow is for people who become embittered from a shattering traumatic experience or who are at odds with their fate. This combination can heal our psychological wounds and give us a more conciliatory, optimistic mood. Possible complementary essences: *Clematis, Crab Apple, Holly, Honeysuckle, Vine, Wild Rose.*

31/32 Vervain/Vine

Total intolerance

Vervain/Vine is for people who are absolutely convinced that their opinions are right and who take it for granted that those around them will adopt their opinions and behave accordingly. They take it as their personal mission to put this belief into action, either by persuasion or compulsion. This form of active intolerance makes life difficult for all involved. This combination makes it easier for us to listen to other opinions and let people live in whatever way they choose. Possible complementary essences: *Crab Apple, Oak, Rock Water, White Chestnut.*

31/35 Vervain/White Chestnut

Fixed ideas

Vervain/White Chestnut is for people who have only their own convictions or ideas in their heads and try to force them on others. Either in the form of fanatical do-gooders or obsessed philosophers, they are a pain for themselves and for others. This combination can free us from the grip of fixed ideas and allow us to lead a normal life. Possible complementary essences: *Cherry Plum, Crab Apple, Holly, Impatiens, Oak, Rock Water, Vine.*

32/35 Vine/White Chestnut

Compulsive dogmatism

Vine/White Chestnut is for people whose thoughts are occupied only with a certain idea or conviction. They are one-sided, intolerant, and often fanatical. This combination can free us from mental obsession and make us more open-minded and tolerant. Possible complementary essences: *Crab Apple, Oak, Pine, Rock Water, Vervain.*

32/38 Vine/Willow

The bitter, domestic tyrant

Vine/Willow is for people who become bitter or offended because something has not turned out the way they wanted. This combination can make us more flexible and willing to compromise and allow us to give up our bitter, offended behavior. Possible complementary essences: *Beech, Crab Apple, Impatiens, Oak, Vervain.*

33/36 Walnut/Wild Oat

Lacking purpose in life

Walnut/Wild Oat is for people who don't know what they want and find themselves pressed into situations they do not wish to be in. They lack the ability to resist the influence of others and therefore find themselves in situations that make them unhappy, such as a bad marriage or a frustrating occupation. This is accentuated even more by the fact that they yearn for happy, fulfilling lives. This combination can give us a certain degree of clarity in finding our own life path and also the conviction and resolve to follow it. It is used when we want to free ourselves from a negative life situation and begin a new life. It must often be taken for months at a time, because such changes occur only in small steps. Possible complementary essences: *Agrimony, Centaury, Cerato, Gentian, Hornbeam, Larch, Mimulus, Scleranthus, Star of Bethlehem.*

34/38 Water Violet/Willow

Bitterness due to restricted freedom

Water Violet/Willow is for people who have a great need for independence and become bitter if they are restricted. They cannot be conciliatory without their freedom. This combination can either normalize an unrealistic need for freedom or help us come to terms with unavoidable dependencies. Possible complementary essences: *Gentian, Holly, Honeysuckle, Star of Bethlehem, Walnut.*

35/38 White Chestnut/Willow

Bitter, obsessive thoughts

White Chestnut/Willow is for people whose thoughts are filled with bitterness stemming from an imagined injustice. They suffer a total mental block. This combination can make us more conciliatory and draw our attention to the more pleasant things in life. Possible complementary essences: *Chicory, Crab Apple, Holly, Honeysuckle, Pine, Rock Water, Star of Bethlehem, Vine, Walnut.*

36/37 Wild Oat/Wild Rose

Lack of drive due to a feeling of pointlessness

Wild Oat/Wild Rose is for people who become resigned because they don't know what the next step in their life should be. Although they've tried this, that, and the other thing to build their future or to find some meaning in life, they have lost their interest in and enjoyment of life. This combination can break down our resignation and apathy and reawaken our interest in life, allowing us to see the way that is right for us. It must be taken over the long term. Possible complementary essences: *Centaury, Gentian, Honeysuckle, Hornbeam, Larch, Olive.*

THREE

REPERTORY: A THERAPEUTIC LEXICON

An arrow (→) indicates that more information about the condition can be found under that entry. Essences linked together by a plus sign (+) should be taken together. An asterisk (*) indicates that the particular combination described is discussed in detail in chapter 2.

Absentmindedness: Clematis (→ Concentration, difficulties with)

Clematis is always the choice when our clear and conscious attention to reality is disturbed.

Accidents → Emergencies

Accomplishment or Performance, acute crisis of *11/17

Accusations

against oneself

    caused by an excessive need for cleanliness and purity: Crab Apple

    due to guilt feelings: Pine

    caused by an excessive need for self-discipline: Rock Water

against others
> due to unfriendliness or spite: Holly
> due to self-righteousness: Vine
> due to bitterness: Willow

Achieve, compulsion to → Ambition

against oneself: Oak, Rock Water

Oak is helpful when we are so involved in our work that we never relax. Rock Water makes us looser and more lenient; it is used when we are too strict with ourselves.

toward others: Vine

Sometimes we need a certain amount of pressure to achieve, but this must be kept in perspective. Vine can be helpful when we make self-righteous, inflexible demands on others.

*compulsion to achieve, with self-abuse *22/27*
*compulsion to achieve, creating stress *22/31*
*compulsion to achieve, with dogmatism *22/32*
*compulsion to achieve, with human contact problems *22/34*

Acne → Skin Conditions

Acquisitiveness → Greed

Act, unable to, due to panic *26/28

Aggression → Cold Emotions → Hate → Rage

Aggression is violent instinctive behavior that functions according to the principle of competition and serves individual self-realization and self-preservation. Depending on our character and the situation, it can manifest itself as hidden and subtle or open and reckless.

general: Holly

Holly helps us against banal, everyday irritability, annoyance, or rage and also against uncontrolled, rash aggression.

with impatience: Impatiens

When we are in a hurry, we quickly become aggressive if we are held up by those slower than we are.

with bitterness: Willow

When bitterness manifests itself in the form of aggressive behavior; take Holly also (15/38); when suppressed bitterness becomes aggression and resentment, take with Agrimony.

aggression due to psychological trauma *15/29
aggressive know-it-all *15/32
aggressive, compulsive thoughts *15/35

Allergy → Intolerance

Allergies are strong defensive reactions that are triggered by certain substances, even when these substances are introduced into the body in small quantities. The organism has at some time had a bad experience with a substance (such as pollen, animal hair, food, or chemicals), becomes sensitized, and cannot tolerate that substance anymore. In unfavorable conditions, these defensive reactions can be very strong and cause severe symptoms. Allergies can also be of a psychic nature in cases where we find a particular person or situation unbearable. (Further remarks → Chapter 1: Beech). Because allergies are signs of psychic or physical intolerance, any essence or combination that is suitable for making us more tolerant will be appropriate.

for people with an inner intolerance: **Beech**
Beech should be used as a basic essence for treating all allergies and conditions related to intolerance. It can be used alone or in concert with other appropriate essences.

for general purifying of the blood: **Crab Apple**
Chronic infections play a role in many allergies. They can poison the body and make it overly sensitive. Crab Apple is the most important detoxifying essence.

with strong immune reaction: **Holly**
Use, for example, in severe fits of sneezing, clear cases of irritation, or allergic shock.

allergic shock reaction *3/15

Altruism, pathological → Good-naturedness

Ambition → Achieve

Ambition is like a spirited horse: as long as we can control it, it takes us where we want to go. When we cannot keep hold of the reins, however, it goes wild, and we run the risk of breaking our necks. Without a certain amount of ambition, we cannot survive in our competitive society, but if our ambition lacks a playful, joyful element (which we also need to withstand our failures), it becomes dangerous.

with respect to social position: **Heather**

Heather suppresses social ambition and enables us to be satisfied with our position.

insatiable and pathogenic: **Oak**

People who cannot give up on something once they have it in their heads need Oak.

Anemia

Anemia is a weakness in or lack of blood. The organism is too weak to generate enough new, healthy blood. The most obvious symptoms are paleness and weakness. Medical treatment can be supplemented by the following essences, which are usually combined.

with hopelessness: **Gorse**

Hope is a basic element of life. Without it, the body cannot heal or regenerate.

with great weakness: **Olive**

with a lack of drive: **Wild Rose**

The body reduces the amount of new blood it produces according to the extent of resignation that we feel. Likewise, weak blood leads to resignation.

Anorexia

Anorexics have a life-negating attitude. They cannot come to terms with life because they feel that they've been treated unfairly or that they are misunderstood or unloved.

due to timidity: **Agrimony + Aspen + Mimulus**

due to self-pity or a need for love: **Chicory**

due to a death wish: **Clematis**

due to contrariness: **Holly**

due to severe exhaustion: **Olive**

due to self-denial: **Rock Water**

due to an unprocessed mental or emotional shock: **Star of Bethlehem**

due to resignation: Wild Rose
due to bitterness: Willow

Apathy → Drive, lack of

Apprehensiveness → Premonitions and Foreboding → Fear

Arrogance: Water Violet (→ Pride)

Arrogance is often a defense mechanism against pushy people rather than a form of contempt. Sometimes it is caused by personal insecurity. (+ Larch *19/34)

Artificiality: Agrimony (→ Facade)

Agrimony helps us behave more naturally when we tend to gloss over our problems or portray ourselves as other than what we really are.
   *artificial friendliness and tolerance *1/3*

Asceticism: Rock Water

Healthy self-discipline means limiting ourselves to what is essential. The strict self-castigation and self-denial of most people who practice asceticism is, however, neurotic. They want to force an increase in personal growth, wisdom, and health or to repay a debt. (+ Pine *24/27)

Asthma (bronchial) → Lung Conditions

Authoritarian Behavior
   due to missionary convictions: Vervain
   due to intolerant closed-mindedness: Vine

Authority, dependence on: Centaury (→ Self-assertiveness)

Centaury is helpful when we do what others tell us to do owing to a weakness in our personality.

Aversion, natural, suppressed: Beech (→ Chapter 1: Beech)

Bechterev's Syndrome → Spinal Problems

Bed-wetting

Sometimes bed-wetting has organic causes, but generally the causes are psychic, especially with childlike sexuality (such as jealousy or the desire for incest). It can also be an unconscious protest against an excessive demand for cleanliness.

due to a lack of attention: **Chicory**

Chicory reduces emotional dependence on the parents so that the child does not fixate his or her burgeoning sexuality on the denying mother or the rejecting father. Chicory is also helpful for cases of childlike jealousy.

against feelings of uncleanliness: **Crab Apple**

Crab Apple counters the learned, embarrassing feeling of filthiness, which is strengthened by the bed-wetter's inner conflict. When a child is ashamed of his own weaknesses, it becomes even harder for him to overcome them.

against the anxiety induced by anticipation: **Mimulus**

Every night, the bed-wetter secretly fears that she will repeat her offense. Mimulus alleviates these fears and counters the actual acting out.

against guilt feelings: **Pine**

It is especially damaging to reproach a bed-wetter for his weakness; when he is overcome with feelings of guilt, he cannot distance himself from them. A humorous, harmless remark will do more good than a serious reprimand.

due to contrariness, resentment, or bitterness: **Willow**

Excessive pressure from a parent or guardian can make a bed-wetter contrary, so that bed-wetting happens exactly because it must not. Disappointments or bitterness stemming from a lack of attention or sexual refusal can call forth such contrary reactions. Willow is always appropriate when a bed-wetter is rebellious, stubborn, or rejecting.

Behavioral Problems → Neuroses

Essentially, all Bach flower essences are used to treat internal and external disorders that affect our relationship with the social realm or with reality. They are appropriate for treating conditions with the following characteristics.

artificiality, dishonesty: **Agrimony**
groundless, delusional timidity or anxiety: **Aspen**
excessive tolerance or generosity: **Beech**

self-injurious cheerfulness: Centaury
insecurity, uncertainty: Cerato
hysteria: Cherry Plum
inattentiveness, learning difficulties: Chestnut Bud
jealousy, excessive mothering and coddling: Chicory
unrealistic fantasies: Clematis
fear of filth, compulsive cleanliness: Crab Apple
sudden feeling of stress and overwork: Elm
weak willed, easily discouraged: Gentian
hopelessness: Gorse
showing off, need for recognition: Heather
unfriendliness, aggressiveness: Holly
homesickness, grieving: Honeysuckle
groundless feelings of stress and overwork: Hornbeam
impatience, restlessness: Impatiens
feelings of inferiority: Larch
excessive timidity or anxiety: Mimulus
depression: Mustard
uncompromising behavior, excessive ambition: Oak
general exhaustion: Olive
guilt complex: Pine
excessive worry and concern: Red Chestnut
panic: Rock Rose
self-abuse, ascetic behavior: Rock Water
indecisiveness, flightiness: Scleranthus
easily insulted, oversensitive: Star of Bethlehem
desperation: Sweet Chestnut
missionary zeal: Vervain
closed-mindedness, dogmatism: Vine
easily influenced, self-alienation: Walnut
human contact problems: Water Violet
restlessness, lack of goals: Wild Oat
resignation, lack of enthusiasm: Wild Rose
bitter and unforgiving: Willow

Beliefs

too strong → **Dogmatism** → **Naïveté**

Vervain when we are obsessed with a conviction or an idea

Oak when we believe too strongly in our abilities and can become overwhelmed

too weak

Gentian when we can't see the possibility of a positive outcome (→ Giving up → Dejection)

Gorse when we have absolutely no hope (→ Hopelessness)

Sweet Chestnut when we feel we are at the end of our rope (→ Desperation)

Birth → Pregnancy

A birth will be more natural and problem-free if the mother-to-be is happy, strong, and relaxed. The following essences can help bring this about. Nature protects mothers during pregnancy by increasing their resistance to pathogens and other disease-causing influences.

for general easing of the discomfort of labor: **Agrimony + Aspen + Chicory + Elm + Impatiens + Mimulus**

This combination can help ease the discomfort of labor and can be used as a general preparation. Agrimony relaxes, Aspen helps instill confidence, Chicory loosens us up and minimizes our sensitivity, Elm imparts strength, Impatiens makes us calm, and Mimulus gives us courage.

premature birth: **Elm + Gentian + Mimulus + Olive + Water Violet**

This combination counters a tendency for premature births and provides strength for the pregnancy.

for postpartum: **Star of Bethlehem**

Star of Bethlehem helps injuries (such as a perineal tear) to heal and helps overcome severe psychic trauma.

with complications: **Rescue Remedy**

For panic, restlessness, or complications of any kind, Rescue Remedy has proved itself useful. (Take often!)

for weakness during labor: **Gentian + Olive + Walnut + Wild Rose**

This combination gives us strength, resolve, and endurance and promotes normal contractions.

Bitterness: Willow (→ Aggression → Influenced, too easily)

The word *bitterness* reminds us of the bitter taste of bile. Bile is often produced when we are too angry, and it is proof that such feelings hurt only ourselves. How else could it be, when we are fighting a battle that cannot be won? Making ourselves angry over something that has already happened and that cannot be undone is sheer foolishness and a sign of mental and emotional immaturity. If we want to live life to the fullest, we draw any positive realizations from all of our experiences and everything we encounter. The world is varied and colorful, and life is an adventure. If it is a cause of anger and rage to us that life does not meet our (unrealistic) expectations, the result is nothing but bitterness, which serves as a constant reminder of our own stupidity. Willow can release us from these feelings and make us more conciliatory, insightful, and understanding; it also helps suppress feelings of self-righteousness.

bitterness caused by rejection or ingratitude *8/38
bitterness due to rage or hate *15/38
bitterness caused by loss *16/38
bitterness causing depression *21/38
bitterness caused by an unprocessed trauma *29/38
bitterness caused by intolerance *32/38
compulsive bitterness *35/38

Blackmail, Extortion, emotional → Family Problems → Partner Problems

It takes two to pull off blackmail: the blackmailer and the blackmailed. Each plays a role, but both can do something about it when they are aware of their roles. Often, someone who has a tendency to be victimized will unconsciously seek out someone to take the role of the blackmailer and, by his anxious, weak, or masochistic behavior, will trigger the blackmailing reflex in the perpetrator. Blackmailers, on the other hand (which means anyone who transmits her will into action through psychic pressure), are always on the lookout for victims. Most cases of psychic blackmail take place in familiar surroundings.

in the passive role: **Centaury**

Centaury gives us more self-assertiveness so that we can stand up to blackmail or to being used and so that we do not provoke anyone to committing blackmail by our passive, obsequious behavior. Pine can also be useful when guilt feelings are involved.

in the active role: **Chicory**

Chicory is effective against the habit of blackmailing people through emotional terror (for example, by provoking in them a guilty conscience or "fishing" for sympathy). Children often have such a tendency when we don't deal with them honestly.

Blood, weak → Anemia

Blood Pressure

The body's performance and efficiency depend on how much oxygen and nutrients can be transported from the blood to the cells. The arteries, like water pipes, need sufficient pressure. When the body is put under too much strain, the pressure is too high; on the other hand, it doesn't perform optimally when the pressure is too low.

low blood pressure (hypotension)

Low blood pressure is often characterized by paleness, weakness, dizziness, or fatigue.

> Clematis if we are not oriented toward success or taking charge of our lives, with a tendency toward daydreaming
>
> Clematis for a tendency toward unconsciousness or fainting, often used when the consciousness is clouded
>
> Olive for general exhaustion
>
> Wild Rose for a general loss of interest; when we just mope though life, we don't need a vigorous blood flow.

high blood pressure (hypertension)

Hypertension is often accompanied by reddening of the skin and increased general activity. It can often lead to headaches, dizziness, a dazed state, insomnia, and, in the long term, calcification, stroke, or angina pectoris.

Aspen for suppressed fears, when we are under constant pressure

Cherry Plum for strong emotional pressure

Holly for rage, irritability, or annoyance, and for when "the blood begins to boil"

Impatiens for severe impatience, haste, or restlessness

Oak for people who cannot give in or give up; they put themselves under pressure and face the danger of hardening of the arteries

Vervain for excessive activity and readiness for action

Willow for bitterness or resentment, with internal pressure

Boils or Abscesses → Skin Conditions

Breakdown, on the verge of: Cherry Plum (→ Obsession → Psychosis)

Cherry Plum is used when we find ourselves on the verge of a breakdown because we have suppressed emotions or drives (such as sexuality).

breakdown caused by panic *6/25

Cancer

Most of us have been misinformed and led to believe that we are all in danger of getting cancer and that cancer is nearly always fatal. Actually, in most cases, the body can heal itself without the need of any special form of treatment. This fact is virtually unknown in scientific medicine, since usually only the most serious cases make it to the therapeutic slag heap. Cancer is an illness like any other; it typically appears in the form of a "normal" illness and disappears just as normally, because the body has focused on healing itself. Every illness is a pivotal experience and has a meaning for us, and every illness can arise only as the result of certain circumstances of life and consciousness. If these conditions don't exist, we don't get sick. Cancer is most probably the body's extreme reaction to a profound psychic or physical injury that hurts us deeply, and it is often an example of the inseparable connection between body and soul. Cancer is essentially a process of destruction and rebuilding, and we can get cancer only if we are somehow in need of rebuilding. The generally accepted belief that we are all susceptible to cancer arises from ignorance regarding the nature of cancer and makes us insecure if we lack insight. Even the suspicion that we might be diagnosed with cancer can affect us so deeply that if we do have cancer, it can be fatal. Most cancer fatalities are the result of foolish, unfeeling, and meaningless treatment. The most important prevention against cancer is staying happy and content, avoiding severe emotional conflict (or resolving conflicts as soon as possible, if they do appear), and keeping mind and spirit in balance. A healthy person does not become ill.

fear of cancer: **Aspen + Mimulus**
This combination strengthens our healing powers and also alleviates the general fear of cancer.

panicky fear: **Cherry Plum + Rock Rose + White Chestnut**
This combination is useful when we are overwhelmed by our own fear of cancer. Cherry Plum allows us to come to terms with our fears so that we are not overwhelmed by them, Rock Rose is for panic, and White Chestnut allows us to think clearly and sensibly.

treatment
Cancer should always be treated by a qualified doctor! Additional Bach flower treatment should employ essences appropriate to the specific condition.

Carefree Facade, seemingly: Agrimony
Pretending that we have no problems can be useful from time to time; in the long term, however, it prevents us from solving our problems, damages relationships, and makes us unhappy.

Carelessness → Scatterbrained Behavior

Caring, excessive: Chicory
When we worry too much about other people, we generally have the need to cling to them. (→ Family Problems)

Change, constant
due to helplessness: **Cerato**
Cerato helps minimize the need to want to make everything right, which often leads to following any advice that we might come across.

due to indecisiveness: **Scleranthus**
Scleranthus is useful when we can't choose among several alternatives and keep changing our minds.

due to having no direction: **Wild Oat**

Wild Oat helps us find our personal style so that we don't have to keep trying everything that comes along.

Clarity, lack of: Wild Oat

Wild Oat is useful when we are unsure how to proceed. It helps us find our way in life.

Cleanliness, obsessive: Crab Apple

cleanliness stemming from moral grounds *10/24
cleanliness and self-discipline, excessive *10/27
fanatical cleanliness *10/32

Clinging, due to fear *8/20

Cold Emotions

We normally describe someone who is not warm or friendly with other people as cold or icy. Actually, this "coldness" is the inability to develop either positive or negative emotions.

due to stubbornness and pigheadedness: **Oak**

When we ambitiously pursue an abstract goal, we risk the danger of becoming a soulless, unfeeling machine and losing our life-affirming contact with the world.

caused by self-negation: **Rock Water**

Often, self-castigation and extreme self-discipline are motivated by the desire to bring a difficult emotional life under control. When this impulse becomes excessive, we impoverish the spirit and become a bloodless, unemotional fanatic or turn to asceticism.

due to psychic trauma: **Star of Bethlehem**

Traumatic experiences sometimes trigger an emotional inflexibility that can be loosened with Star of Bethlehem.

due to excessive emotional distance: **Water Violet**

due to resignation: **Wild Rose**

When we have no more interest in life, our emotions wither away.

Collapse → Nervous Collapse

on the verge of a psychic and physical collapse *6/11
collapse caused by a mental or emotional trauma *11/29

Companionship → Aversion → Distance → Loneliness → Talkativeness

a need for

Agrimony to distract us from our problems and worries

Chicory when we have a strong craving for attention

aversion toward

Impatiens when others are too slow

Water Violet to pursue our own interests in quiet

the company of others making us aggressive *15/34

Compete, inability to

The struggle for survival is one of the fundamental principles of nature. This struggle helps us become stronger and helps us achieve. Even human beings become caught up in this struggle whether we want to or not, each of us in his own way. Because there is a limited amount of territory on Earth, any victory we win for ourselves usually represents someone else's downfall, and any time we act to ensure our survival, we are often inflicting the opposite result on another creature. Only in the mental or spiritual dimensions are we free of this struggle. We can share the same thoughts without the fear of anyone taking them away from us. We can consciously try to limit the damage we do to others in our actions, but we are still faced with the necessity of providing for our own needs. Unhappiness results when we are unable to face this struggle for survival, or if we are unsuccessful. The effects appear in our animal nature as well as in our transcendent soul. We all know the feeling of well-being that arises when we are successful in fulfilling our needs, whether it be satiating our hunger, thirst, or sexual drives or through love, success, social recognition, or power. There are many Bach flower essences used to treat various forms of weakness that impede our ability to compete successfully.

from general timidity: **Aspen**

People who shy away from life owing to vague, generalized fears or the fear of some unknown misfortune can benefit from Aspen.

from giving up: **Centaury**

Centaury increases our self-assertiveness and self-confidence when we allow ourselves to be used.

weak will: **Gentian**

We are not meant to overcome every obstacle in our path. Sometimes perseverance is required, and Gentian can strengthen it.

due to total hopelessness: **Gorse**

due to feelings of stress and overwork: **Hornbeam**

due to a lack of self-confidence: **Larch**

caused by fear: **Mimulus**

Mimulus is helpful when we stray from our path because we fear a test of our strength. It is often used in combination with Agrimony.

due to melancholy: **Mustard**

Mustard is useful in treating melancholy that seems to arise for no apparent reason and makes everything seem pointless.

due to exhaustion: **Olive**

due to resignation: **Wild Rose**

Wild Rose helps restore our drive and enthusiasm and strengthens our interest in an active life.

Complaining

insufficient

Complaining about misfortune is such a widespread phenomenon that it almost seems abnormal when we keep our mouths shut despite having an obvious reason for being unhappy. This reticence is normally caused by a disturbed relationship with life or with other people.

> Agrimony when we act as if everything is fine, even though we suffer inside
>
> Water Violet for people who keep such a great distance from those around them that they can't share their feelings
>
> Wild Rose when we are so shut off from others that we can't bring ourselves to bemoan our misfortune

too much

Stop complaining! When we complain about misfortune or suffering, we normally can't accept that we played a role in bringing it about or that it's within our power to end our misery. Instead, many of us act like children who cry until their mothers do what they want. This behavior at least allows us to vent our negative emotions, but in the end it does nothing to relieve our suffering. Unlike a mother, fate will not allow itself to be blackmailed. Instead, it demands—in our own interests—absolute honesty and resolve.

> Chicory for self-pitying whining and complaining caused by a craving for attention
>
> Heather for people who always try to make themselves the center of attention, even by whining and complaining if necessary
>
> Willow to relieve the bitterness that is so often the cause for complaining

Compulsions

compulsive thoughts: **White Chestnut** (→ **Expectations**)
White Chestnut helps when we can't get rid of unwanted thoughts that tyrannize us and make us unable to think clearly.

compulsive thoughts making us inattentive *7/35
obsessed with love *8/35
obsessive dreams of the future *9/35
compulsive thoughts of filth *10/35
compulsive thoughts due to vanity *12/35
compulsive, aggressive thoughts *15/35
obsessive memories *16/35
compulsive thoughts filled with fear *20/35
compulsive thoughts, oriented toward success *22/35
obsessive perfectionism *24/27
compulsive thoughts caused by guilt feelings *24/35
obsessive, worried thoughts *25/33
compulsive, traumatic thoughts *29/35
obsessive dogmatism *32/35
compulsive thoughts caused by bitterness *35/38

Compulsive Character

when we can't stand any sort of disorder or filth: **Crab Apple** *when fear or guilt makes us behave other than we would like:* Pine

when we place excessively strict demands on ourselves and restrict our own freedom: Rock Water

Compulsive Chattering → Talkativeness

Concentration, difficulties with

affecting our ability to learn: Chestnut Bud

Chestnut Bud improves our ability to learn and awakens our interest in whatever we're studying. Recommended combinations: Scleranthus (7/28), Wild Oat (7/36), Clematis (7/9), and Honeysuckle (7/16).

due to strong emotions: Cherry Plum

due to daydreaming: Clematis, Honeysuckle

Clematis improves our concentration when we can't restrain our imagination, and Honeysuckle when we're plagued by too many memories. Often combined with White Chestnut (9/35 or 16/35).

due to restlessness or impatience: Impatiens

due to depression: Mustard

due to exhaustion: Olive

due to tic, distracted behavior: Scleranthus

due to a traumatic experience: Star of Bethlehem

Star of Bethlehem is useful when a mental or emotional trauma or very unfavorable circumstances cause us to lose our inner balance and ability to concentrate.

due to obsessive thoughts: White Chestnut

White Chestnut is appropriate when certain thoughts persistently plague our consciousness, making it impossible for us to concentrate on anything else.

Conflict → Tension

Conformity

When we are working from a position of weakness, we must conform; when we are working from a position of strength, we may not. This is a principle of nature; we know instinctively how we must behave.

excessive, from a lack of will: **Centaury**
Centaury reduces a tendency to conform unnecessarily.

insufficient, due to feeling rushed: **Impatiens**
When we are in too much of a hurry, we become clumsy and cannot adapt sufficiently to the circumstances.

insufficient, due to idealism: **Vervain**
Ideals, just like prejudices, make us blind and prevent us from behaving realistically.

insufficient, due to stubbornness: **Vine**
Stubborn opinions and behavior make us unable to react to life's unpredictability. We proceed straight ahead, even though the road is curved.

excessive due to being easily influenced: **Walnut**
Walnut helps us remain true to ourselves and follow our own path.

Conscience, guilty → Guilt Feelings → Self-blame
conscience, guilty, leading to insecurity *5/24

Consolation
need for: **Chicory**
The more we depend on other people, the more we need consolation and comfort from them in times of misfortune. It is, to a certain extent, proof that we are not alone. When the need for consolation makes us too weak or makes us a burden on other people, we need Chicory. If the source of our pain has been a shocking experience, combine with Star of Bethlehem.

rejection of: **Water Violet**
Very independent people often would prefer not to be comforted during a time of misfortune; they would rather get through it alone. This rejection can become so strong that it can create a chasm between us and our sympathetic friends and make us lonely.

Conspiracy, obsession with: Aspen
Aspen is indicated when we make inexplicable connections between seemingly unrelated events or facts—especially when they are somehow a cause for fear.

Contact, excessive need for → Pushiness

We all have a need for human contact that varies according to our dispositions. When a weakness of character makes this need too strong, the effect is often the opposite of what we need: we push people away and become isolated.

with a craving for emotional relationships: Chicory

Chicory is useful when we want to cling too tightly to those we love and push them away from us.

due to a need for recognition: Heather

Heather helps break the habit of trying to be the center of attention and using contact with other people as a means of self-projection.

Contact Problems → Loneliness → Isolation → Inhibitions → Partner Problems

The secret of harmonious relationships lies in knowing the proper amount of distance to maintain and allowing for the interplay of commonalities that unite us and opposites that pull us apart. When we are compelled to share a limited space with someone with whom we are not compatible, the result is an irremediable hostility; on the other hand, we may enjoy each other's company if we allow each other enough space. We each have our own limits and needs for distance as well; some of us need constant companionship, while others prefer to be alone.

due to a fear of openness: Agrimony

When we're afraid to show who and what we are, it's difficult to form meaningful relationships. Agrimony allows us to express ourselves more naturally, spontaneously, and openly.

due to a fear of dirt and filth: Crab Apple

Crab Apple is indicated when an extreme need for cleanliness makes it impossible for us to be in contact with others.

due to an inferiority complex: Larch

Open and enriching communication is possible only among equals. This is not a question of social status but of a feeling of self-worth and self-confidence. When we feel inferior to others, we cannot establish successful contact.

due to depression: Mustard

No one likes to spend time with grouchy, moody people. Mustard limits the frequency and severity of depressions.

due to negative experiences: **Star of Bethlehem**

Star of Bethlehem helps us forget and come to terms with negative experiences and allows us to regain our trust in people. It is often used in combination with Willow (29/38).

due to keeping one's distance: **Water Violet**

Sometimes fear, misunderstandings, or oversensitivity will cause us to keep such a distance from other people that we feel lonely. We'd like to get closer, but we can't bridge the gulf that separates us. (This often happens with shy lovers.) Water Violet helps us jump the hurdles and bridge the gap. It is also helpful for brittle, fragile, shy people.

due to bitterness: **Willow**

Bitterness increases our distance from other people. We want nothing to do with those who have disappointed us, and this in itself makes us unhappy. Willow can restore our conciliatory mood and helps us reestablish contact. Often used in combination with Star of Bethlehem (29/38).

contact problems due to a lack of openness *1/34

fear of contact, extreme *1/34

contact problems caused by fears and anxieties *2/34

contact problems with aggression *15/34

contact problems due to an inferiority complex *19/34

contact problems due to depression *21/34

contact problems due to a mental or emotional trauma *29/34

Contagion, protection against → Flu

As long as the body is engaged in the fight against harmful agents and pathogens, it is immune to the infection that these ubiquitous pathogens carry. An infection (the activation of contagion) is a sign that the body is occupied with detoxifying or repairing itself. When a contagion becomes active, we find ourselves in the parasympathetic healing phase. The best safeguards against infection are mental and emotional health, inner peace, and optimism: a healthy person does not become ill!

due to blood purification: **Crab Apple**

Harmful materials are eliminated in increased numbers. Crab Apple is particularly effective for people who feel themselves poisoned or contaminated.

by a strengthening of defenses against negative influences:
Walnut

Walnut helps us maintain a healthy inner balance.

Convalescence, stalled *12/28

Convictions → Dogmatism → Beliefs

Coughing → Lung Conditions

Cowardice

Cowardice is a practiced form of fear. The term is normally used to belittle someone who tries to avoid danger. In doing this, we judge others (which is always a mistake) and believe that everyone should act just as courageously in the same situation as we do. We forget, however, that we are all cowards in certain situations. (Courage, by the way, is not just the naive and thoughtless risking of life and limb but the process of consciously overcoming fear. We can only be courageous if we are afraid.) We should try to avoid calling anyone a coward, especially if we don't know all the reasons for his or her behavior. Generally, we all have sensible reasons and act as we do to ensure our survival.

due to fear: **Aspen, Mimulus**

Aspen is used to treat vague fears, and Mimulus is given for specific fears. Fears are often groundless and can be countered if we try to confront them consciously or with practical experience.

due to a weak personality: **Centaury**

People who let themselves be used often appear to be cowards because they frequently give up their rights for no apparent reason. Centaury gives them more courage.

due to feelings of stress and overwork: **Hornbeam**

Hornbeam is useful when we feel overworked and try to avoid a potential strain or responsibility.

due to feelings of inferiority: **Larch**

When we lack confidence in ourselves, we also tend to feel too much pressure from our responsibilities. Larch strengthens self-confidence and is often used for children.

due to a negative experience: **Star of Bethlehem**

"Once burned, twice shy." If we've had a negative experience, we tend to be overly cautious or even to avoid similar subsequent situations. Star of

Bethlehem helps when we can no longer differentiate when we need to be cautious, and we develop a fundamental (and often unjustified) defensive posture. Sensitive children often have this tendency.

Craving for Food → Anorexia

People who crave food suffer from severe frustration that usually stems from an unfulfilled or excessive need for love and happiness. Eating provides oral gratification and is an attempt to compensate for the things they lack.

for fears that are displaced by eating: Aspen + Mimulus
for a strong, unfulfilled need for attention: Chicory
for dissatisfaction with oneself: Gentian + Hornbeam + Larch
for contrariness and aggression: Holly
for severe frustration or unresolved psychic shock: Star of
   Bethlehem

Crisis: Walnut

In a life crisis, life change, or at the beginning of a new life phase, Walnut can help us stay true to ourselves and find our true nature.

Criticism

of others → Know-it-all → Dogmatism → Domestic Tyrant
of oneself → Guilt Feelings

Daydreams → Sentimentality

daydreaming making us inattentive and distracted *7/9
daydreaming, with a weak will *9/12
daydreaming, total *9/16
daydreaming undermining our ability to make decisions
   *9/28

Death

fear of: Aspen + Rock Rose
These essences help lessen the fear of death.
longing for death: Clematis
People who find little happiness in the present and seek comfort in the future often hope for a final solution in death (especially during an illness).

easing the process of dying: Oak + Walnut

Oak shortens a futile struggle with death, and Walnut brings an inner tranquillity.

longing for death caused by exhaustion *9/23
longing for death with general resignation *9/37

Defense, weak, against accusations *24/33

Dejection → Fear

dejection accompanying feelings of stress and overwork *11/12

Delusions → Poisoning, fear of

fearful: Aspen
psychotic: Cherry Plum

Demands on oneself leading to feelings of inferiority *19/27

Dependence → Fear → Insecurity

dependence due to a weak personality *4/5
dependence leading to feelings of stress and overwork *4/17
dependent and easily influenced *4/33
dependence caused by self-abuse *5/27

Dependence on others

Dependence can be treated when it creates suffering or other negative emotions. These emotions show that our need for independence is being restricted.

from a weak personality: Centaury

Centaury strengthens the personality and minimizes mental dependence.

from a need for attention: Chicory

Chicory helps temper a pathological need for emotional relationships; when we allow other people to be free, we become more independent.

from a need for recognition: Heather

This essence is used when we are not aware of our own worth and need the validation of other people.

from fear: Mimulus

Mimulus mitigates an excessive need for protection.

from guilt: **Pine**

Pine lessens guilt feelings and frees us from the dependency-inducing need for forgiveness.

from being easily influenced: **Walnut**

Walnut makes us more independent by helping us be true to ourselves.

Dependence and Insecurity: Cerato

Cerato is for people who constantly seek advice because they don't know how they should behave.

Depression → Chapter 1: Mustard

basic treatment: **Mustard**

Depression results when important life-affirming impulses or needs that are crucial to our happiness are suppressed. The extent of the depression is determined by the force of the suppression. You might say that the most depressed people have the potential for the most happiness. When we know and understand the reasons for our depression, we call it reactive depression (meaning a reaction to unhappy circumstances), and when it seems inexplicable, we call it endogenous depression (stemming from the mind or psyche). Often, reactive depression can be countered by treating the conditions creating the depressed state, while endogenous depression demands a profound rehabilitation of our total worldview and assumptions. This cannot be achieved when the depressed person will not allow the therapist access to his inner mind or when he is mentally broken.

The role of one's physical condition should not be underestimated: liver conditions especially can create a depressive state (melancholia). Mustard is the basic treatment and should be combined with the following essences, as needed.

caused by fear: **Aspen**

Aspen helps when we have lost joy in life because of vague, groundless fears.

due to helplessness: **Cerato**

Cerato is for people who are depressed or discontented because they don't trust their own opinions and do not know how to act.

due to self-denial: **Crab Apple**

Crab Apple is appropriate when we are depressed because we feel unclean, poisoned, or besmirched.

due to failure (reactive): Gentian

Gentian is helpful for any depression caused by failure or humiliation. It helps restore our optimism.

due to lack of recognition: Heather

Heather helps us when our need for recognition or popularity is so excessive that it can never be satisfied, and this makes us sad.

due to suppressed aggression: Holly

When aggression or rage is suppressed, depression is often the result. Holly suppresses our aggressive feelings.

due to a fear of failure: Hornbeam

Hornbeam counters the (often melancholy) feeling that we are not up to the challenges of everyday life.

due to insufficient self-confidence: Larch

When we lack self-confidence and often deny ourselves, often the result is that we eventually become morose, sad, or depressed. Larch helps restore our self-confidence.

without apparent cause (endogenous): Mustard

Mustard is appropriate for the endogenous, inexplicable depression that seems to come over us out of the blue.

due to weakness: Olive

Exhaustion (especially a weakness of the heart) promotes the development of depression. Olive improves our mood and increases our strength.

due to guilt feelings: Pine

Feelings of guilt poison our thoughts and mood and make us depressed.

due to excessive worries: Red Chestnut
due to an unresolved shock or unbearable problem: Star of Bethlehem

If we cannot reach a state of closure with a distressing life experience or living conditions, we cannot proceed with a feeling of optimism. Star of Bethlehem helps us see our unpleasant experiences in a more positive light.

due to extreme desperation: Sweet Chestnut
due to a lack of purpose in life: Wild Oat
with resignation and lack of interest: Wild Rose

Our consciousness demands that we put life in a meaningful context; otherwise, we lack positive motivation and optimism. Wild Oat helps us find meaning in our lives.

depression due to unrequited love *8/21*
depression and disgruntlement *12/21*
depression due to hopelessness *13/21*
depression due to rejection and loneliness *14/21*
depression due to a loss *16/21*
depression due to exhaustion *21/23*
depression due to guilt feelings *21/24*
depression due to psychic trauma *21/29*
antisocial behavior caused by depression *21/34*
depression due to a feeling of meaninglessness *21/36*
depressive resignation *21/37*
depression due to bitterness *21/38*

Despair Accompanying a Life Change *12/33

Desperation, absolute: Sweet Chestnut

Sweet Chestnut is used when we've reached a point when we feel we just can't go on (generally because we've been struggling against fate), when we've lost all hope, when we can no longer think or speak. If taken in a timely manner and in combination with other appropriate essences, Sweet Chestnut can help get us out of this black hole.

premonitions, secret *1/2*
desperation caused by emotional stress *6/30*
desperation due to stress and overwork *11/30*
desperation, absolutely hopeless *13/20*
terrified and exhausted *20/23*
desperation caused by panic and fear *26/30*
desperation caused by mental and emotional trauma *29/30*

Developmental Difficulties

When children don't develop correctly, it is a sign that they are lacking something or being suppressed or impeded in some way. Possible causes can include, but are not limited to, improper nutrition or an unfavorable environment as well as the psychic constitution. The psyche is positively or negatively influenced by everything it perceives and experiences and transmits all harmful experiences to the body. Physical health is impossible without mental and psychic well-being.

due to fear: **Aspen, Mimulus**

Fear can inhibit our natural development because it forces us to be cautious and tentative. Aspen is for vague, nebulous fears, and Mimulus is for specific, nameable fears.

due to a relapse in an illness: **Gentian**

Gentian promotes healing and convalescence by increasing the body's endurance, thus avoiding relapses.

due to an inferiority complex: **Larch**

A child who feels himself inferior tends to hold himself back and to hide himself, which can impede physical development. Larch helps him regain his proper posture and promotes the development of an erect bearing.

due to exhaustion: **Olive**

Development and growth mean strength. Olive is a good choice for chronic exhaustion that can hinder normal development.

due to a traumatic experience: **Star of Bethlehem**

Shocking experiences can so undermine our courage and trust in fate that the development of body and psyche can be disrupted. This essence can be combined with Mimulus (20/29).

Disappointment

When we can recognize that a disappointment frees us from illusion (which makes it essentially something positive), we can overcome it more quickly and will perhaps not be so easily disappointed in the future.

due to failure: **Gentian**

Gentian makes us more optimistic so that we won't throw in the towel at the first sign of failure.

with bitterness: **Willow**

When a disappointment makes us bitter, Willow can make us more optimistic.

Discipline (too severe and remote)

The purpose of discipline is to sustain and improve our lives and to promote our happiness. It should not be practiced as an end unto itself and it should be carried out with a certain amount of compassion and flexibility.

with oneself: **Rock Water**

People who put themselves under so much pressure that they do not allow themselves or others any pleasure need Rock Water.

toward others: Vine

When we are too strict with others, we need Vine. It is good for teachers who can only see their charges as objects, not as subjects, and for parents who demand excessive order or morality from their children.

Discontentment → Depression → Moodiness → Ungratefulness → Enthusiasm, lack of

due to insatiability: Chicory

Chicory is for people who can never get enough of anything (especially emotional attention).

caused by failure: Gentian

To a certain extent, it's perfectly normal to be discontented when things don't go as we plan or as we would like them to go. Gentian prevents our discontentment from becoming a crippling permanent condition and helps us adjust our expectations.

for no recognizable cause: Mustard

Vague, general discontentment is a mild form of depression, which can be improved with Mustard.

with life: Wild Oat (→ Vocation)

It is impossible to be content if we have no meaning in our lives. This doesn't have to entail a grand philosophical design or a moral ideal; it could be a pleasant daily plan or work that is done carefully and thoughtfully—anything that helps us get through life with a sense of purpose. Some people need a long-term plan or a great life goal, while others just need to live from day to day. As long as no important needs or drives are suppressed or ignored, we can be content; otherwise, we'll never be at peace, and our restlessness will prevent us from taking care of our own needs. Wild Oat helps us set our priorities straight.

Discouraged and exhausted *12/23

Disloyalty → Unreliability

Disorder

not tolerated

Crab Apple for a compulsive need for order and cleanliness

Rock Water for excessive discipline

Vine for mental and emotional inflexibility

excessive

Clematis with an excessive tendency to daydream

Honeysuckle when we are too overcome with nostalgia or heartache to concern ourselves with anything else

Scleranthus when we can never make a clear decision

Wild Oat when we don't know how to behave

Distance, emotional → Pushiness → Loneliness → Loner → Contact, excessive need for → Contact Problems

Distraction

When we are distracted, we are unable to devote our hearts and souls to a situation, a thought, or an activity. We can't think things through thoroughly, and we are never totally content.

from inattentiveness: **Chestnut Bud**

from indecisiveness: **Scleranthus**

We cannot choose among possible alternatives and follow every whim.

from our own goals: **Walnut**

We can't defend ourselves from outside influences and are always diverted from our own path.

from interest in too many possibilities: **Wild Oat**

Because we are always on the lookout and interested in everything, we cannot concentrate on one thing.

distracted behavior leading to learning difficultiess *7/28

Distress → Shock

frozen in panic *1/26

distress causes aggression *15/29

distress, mental, leads to desperation *29/30

Do-gooder

When we feel the need to improve the world, we believe that we alone possess the truth or that we are better than other people. Seen in absolute terms, this is mere foolishness; we're all part of a greater whole, a part that cannot change or improve the whole by itself. We can fulfill only our allotted function. Subjectively, however, we must behave in the way that seems right to us. When things don't seem right, we must change them appropriately, and this is how we each fulfill our mission to change the world. As long as the result is positive for us and for the rest of the world, this is all well and good, but as soon as our actions cause suffering, some kind of adjustment is necessary—not an adjustment with the world, but with ourselves.

due to self-abuse: **Rock Water**

When we torment ourselves or feel compelled to practice self-denial to serve as an example for others, we need Rock Water.

caused by dogmatic convictions: **Vine**

Vine helps eliminate the habit of expecting others to behave as we do.

aggressive do-gooder *15/31

Dogmatism

A dogma is an idea that is put forth as a general guideline that should be followed by all. It exercises a strong (and even seductive) compulsion that removes some of life's diversity, variety, and complexity and saves us the hard work of finding our own truth. It has the effect of putting on blinders. Blindly accepting a dogma is often easier than finding our way unprotected through the confusing complexity that reality offers us. This advantage— when seen from the perspective of personal development—becomes a disadvantage because it results in a diminution of personal responsibility and our ability to have autonomous feelings and an independent life. Dogmas are often the result of a mental or psychological disruption—in those who follow them as much as in those who impose them on others. For the followers, there is a lack of maturity, and for the leaders, there is mental inflexibility, one-sidedness, and insufficient self-criticism. With the following essences and combinations, we can try to counter the tendency toward dogmatism.

accepting dogma: **Centaury, Pine**

Centaury is for people who have no life experience or concept and are used to following others. Dogmas play a major role in providing important order in their lives.

Pine helps those who feel guilty when they rebel against authority. Dogma demands our unconditional surrender and is generally linked with some sort of punishment for those who don't follow the rules. Pine diminishes the compulsion to be responsible for others.

dogma is practiced: **Rock Water, Vine**

Rock Water frees us from an inner pressure to discipline ourselves with rules and dogmas. It allows us to live according to our own needs rather than by following theoretical attitudes or ideals.

Vine is for obstinate, closed-minded people who take their own opinions and ideas for the last word, and who impose them on others. They become more flexible, tolerant, and pragmatic.

dogmatic need to achieve *22/32
dogmatic compulsive thoughts *32/35

Domestic Tyrant: Vine

People who tyrannize and bully their relatives with their own inflexible, intolerant ideas and believe themselves to be infallible role models should take Vine.

domestic tyrant, aggressive or irritable *15/32
domestic tyrant, embittered *32/38

Dominate, need to → Emotional Tyrant → Domestic Tyrant

Doting Mother: Chicory

When a mother worries too much about her child, she only makes the child more dependent and becomes the dominant person in the child's life. The mother's strength causes weakness in her child.

Doubt → Insecurity → Turmoil, inner

Dreams → Nightmares → Sentimentality

Drive, lack of → Weakness

When a lack of drive is evident after a stress or strain, it generally signals the beginning of the parasympathetic healing phase, which should not be disrupted by forceful means, such as stimulants. Long-lasting bouts of listlessness, on the other hand, signal some kind of damage. (→ Anemia → Illness)

due to a lack of self-confidence: **Larch**

with depression: **Mustard**

Depression is suppressed aggression. Listlessness is a consequence of this self-suppression.

due to exhaustion: **Olive**

general: **Wild Rose**

Wild Rose is called for in cases of general resignation, which is usually a dangerous sign. Wild Rose is best combined with Olive (→ 23/37).

Drowsiness → Apathy → Fatigue → Resignation

Drug Abuse

Drugs can elicit unusual states of mind and illusions. People use them when they are unable to cope with life or are dissatisfied. Alcohol and psycho-pharmaceuticals are drugs in this sense, when we find life unbearable without them.

to compensate for urgent inner needs: **Agrimony**

Agrimony helps us give full expression to personal problems. People who cannot do so are often plagued by inner torment and try to lessen the effects by taking drugs, especially alcohol. Alcohol helps us displace our problems and see the world through rose-colored glasses.

and flight into fantasy: **Clematis**

Clematis works against the temptation to replace sobering reality with pleasant fantasies, often with the "help" of drugs.

to make life bearable: **Star of Bethlehem**

Star of Bethlehem helps us endure difficult circumstances or terrible experiences that we might otherwise try to suppress or gloss over with the help of drugs or alcohol. It can be combined with Agrimony.

Eagerness to Help Others, due to feelings of inferiority → 4/19

Ear Problems

itchiness in the ear (eczema): **Crab Apple + Impatiens**

hearing difficulties: **Agrimony + Clematis + Mimulus + Oak**

Eczema → Skin Conditions

Egocentrism → Egotism

Egocentric people consider themselves to be the center of the world, and they relate everything they see or experience to themselves. While this is natural to a certain extent—our consciousness can comprehend only what happens to us directly and understand in those around us only the experiences we have in common—the balance between "me" and "you" can swing too far in the direction "me." Our mental lives are impoverished from a lack of communication, and our relationships become cold or hostile from insufficient interest in other people.

***too concerned with our own image:* Heather**

For anyone who regards other people as an accessory to his own life, or expects them to be an adoring audience.

***excessive interest in ourselves:* Rock Water**

Rock Water is needed when we are too concerned with ourselves and lose our feeling for the relativity of all values.

***too obsessed with our own ideas:* Vervain**

Vervain is for people who overestimate their own ideas and constantly try to impose them on others.

***too self-satisfied:* Vine**

When we cannot listen to anyone's opinion but our own, we need Vine.

***too frugal or lacking contact:* Water Violet**

Water Violet is called for when we have retreated so far into our own world that we have virtually no human contact. It is sometimes combined with Rock Water (27/34).

Egotism → Egocentrism → Self-denial

The term *egotism* has both a positive and a negative meaning. In the positive sense, it means that we recognize our rights and needs in a natural way, and, if they are threatened, we defend them. In addition, we take into consideration the rights and needs of others, as long as they do not threaten our own. In its negative form, it causes us to ignore the needs of others and have no feelings for their happiness. The typical egotist thinks only of herself and demands more than that to which she is entitled or needs. This behavior is unnatural, senseless, and not genuine, and it causes suffering. It makes us discontent and also creates hate and envy. For this reason, we must be careful when receiving (and giving!) to keep our sense of proportion.

insufficient: **Centaury, Larch, Star of Bethlehem**

Centaury is good for anyone who has lost the feeling for her own rights, and who serves others without deriving any benefit for herself. Her selflessness arises predominately from a weak personality and not from an aware, energetic openness to others; her character becomes weak and incites a thoughtless egotism in those with whom she comes in contact (→ Blackmail).

Larch is helpful when we do not have sufficient self-confidence or enough healthy egotism to take what we need from life.

Star of Bethlehem can be combined with Larch or Centaury when an unresolved trauma is partly the cause.

excessive: **Chicory**

Chicory works against selfish egotism that is caused by jealousy, envy, and resentment. Anyone who has the feeling that she does not have enough needs Chicory. This is especially true for emotional needs. It can be combined with Holly in the case of aggressive reactions or with Willow if the cause is resentment or bitterness.

Embarrassment

because we want to hide something from ourselves or portray
ourselves as other than we actually are: Agrimony
because we have no self-confidence: Larch
because we suffer from a guilty conscience: Pine

Emergencies: Rescue Remedy (see chapter 2)

Emotional Pressure → Obsession

Emotional Tyrant: Chicory

In almost every family (→ Family Problems) there is someone who tyrannizes the others with skillful emotional manipulation and blackmail. This normally takes place through displays of suffering, which trigger sympathy or guilt (→ Guilt Feelings) and brings them the attention they need or other advantages. We often see this behavior in spoiled, egotistical, or self-pitying children who incessantly torment their parents, and also in parents who try to prevent their children from leading their own lives. Chicory promotes emotional independence.

Endurance

insufficient: **Gentian**

Gentian acts against pessimism and faintheartedness and prevents us from giving up unnecessarily or prematurely.

excessive: **Oak**

Oak helps when our ability to withstand difficult circumstances becomes a senseless compulsion. It enables us to give up if the balance between costs and benefits isn't favorable.

Enthusiasm

lack of: **Mustard** (→ **Depression**)

Lack of enthusiasm is a mild form of depression. Mustard helps us overcome these feelings, especially when they seem to have no cause.

exaggerated: **Vervain**

When we become too one-sided or enthusiastic about one particular thing, Vervain prevents us from neglecting our other needs and interests and from losing our sense of proportion.

unenthusiastic and discouraged ***12/17**

Envy → Egotism → Jealousy

Epilepsy: Agrimony + Clematis + Rock Rose + Star of Bethlehem

An epileptic seizure is generally characterized by a disruption of consciousness with convulsions that result from a mental overload or a shocking experience. In addition to the usual medical treatment, this combination can be used for prevention and treatment. These essences should be given during a seizure by dropping on the lips or by rubbing into the forehead.

for convulsions: **Agrimony**
for the premonition of a seizure: **Aspen**
for the loss of consciousness: **Clematis**
for panic: **Rock Rose**
to treat psychic (and possible physical) trauma: **Star of Bethlehem**

Erratic Behavior → Unreliability

Excitement, arousal → Obsession

When excitement is not redirected in the form of actions, it can cause blockages and complex disruptions in the body.

suppressed and glossed over: **Agrimony**

Agrimony helps us express feelings that would otherwise bring forth a tormenting inner pressure.

strong, internal: **Cherry Plum**

Cherry Plum is the basic essence for intense, difficult emotions.

aggressive: **Holly**

If pent-up mental or physical stimulation makes us irritable, angry, or violent, Holly can help us let off steam.

restless, impatient: **Impatiens**

When we suffer from restlessness, impatience, or haste, Impatiens can help ease the situation and allow us to better master our need for constant stimulation.

due to excessive ambition: **Vervain**

Vervain is for those who inflict themselves with stress owing to excessive enthusiasm and hyperactivity.

Exemplary Behavior

when we want to be a good example: **Rock Water**
when we take ourselves to be a good example: **Vine**

Exhaustion

Exhaustion means that we require more strength than we are able to muster at a given time. Ideally, we should have the sense to rest as soon as we notice that we are tiring. Our organism can endure nearly every stress as long as it has a chance to rest, but long-term stress with no chance to rest can be harmful.

from excessive stress: **Elm**

When we create our own stress by putting ourselves under too much pressure to achieve, we need Elm to help put us back on our feet.

due to hopelessness: **Gorse**

When we have no more hope, the organism can no longer mobilize its strength: "It's no use!" Gorse can help on such occasions.

due to pessimism: **Hornbeam**

Hornbeam is effective against the crippling feeling that we are not up to our daily work.

due to physical exhaustion: **Olive**

Olive is the great giver of strength if we are drained after a long illness or periods of hard work.

due to resignation: **Wild Rose**

Wild Rose gives us more enthusiasm when we drag through the day, tired and without initiative.

> *exhaustion causing absentmindedness or unconsciousness* *9/23
>
> *exhaustion, serious physical and mental* *11/23
>
> *exhausted and discouraged* *12/23
>
> *exhaustion causing hopelessness* *13/23
>
> *exhaustion causing a flight into the past* *16/23
>
> *exhaustion undermining self-confidence* *19/23
>
> *exhaustion creating fear* *20/23
>
> *exhaustion making us depressed* *21/23
>
> *exhaustion causing psychic instability* *23/29
>
> *exhaustion causing us to be easily influenced* *23/33
>
> *exhaustion making us unsociable* *23/34
>
> *exhaustion leading to resignation* *23/38

Expectations

Expectations are merely fantasies and should be treated as such. Confusing them with reality brings disaster.

fantasies of the future: **Clematis**

Clematis is useful when we live too much in our fantasies and lose touch with reality.

creating fear: **Mimulus**

When we always expect that bad things will happen to us, we are subject to a particularly tormenting variety of fear, because these problems are not real and not solvable.

Eye Conditions

The eyes are greatly influenced by the psyche. The following essences or combinations are often used to treat eye conditions. There are also exercises that we can practice to keep our eyes healthy or restore them to health.

1. Keep alternating the focus by gazing from near to distant objects.
2. Move the eyeballs in wide circles both to the right and left.
3. Standing in front of a strong light source with eyes closed, keep covering and uncovering your eyes with your hands.

poor eyesight

As with any organ, the eyes lose some of their strength and functioning abilities when they are not used very much. If we do not use them enough, there is a danger that either the eyes or the part of the brain that controls them will deteriorate.

Aspen for general fears, when we close our eyes to reality

Clematis for dreaminess and fantasy, when we have little interest in what's going on around us and look only at what is inside, such as illusions or dreams of the future

Honeysuckle for sadness or nostalgia, instead of reality—when all we can see are pictures and images from the past

Mimulus for the fear of something specific at which we do not dare to look (generally combined with Aspen)

conjunctivitis: Crab Apple

Conjunctivitis is often caused by a sinus infection. In such cases, the blood-purifying effects of Crab Apple can help strengthen the effects of appropriate medications. When caused by allergies → Allergies.

cataracts: Oak

glaucoma

Glaucoma is caused by a blockage of fluid exchange in the eye, which can arise during times of stress (Crab Apple) and tension. Relaxing meditation or biofeedback have been proven to have positive effects.

Agrimony for inner tension, when we want to hide something

Elm for sudden stress

Holly for rage

Mimulus or Aspen for tension related to fear

Oak for grimness and inflexibility

Vervain for long-term, self-induced stress

Willow for bitterness

Facade: Agrimony

Agrimony gives us the courage to take off the facade or mask behind which we hide our feelings, fears, or problems and allows us to show ourselves as we really are.

Failure → Fear

failure caused by a weak will and lack of attentiveness *7/12

Family Problems → Partner Problems

A family has two fundamental functions: on the one hand, it is a voluntary partnership between two people, based on mutual affection, and, on the other hand, it provides optimal conditions for the development of the off-spring that the partnership creates; it provides love, nourishment, protection, and education to prepare the child for life. When these requirements are not fulfilled properly and the family unit turns into a vehicle for power, obsessions, or compulsions, when there is no love between the parents, or when the children are neglected, or emotionally or physically abused, then well-known, complex family problems arise. Because such fundamental needs of our existence are involved, these problems can often end in a deadly battle or in a lifelong illness. With most chronic illnesses, the family relationships must be totally overhauled, which is extremely difficult and usually means breaking up the family unit. It would be much better if we could avoid the "family plague" (from W. Reich) entirely by not entering bad marriages and making sure not to have any children if we are in a bad marriage.

by allowing oneself to be used: Centaury

People who are prevented from becoming independent and self-confident in their childhood often develop a tendency toward self-denial and self-sacrificing, obsequious behavior. They let themselves be used and often place themselves at the disposal of their parents. This is an unnatural situation (in nature, the task of caring for someone is always a parental function; the parents take care of the children, not the other way around), and it can cause unhappiness and illness: the child misses out on her own life, and the parents are denied the joy of seeing their child be happy. A similar situation exists with couples, when one partner gives up his or her happiness to serve the other. This behavior is not motivated by love; it poisons the relationship and creates a subconscious hate. Centaury promotes the awareness that we have the right to our own lives and that we serve no moral purpose by allowing ourselves to be blackmailed or used.

through emotional tyranny or laying claim to someone:
Chicory

Chicory is used to treat a strong desire for attachment, when parents can't let their children go, or children are not able to leave their parents. The natural course of events is that in puberty a person will begin to lead her own life, which means that she finds a place in a new functioning partnership. This is impossible when parents (the mother for the daughter, and the father for the son) won't let go of their children, when they are overcome by jealousy, or when they use illness to cling or through emotional castration make it impossible for the child to establish a normal sexual relationship. The consequences of such pathological parent-child relationships are often impotence, frigidity, and homosexuality; moreover, the children can become too attached to the guardian through the latter's demands for love or as the result of jealousy. These widespread neurotic dependencies between parents and children of the opposite sex are unnatural and can never be satisfied, and they can generate hatred and destroy the lives of all involved. These tendencies will arise again in the relationship of marriage or life partnerships. Chicory must be taken over a long period of time, often in combination with Holly (8/15), Walnut (8/33), or Willow (8/38).

with jealousy: Chicory, Holly

Some people take severe jealousy as a sign of love. In fact, it indicates only a strong need for possession. True love strives for happiness, not ownership.

with hate and jealousy: Holly

The complex and usually unsatisfied demands within the family often bring forth such negative emotions as hate, envy, mistrust, or lust for revenge.

due to guilt feelings: Pine

Guilt causes hate and can poison any human relationship. It is often employed in familial power struggles. Pine can assuage guilt. It promotes the realization that neither parents (because of the wrongs they have inflicted on their children) nor children (because of their inability to fulfill their parents' expectations) are guilty. All of us do the best we can under the circumstances. Human error is just that—human. We all get along much better when there is no guilt involved.

with psychic trauma: **Star of Bethlehem**

Star of Bethlehem helps overcome psychic injuries that are caused by family power struggles and severe relationship disruptions. It is the basic essence used to treat all neurotic problems in social relationships.

due to a lack of distance and tolerance: **Water Violet**

We often think that a blood relationship means a mental and emotional relationship. Actually, most family members have very different and even opposite characters. Even between parents and children there is often alienation or incompatibility. When we refuse to accept this, the family community can become a family prison. A certain distance (→ Distance) is required in every human relationship, and this distance must not be too great or too small. Water Violet can normalize relationships when a family member, for whatever reason, has put too much distance between herself and others and is feeling isolated. It is often combined with Agrimony (1/34), Star of Bethlehem (29/34), or Willow (34/38).

due to intolerance or imposing one's will: **Vine**

When someone (generally a parent) imposes his personal views on family members and doesn't take the opinions of others into account, he needs Vine. Vine is effective against the authoritarian, closed-minded superiority and bossiness that often plague family relationships.

due to being too easily offended: **Willow**

Fanaticism → Obsession → Dogmatism

related to cleanliness: **Crab Apple**

Crab Apple is for clean freaks who see dirt and filth everywhere and feel the need to do something about it.

in leading our own lives: **Rock Water**

Rock Water is for people who put themselves under obsessive (and forceful), strict, narrow-minded rules.

in do-gooders: **Vervain**

and dogmatism: **Vine**

and mental obsession: **White Chestnut**

Fanatics can think only about their own goals. White Chestnut frees us from this mental narrow-mindedness. It can be combined with Vervain (31/35) or Vine (32/35).

Fantasies, anxious: Aspen

Fantasies are harmful because they displace our clear view of reality and adversely influence our ability to deal with life. They come about from a condition of the brain or from emotional stress.

Fantasy and Imagination, excessive: Clematis

Clematis clears our view of reality when it is clouded by our fantasies.

Fatalism → Resignation

Fatigue → Weakness

Fear

Fear is a constricting physical feeling, which can affect, above all, the vicinity of the heart and the upper abdomen. It is caused when we try to resist—more or less unconsciously—an event that we know or assume will cause us pain or suffering. Essentially, we attempt to fight against fate. As soon as we can find another focus, give up our tense defensive posture, and trust fate, our inner constriction disappears along with our fear. This must be accomplished in small increments at every possible opportunity; the following essences are helpful. (Further remarks → Chapter 1: Aspen and Mimulus)

of being seen through: **Agrimony**
Agrimony is for people who do not dare to show their feelings or admit the truth about themselves.

vague fears: **Aspen** (→ **Premonitions**)
Aspen is helpful when we suffer from terrible, anxious, and seemingly groundless fears. It is generally combined with Mimulus.

of making the wrong decision: **Cerato**
We always want to be right and fear making mistakes.

of going insane: **Cherry Plum**
When strong emotions are suppressed, there is the danger of a resulting emotional short circuit.

of loss: **Chicory**
The more our hearts become attached to something, the more we fear losing it. Chicory helps us let go and allows us to be free.

of impurities, sins, or contagion: **Crab Apple**

Crab Apple is for people who have an excessive fear of the consequences of a "sin" or an impure act.

of disgrace: **Heather (→ Recognition → Inferiority, feelings of)**

People with low self-esteem live with a constant fear of making fools of themselves. Heather tempers vanity and the craving for recognition.

of failure: **Hornbeam**

Hornbeam helps if a task seems too difficult before we even begin.

of failure: **Elm + Hornbeam + Larch**

Fear of failure is characterized by the interplay of several factors. Larch helps with undeveloped self-confidence, Hornbeam helps with feelings of overexertion, and Elm helps with the danger of an acute collapse.

of particular things: **Mimulus**

Mimulus is suitable for specific fears as well as for treating the general constitution of anxious individuals.

of punishment: **Pine (→ Guilt Feelings)**

Guilt feelings or a bad conscience are both manifestations of a fear of punishment. Pine frees us from guilty thoughts.

for others: **Red Chestnut**

When we fear for the sake of others, we are projecting our own fears on them.

with feelings of panic: **Rock Rose, Aspen**

Rock Rose is appropriate in sudden and unusual situations when we can lose our sense of perspective. Aspen helps when submerged fears suddenly take on a paniclike urgency. When in doubt, take a combination of the essences (→ 2/26).

due to unresolved shock: **Star of Bethlehem**

Fear is a defense mechanism. Unresolved traumas or shocks are essentially psychic allergies: they make us unstable, and even the most seemingly insignificant memories can trigger a massive defensive reaction.

of intimate contact: **Water Violet**

Water Violet is for loners or people for whom contact with other people is too much.

anxious depression *2/21
anxious obsequiousness *4/20

anxious insecurity *5/20
anxious clinging *8/20
anxious irritability *15/20
anxious restlessness *18/20
anxious worry about others *20/25
anxious obsessive thoughts *20/35
fear of cancer → Cancer
fears, secret *1/2
fears that are covered up or suppressed *1/2
fear is covered up or kept secret *1/20
fear with the danger of a short circuit *2/6
panic, absolute, caused by fear *2/26
fears causing problems with human contact *2/34
fear-related conflict, serious *6/20
fear of dirtiness *10/20
fear of failure, sudden *11/20
fear of loneliness making us pushy and insistent *14/20
fear of the future provoking an escape into the past *16/20
fear of failure *17/20
fear due to a lack of self-confidence *19/20
fear and exhaustion *20/23
fear of guilt *20/24
fear of an impaired ability to make decisions *20/28
easily influenced due to fear *20/33
timidity, general: Mimulus
timidity, total *2/20
timidity causing an unnatural tolerance *3/20
timidity with a tendency to panic *20/26
timidity due to psychic trauma *20/29

Fearful: Aspen + Gentian + Larch + Mustard (→ Fear)

This combination makes life more bearable by minimizing our frightened premonitions and negative expectations. It should be taken over a long period of time, and is often used for children.

Fidgetiness: Impatiens + Scleranthus + Wild Oat

Filth, feelings of, with self-loathing *10/19

Finickiness → Indecisiveness

when we don't know what's right: Cerato
when we cannot make decisions: Scleranthus
when we don't know what we want: Wild Oat

Fixations → Obsession

*fixations *31/35*

Fleeing → Cowardice

When we are faced with danger, there are two choices: fight or run. Both are equally effective as survival tactics. Which act is the better of the two depends on our dispositions and on the specific situation. Flight becomes bad only when it is not necessary. In that case, we should look for ground-less fears that cause us to react inappropriately.

from ourselves: **Agrimony**

Agrimony helps when we cannot stand our own problems and weaknesses.

from reality into dreams: **Clematis, Honeysuckle**

For people who find reality too unpleasant or uninteresting and take refuge in dreaming of the past (Honeysuckle) or in the prospect of a better future (Clematis). Honeysuckle and Clematis are often used to treat children.

escape into illness: **Hornbeam**

An illness will often provide a way out and save us from a situation that we feel we cannot handle. Hornbeam alleviates our fear of failure.

*escape into the past due to stress and overwork *16/17*
*escape into the past caused by a lack of self-confidence *16/19*
*escape into the past caused by fear of the present or future
   16/20
*flight into the past caused by exhaustion *16/23*

Flexibility

If we are flexible and malleable, we have no clear limits to our actions. If we're too rigid and inflexible, we run the danger of "breaking."

too much: **Scleranthus**

Scleranthus eases excess mental agility, erratic behavior, and a tendency to shy away from important decisions.

too little

Oak when we don't know how to give up

Rock Water to broaden our intellectual horizons if we are rigidly self-disciplined

Vervain for people who are narrow-minded and tend to pursue one specific idea

Vine against inflexible, rigid dogmatism

Flighty and Impatient → 18/28

Flu → Contagion

prevention: Clematis + Crab Apple + Olive + Walnut

Clematis for strengthening our resolve to stay healthy

Crab Apple for promoting purification of the blood and helping divert contagions

Olive to give us reserves of strength

Walnut for strengthening our immune system against pathogens

This combination provides us with some preventive protection. It must be taken at the first sign of an illness and complemented with another essence, such as those listed below.

Chicory for a conspicuous craving for love or comfort

Elm for sudden exhaustion

Holly for groundless irritability

Mustard for an inexplicable bad mood

Water Violet to treat the need for quiet and the need to be left alone

treatment

Use those essences listed under *prevention* that are appropriate for the psychic or physical condition. Also use Gentian in case of a prolonged illness or a relapse.

Forgetfulness

caused by suppression: Agrimony

Suppression is a kind of deliberate forgetfulness and is sometimes necessary to maintain inner peace. This capability is useful, however, only when it is employed consciously; otherwise it can lead to destructive habits.

caused by learning difficulties: **Chestnut Bud**
caused by daydreaming: **Clematis, Honeysuckle**

Clematis is useful when the mind is dominated by fantasy and speculation, and Heather when the mind is dominated by memories.

caused by difficulties with concentration: **Scleranthus**

Scleranthus improves the ability to think clearly and decisively.

due to exhaustion: **Star of Bethlehem**

Sometimes the psyche causes us to be forgetful in order to protect itself from a traumatic experience. This type of forgetfulness (amnesia) also occurs in cases of head trauma.

Frantic Activity: Vervain

Vervain is useful when we become too active because of some conviction or enthusiasm.

Frigidity → Sexual Dysfunction

Frustration → Discontentment

Gall Conditions → Liver Conditions

Giving Up (prematurely)

with acute feelings of overexertion: **Elm**
from a lack of endurance: **Gentian**
due to anxiety: **Mimulus**
due to exhaustion: **Olive**

Glaucoma → Eye Conditions

Glossing Over: Agrimony + Beech (*1/3)

Some people have a cheerful, even temperament and seem to have no problems, while others act as they do only because they do not want to face their problems. They internalize their problems and make themselves suffer even more. The spirit will not allow itself to be deceived—it accepts only the truth.

Goal Orientation, too strong

when we need to finish everything as quickly as possible and are in a constant rush: **Impatiens** *when we are so engrossed in pursuing our goals that we are on the verge of tearing ourselves apart:* Oak

when we are obsessed with an idea: Vervain

Going Crazy (danger of): Cherry Plum

Good-naturedness, affability, excessive: Centaury (→ Conformity)

Affability loses its value when it makes us unable to protect our own interests. Thinking of ourselves is a natural instinct. It doesn't mean being egotistical or coldhearted, but prudently ensuring everyone's well-being. "Love your neighbor as you would yourself"; if we can't help ourselves, we certainly can't help anyone else. Centaury helps counter pathological good cheer.

affability, pathological *1/4

Gratitude → Ingratitude

True gratitude means spontaneously being happy over a gift or a good deed without feeling obligated to return the favor. This is more difficult than we might think, since in our society, most gifts are given with the intention of making the recipient dependent or of obliging them to respond with a counter gesture. This is the spirit that gives rise to run-of-the-mill false gratitude—the feeling that one has not earned the right to be happy and that the gift might be taken away from us if we don't act gratefully and obsequiously.

feigned: Agrimony

When we feign gratitude because we are afraid or because we need a favor, we need Agrimony. It helps us to be more open and honest.

false: Pine

The person brought up in a "Christian" manner, with deeply ingrained guilt feelings, constantly feels the need to express some kind of thanks (either through obsequious behavior or in returning the favor); he fears that his "God" will be angry with him otherwise. This behavior makes it difficult for him to experience true, free happiness (which is identical to true gratitude). Pine lessens the guilt feelings that cause this false gratitude.

Greed → Egotism

Grief → Separation → Loss

Grieving means not being able to accept reality; it is the untimely appreciation of someone or something precious and the concurrent reaction to its loss, which a lack of mental and emotional maturity makes extremely difficult. Instead of focusing positively on whatever has replaced what we've lost, we're stuck in a melancholy past. The dynamic progress of life loses its continuity and dissolves (like a movie that is running too slowly through a projector) into single frames of aspects and emotions taken out of life. We lose the ability to recognize the positive and beautiful aspects of life. Often, the standard grief that we think of is artificial and neurotic; it is instilled in us as we grow up and teaches us emotional dependence. We learn to suffer a guilty conscience if we don't grieve when we lose someone close to us. A unique example of the social significance of grief is the existence of professional mourners in many cultures, whose job it is to keep up appearances, both for society (the public) and for the deceased, whose wrath they fear (and who can still dominate and manipulate us from the grave). Self-pity is a "truer" form of grief, when we feel sad for ourselves and for the beautiful thing that we've lost. Not grieving is not necessarily a sign of coldness, but it can signify either that we've lost nothing significant or—and this is the "art" of life—that we cannot truly "lose" anything.

with self-pity: **Chicory**

The more we demand, the more we stand to lose. Chicory is for people who live off the emotions of other people, and it helps us become more independent and allows us to bear a blow with our own strength.

due to losing touch with reality: **Honeysuckle**

Honeysuckle helps us when we mourn a loss and cannot come to terms with the present. It can help us distance ourselves from the past.

with bitterness: **Willow**

People whose grief is mixed with bitterness are not capable of accepting their fate.

grief caused by the loss of love *8/16

Guilt Feelings → Conscience → Chapter 1: Pine

Guilt arises when we break a rule or a commandment; it is caused by the fear of punishment. Since all rules and prohibitions (even the so-called divine ones) are set down by people who are trying to defend their rights or privileges, guilt is essentially only an instrument used in the social struggle for power. When we look at guilt in this way, it loses its mystical "taboo" connotation, and it becomes easier to deal with. We get a clearer view of how we should act, and, if we've gone too far, we can try to right any wrongs we've committed or save ourselves. The demoralizing, "wrath of God" sort of guilt, which is a very popular weapon among moralists who despise the rest of us, simply does not exist. We all act the best we are able under particular circumstances. We are inextricably caught up in a lattice of joy and sorrow, right and wrong. These are the facts, and we're free to look at them in a positive or negative light. If we want to suffer, we judge ourselves; if we want happiness, we speak of fate, destiny, or misfortune and do not take on the responsibility for everything that happens in the world.

guilty conscience: **Pine**
Pine relieves a guilty conscience and makes us immune to people who want us to feel guilty.

causing in others: **Vine**
People who take their beliefs to be the absolute truth often try to make those who believe otherwise feel guilty.

guilt leading to self-sacrifice *4/24
guilt leading to insecurity *5/24
guilt creating fears *20/24
guilt causing depression *21/24
guilt complex, debilitating *23/24
guilt creating worries *24/25
guilt making us easily influenced *24/33
guilty compulsive thoughts *24/35

Habits and Routines

Habits are useful for establishing a certain amount of order in our lives, but they can be harmful when they become a meaningless routine or when they prevent us from making much-needed changes.

personal: **Chestnut Bud**
Chestnut Bud helps us when we are so thoughtlessly entrenched in our routines that we continually make the same mistakes.

collective habits or routines: **Walnut**

Walnut helps us find our own way when we are hindered by the pressure of tradition.

Hallucinations

terrifying fantasies or premonitions: **Aspen**
illusions and fantasies: **Clematis**

Harshness

against ourselves

> Oak for when our ambition causes us to place unrealistic or excessive demands and expectations on ourselves
>
> Rock Water for people who cannot reward themselves and who impose excessive self-discipline to be more "healthy" or to make examples of themselves

against others

> Holly when rage, envy, or the lust for revenge makes us treat others harshly
>
> Vine to make tyrants or dogmatic types more tolerant and tractable

Haste → Nervousness

due to fear: **Aspen, Mimulus**

Aspen helps with generalized fear that causes us to be nervous. Mimulus helps with specific fears.

due to impatience: **Impatiens**

Impatiens is for people who find that nothing happens quickly enough or that they are always rushing.

caused by indecisiveness: **Scleranthus**

When we can't figure out what we should do, we often find ourselves rushed or stressed. Scleranthus makes it easier for us to make decisions.

Hate → Aggression → Cold Emotions → Rage → Chapter 1: Holly

Aggressive behavior is natural and instinctive, and it serves to overcome any obstacles to achieving self-realization. If it is suppressed for a long period of time, it can turn into hate, which loses some of the competitive, gamelike aspect of aggression and is always somewhat destructive. There is a reason that we often speak of "deadly" hate. Of course, each individual's personality plays a role. Introverted, emotional people are just as capable of hating as more extroverted, rational types; the more intensively we're able to love, the more intensively we can hate as well. It is always better to stand up for our rights when someone treats us unjustly, instead of swallowing our rage and allowing it to ferment and turn into bitter hate. Likewise, we should never treat anyone (without having a good reason to do so) so as to arouse hate in them (keeping in mind that everyone feels justified where their own interests are concerned).

love-hate *8/15
hate and bitterness *15/38

Headaches

The following essences can be combined as needed.

for tension: Agrimony
for problems with concentration: Clematis
for feelings of stress and overwork and fear of failure: Elm
for nervousness or impatience: Impatiens
for grimness and stress-related tension: Oak
for guilt feelings: Pine
for excessive activity: Vervain
when we are thinking too strenuously: White Chestnut

Heart Conditions

All serious or recurring heart conditions should receive medical treatment and diagnosis. Bach flower treatment is meant to support proper medical treatment.

vague fears affecting the chest: Aspen

This type of fear is a warning sign and can signal an impending heart attack. Aspen can ease this fear (and the underlying complaint). When this fear appears frequently, special medical examinations are imperative. If the onset is sudden and severe → *heart attack.*

heart attack: Rescue Remedy + Elm + Holly + Willow

A heart attack can be relatively severe or light. Less severe ones can occur without us even noticing them. They cause a certain amount of pain in the area of the heart that passes with time. Special medical examinations are recommended when the pain or discomfort increases under strenuous (emotional or physical) conditions. When the body is under physical strain and the symptoms disappear, the condition is relatively harmless. A more serious heart attack causes more severe, often debilitating pain in the chest. We feel as if we are about to die. See a doctor immediately. Keep quiet and comfortable—half sitting—breathe comfortably, and take Rescue Remedy (if possible, together with Elm), three drops every five to twenty minutes on the tongue or the lips. After the acute symptoms pass, take Holly and Willow, because a heart attack is generally the result of some kind of anger, aggravation, insult, or defeat.

palpitations

Agrimony + Impatiens + Oak + Vervain with stress

Aspen + Impatiens + Rock Rose with panic

irregular heartbeats or arrhythmia

Any sign of an irregular heartbeat is cause for a thorough medical examination. The following essences are recommended for less severe cases or to supplement medical treatment.

Crab Apple for purification of the blood

Many cases of irregular heart rhythms are caused by chronic infections.

Olive to lend more strength to the heart

Rescue Remedy to prevent a deterioration of the condition for severe cases

Scleranthus for normalization

weak heart: Olive

Olive is an excellent choice for any kind of general weakness, even when related to the heart. Signs of a weak heart are shortness of breath with physical exertion, swollen legs in the evening, or the necessity to sleep with the trunk elevated.

Heartbreak → Partner Problems

There are two forms of love: requited, where we love and are loved in return, and unrequited, where we love and are not loved in return. In both forms, the feelings of love start from within and cannot be aroused or fed from outside sources; because of this, they make us happy—each in his or her own way. As soon as we begin to demand love, however, instead of merely giving it, it causes heartbreak and becomes a thing to be coveted. When we covet, it means we want to possess, and we become unhappy when we want to possess something we can't have. Heartbreak is not a sign of love but a sign that we covet something that we can't have. We expect from someone something that they can't give us (love cannot be switched on and off at will), and the resulting disappointment makes us ill. Instead of learning from this suffering that we've had the wrong attitude and trying to adjust, our unhappiness increases, and we are stricken with feelings of "unrequited love." The solution is either that we set the object of our desire free or that we allow ourselves to be happy with the well-being and happiness of our beloved without feeling possessiveness.

hidden and ignored: **Agrimony**
Agrimony helps us when we suffer from unrequited love but try to keep it hidden, which only strengthens our suffering and prevents a resolution.

with hysterical symptoms: **Cherry Plum**
Passion that is suppressed or kept secret can create such strong emotional pressure that we can become downright "possessed" or crazy, or at least on the verge of hysteria (→ Hysteria).

with possessiveness and self-pity: **Chicory**
Chicory is helpful when love is characterized by possessiveness and turns into self-pity.

with discouragement: **Gentian**
When we become discouraged from misunderstandings in the process of "wooing" someone, Gentian can bolster our perseverance.

leading to hopelessness: **Gorse**
Gentian is appropriate when a disappointment in love has made us lose hope that we'll ever love again.

with compulsive thoughts: **White Chestnut**
When we can think only about our love problems and cannot concentrate on anything else, White Chestnut can clear the mind and spirit.

with resentment and bitterness: **Willow**
Willow helps us weather disappointments in love without bitterness.

heartbreak making us depressed *8/21

Heartbreak, secret: Agrimony (→ Depression → Worries)

Agrimony helps people who try to hide or suppress their worries, needs, or pain and suffer silently. It allows us to express ourselves, lighten our load, and find the way to solve our problems. It is often combined with Walnut (1/33).

Helplessness: Cerato

helplessness due to inattentiveness *5/7

Hesitation

due to insecurity: Cerato
due to indecisiveness: Scleranthus
due to timidity: Mimulus

Homesickness: Honeysuckle

Honeysuckle lets our pleasant memories fade away when they prevent us from finding happiness in the present or from being grounded in reality.

Hope, lack of → Pessimism

If only we could learn to expect nothing, to be able to give up our hopes when necessary, and to realize how insignificant our daily fears and problems really are. Normally, though, we're not able to do this. Instead of soaring like eagles, we crawl drearily through life like lowly earthworms, drawn slowly forward by the hope of better times. Hope signifies progress and growth and provides our inspiration for living. It gives us optimism and strength, and losing it is perilous. Hope is especially important during an illness. When we're ill and without hope, we're almost certain not to recover.

due to failure: Gentian

Failure and setbacks give us the opportunity to exercise our strengths and abilities. Understood properly, they can help us to make our future better, but when they cause us to be discouraged, Gentian can help by making us more optimistic and able to ride out the bad times. Combined with Chestnut Bud, it can help improve the learning process.

total: Gorse

People who have lost all hope and live only for the sake of their friends and family need Gentian. It is especially helpful for serious, hopeless illnesses.

due to depression: Mustard

When the black clouds of depression follow us everywhere and we lose hope of improvement, Mustard can help us become happier and more optimistic.

and absolute desperation: **Sweet Chestnut**

Sweet Chestnut is needed when we are desperate and hopeless and everything seems to have lost its meaning.

with resignation: **Wild Rose**

Hopelessness can be the manifestation of a general sense of resignation. We merely exist, lose all our hopes, and are not interested in anything. Wild Rose can reawaken our hopes and our interest in life.

hopelessness making us compliant and tractable *4/13
hopelessness, sudden, caused by stress and overwork *11/13
hopelessness and weak will *12/13
hopelessness making us depressed *13/21
hopelessness due to exhaustion *13/23
hopelessness due to a severe trauma *13/29

Hopelessness: Sweet Chestnut

Sweet Chestnut helps in the case of absolute desperation, when we feel we just can't go on. Combine with Rock Rose (*26/30) for accompanying feelings of panic and Elm (*11/30) when preceded by excessive stress.

Horror → Premonitions and Foreboding → Fear → Panic → Shock

Humiliation, consequences of: Heather

When we are vain, we can easily be humiliated. Heather suppresses vanity, and is often combined with Larch.

humiliation leaving behind a psychic trauma *14/29

Humility, false → Servility → Obsequiousness

True humility means giving ourselves up to and trusting, joyfully and willingly, a "divine" authority that orders and connects all things, because we know that the intentions of this higher authority are good and we recognize our own limitations. False humility, on the other hand, is a type of subjugation that takes place only through our own weaknesses; we want to buy ourselves the good graces of those to whom we subjugate ourselves (God, for example).

due to an undeveloped personality: **Centaury**
Centaury allows us to develop the consciousness of our rights and needs; only then is true, free humility possible.

due to guilt feelings: **Pine**
Pine alleviates our guilt feelings, which bring forth false humility.

demanded of others: **Vine**
Dogmatically religious types who demand humility in others essentially want other people to submit to their own convictions.

due to apathy and resignation: **Wild Rose**
Wild Rose is effective against stifled, resigned devotion, which is often misconstrued for humility.

Humorlessness

Having a sense of humor is being able to laugh in spite of everything. Certain people lose their sense of humor quite easily. It becomes difficult for them to laugh (especially about themselves) because they are too sensitive or too stubborn. They should, however, make a conscious effort to ensure that their tendency to take things too seriously doesn't become a habit.

due to being overly sensitive: **Chicory**
People who are overly sensitive generally cannot laugh about pain, sorrow, or unhappiness. Chicory can assuage self-pitying melancholy, give us a little distance from our pain, and ensure that we don't become mired in negativity.

with melancholy: **Mustard**

with a tendency to make our lives too hard: **Rock Water**
Rock Water is for people who inflict severe self-discipline on themselves and lose the ability to laugh at their own mistakes.

dogmatic: **Vine**
People who insist that everything must go according to their plans often find it difficult to laugh when things go wrong.

from being offended or insulted: **Willow**
Willow can prevent us from being too easily offended and keep us from losing our sense of humor when we are faced with unpleasant surprises.

Hyperactivity → Obsession → Impatience
hyperactivity, mental *18/35

Hypersensitivity, psychic (physical → Allergies)

Oversensitivity usually serves a protective function (it's often said that the best defense is a good offense). It also indicates a personal weakness.

caused by a lack of love: **Chicory, Heather**

Chicory helps mitigate an excessive need for attention; it's helpful for anyone, especially children, who take even the most normal, trivial lapses of attention as signs of the loss of love.

Heather is for people who always want to be popular.

to failure: **Gentian**

Gentian is helpful when we take failure or problems too seriously.

caused by disregard: **Heather**

People who suffer from a pathological need for recognition cannot stand it when they don't receive attention.

to belittlement: **Larch**

When we feel inferior, we are especially hurt when we feel left out or undervalued.

to criticism: **Pine**

Pine minimizes the tendency to suffer from a guilty conscience and to overreact to accusations of any kind.

to negative experiences: **Star of Bethlehem**

When we are too easily shaken from a traumatic experience, Star of Bethlehem is helpful.

to being influenced: **Walnut**

Walnut helps us become more thick-skinned.

Hypertension → (High) Blood Pressure

Hypocrisy → Artificiality

Hypotension → (Low) Blood Pressure

Hysteria: Cherry Plum (→ Menopause)

Hysteria is extreme (and inappropriate) emotional behavior, which can serve as a release valve for pent-up emotions or drives. You could look at it as a raging stream that has been dammed up and needs an appropriate outlet. Often, there are sexual drives at work (the word *hyster* means "womb"), but fears and anxieties can also be important factors. Both women and men are susceptible to hysteria.

Idealism, extreme

when we see the world through rose-colored glasses: Beech
when we deny ourselves for some "higher" ideal: Rock Water
when we want to impose our ideals on others: Vervain

Illness

We must keep two things in mind if we want to use Bach flowers properly: the current psychic condition and the underlying causes for that condition.

with fear or panic: Aspen, Mimulus, Rock Rose
Emotional factors give rise to illness or a toxic reaction.

with a need for attention or sympathy: Chicory
Some people (especially children) become ill because they aren't receiving enough attention or because they need sympathy. By being ill, they hope to receive the love and attention that they feel is being withheld from them.

with a death wish: Clematis
People who find the struggle for survival too difficult often hope for a solution in death.

due to excessive stress: Elm
Psychic stress is harmful when it exceeds our tolerance. As a built-in protective mechanism, the psyche then transforms psychic stress into a physical form. Elm helps mitigate pathological stress and gives us the strength to endure an illness. Elm is used as a basic treatment for all serious, acute illnesses.

with hopelessness: Gorse
Hopelessness impairs the immune system.

due to humiliation and embarrassment: Heather
Humiliation can cut some people so deeply that they can become seriously—even fatally—ill, especially with heart and lung conditions (→ Heart Conditions → Lung Conditions).

hot-tempered and aggressive: Holly
An illness can strike violently and suddenly and/or we can become noticeably irritated or unbearable or angry.

due to rage or anger: Holly
Aggression can cause physical symptoms if it is not released immediately.

due to overexertion and exhaustion: Olive

Illness serves the function of taking us out of circulation when our strength is drained, allowing us an opportunity to recuperate.

due to guilt feelings: Pine

A bad conscience can weaken our immunity to the point that we become ill. This is often seen as a kind of penance. An illness can also be a way of avoiding an unpleasant penalty.

due to worry: Red Chestnut

We really can worry ourselves sick. Lung conditions are especially common in people who worry excessively.

shocking experience: Star of Bethlehem

Unprocessed shock or trauma can trigger an illness or remain as inner wounds, which the organism will try to neutralize or divert in the form of physical or psychic symptoms.

with a tendency to withdrawal: Water Violet

Certain types of people don't want sympathy or tend to withdraw when they're ill or are experiencing problems. Water Violet is the right choice for any illness for these types.

with resignation: Wild Rose

Resignation signifies the loss of the will to become healthy, and it can impede the healing process. It plays a decisive role in life-threatening illnesses and is one of the real (albeit hidden) causes of cancer.

due to disappointment: Willow

Severe disappointment can undermine the will to live. Sometimes an illness will be a way of getting back at someone.

chronic illnesses

When an illness becomes chronic, it's a sign that the organism is under heavy attack. Some chronic illnesses can last for years, or even a lifetime, and lead to a loss of strength and happiness. Often, it is a sign that we're unable to come to terms with life. Healing requires not just the restoration of physical health but also increasing our awareness, wisdom, and insight into our own fate. In the end, an illness can bring about a fundamental change and the realization of the transcendent self within us.

Crab Apple for general purification of the blood

Crab Apple stimulates the elimination of pathogens and toxins that can accumulate during an illness and can serve to worsen the situation. In any chronic conditions, the function of the detoxification organs is impaired, which causes a vicious cycle:

- reduced ability to eliminate toxins
- worsening of the illness
- deterioration of the detoxifying organs

The body will often attempt to detoxify through the skin in the form of rashes, eczema, pimples, or pus. Crab Apple must be taken for a long period of time for detoxification. It is especially useful when the patient feels herself to be impure or "poisoned."

> Gentian + Gorse + Mustard + Olive + Wild Rose for long-lasting illnesses that resist treatment

This combination can help restore our will to live and our healing powers, especially when we no longer have the strength to recuperate.

Illusions → Fantasies

Immodesty: Chicory (→ Modesty)

Chicory is for people who have such a great need for attention and for emotional relationships that they can't keep a proper sense of proportion with regard to their demands.

Impatience: Impatiens (→ Uneasiness)

impatient and irritable *15/18
impatient and flighty *18/28

Imposing One's Will → Know-it-all

Impotence → Sexual Dysfunction

Impurity, thoughts of, oppressive *10/35

Inattentiveness → Learning Difficulties → Daydreams

inattentiveness causing helplessness *5/7
inattentiveness with daydreaming *7/9

inattentiveness with weak will *7/12*
inattentiveness due to nostalgic dreaminess *7/16*
inattentiveness caused by compulsive thoughts *7/35*
inattentiveness preventing formation of clear life goals *7/36*

Inconsistency

caused by an inability to make decisions: Scleranthus
caused by being too easily influenced: Walnut
caused by lack of life goals: Wild Oat

Indecisiveness

Some people by nature find it difficult to make a definite decision because they have the ability to see the various and contradictory sides of a problem or situation. They can bring themselves to make a firm decision, or at least to reach a compromise, only after a complicated mental process. They embody the principle of justice, which painstakingly weighs all the pros and cons before reaching a judgment. Eventually, the scales must tip in one direction or the other; life is impossible without making decisions.

due to a lack of clarity: Cerato
Cerato is for people whose fear of making mistakes is so great that they don't trust their own feelings, and thus they try to cover their bases in every conceivable way. In doing so, they are confronted with so many contradictory opinions that they have no idea what they should do.

due to pessimism: Gentian
Gentian prevents us from becoming too discouraged from failure (and thereby becoming unable to decide how to act).

due to a lack of self-confidence: Larch
Insufficient self-confidence in our own ability to think critically and to act often leads us to not dare to make decisions.

due to mental instability: Scleranthus
Scleranthus is a basic treatment for problems with decision making. It is especially helpful when we are not able to choose from many possibilities.

with the lack of a life concept: Wild Oat
When we lack a grasp of life's "big picture," we often find ourselves unable to know which path to choose or unable to make a decision. Wild Oat brings us more clarity.

*indecisiveness due to general fears *2/28*
*indecisiveness due to insecurity *5/28*
*indecisiveness due to specific fear *20/28*

Indifference → Giving up → Interest, lack of → Resignation

Infallibility → Dogmatism

Infection → Contagion → Flu

Inferiority, feelings of: Larch (→ Vanity → Recognition, need for → Compete, inability to)

Social standing plays an important role in the human struggle for survival, because it determines which of life's advantages we are entitled to. The desire for a "higher" position in society is the expression of a natural vitality; to claim and maintain this position requires a certain amount of self-confidence. If we don't feel strong or superior, we won't have the strength of will to claim what is ours. People who lack confidence in themselves, especially children, will never be able to assert themselves in this way. Parents should take special care not to undermine a child's self-confidence through humiliation or suppression. Larch is the main essence for treating a lack of self-confidence or an inferiority complex.

triggering excessive need for recognition: Heather + Larch (*14/19)
*suppressed feelings of inferiority *1/19*
*feelings of inferiority making us unnaturally tolerant *3/19*
*feelings of inferiority causing an excessive willingness or need to help *4/19*
*feelings of inferiority leading to insecurity *5/19*
*feelings of inferiority causing us to feel unclean *10/19*
*feelings of inferiority suppressed to show off *14/19*
*feelings of inferiority and fleeing into the past *16/19*
*feelings of inferiority leading to stress and overwork *17/19*
*feelings of inferiority due to moral scruples *19/24*

feelings of inferiority due to placing idealistic demands on oneself *19/27*

feelings of inferiority leading to problems with human contact *19/34*

Inflexibility → Stubbornness

Influenced, too easily

with an undeveloped personality: Centaury

Centaury prevents us from being used by others.

due to insecurity: Cerato

Cerato gives us more faith in our own feelings and makes us less dependent on the opinions of others.

even though we really know what we want: Walnut

Walnut helps us set limits against outside influences and allows us to follow our own path.

easily influenced and dependent *4/33*
easily influenced from a lack of self-confidence *19/33*
easily influenced owing to anxiety *20/33*
easily influenced as the result of exhaustion *23/33*
due to insecurity *5/33*

Inhibitions → Distance

due to feelings of inferiority: Larch

Larch helps strengthen our self-confidence when we are inhibited because we feel ourselves to be inferior or less capable than others.

due to difficulties with human contact: Water Violet

Water Violet helps us when we are inhibited in social situations and when our introverted nature makes it difficult for us to make social contact.

Initiative, insufficient

caused by failure: Gentian

Gentian restores our enthusiasm when we become discouraged by difficulties or failure.

due to stress and overwork: Hornbeam

Hornbeam counters the crippling feeling that we are not up to meeting the challenges of everyday life.

due to a lack of self-confidence: **Larch**

Larch brings us more enthusiasm by restoring our confidence in our abilities.

due to depression: **Mustard**

due to a general feeling of resignation: **Wild Rose**

Wild Rose awakens the life spirit when we have lost our enthusiasm and just plod through life.

Injuries: Star of Bethlehem (→ Emergencies)

Star of Bethlehem helps treat the consequences of an accident, whether they are physical or spiritual in nature. It should always be used when a disruption occurs as the result of a traumatic event, accident, or shock. For acute injuries, it's best to use Rescue Remedy (which contains Star of Bethlehem).

vulnerability caused by excessive timidity *2/29

emotional injury leading to psychosis *6/29

Insecurity → Fear → Instability

glossed over: **Agrimony**

Sometimes we need to pretend that we're secure even though we're quaking in our boots. In the long term, this will result in harmful stress because we have to deal with our own stress as well as the suspicions of others. Agrimony allows us to show our insecurity.

due to a lack of self-confidence: **Cerato**

Cerato helps when we don't trust our own instincts and look for help and advice wherever we can find it.

due to a need for recognition: **Heather**

A strong need for recognition is often motivated by an equally strong fear of disrespect, which can cause insecurity. Heather helps us acknowledge that we don't need to seem so high and mighty.

due to feelings of inferiority: **Larch**

We can be relaxed and at peace only when we feel that we are confident and capable. Larch helps restore our self-confidence.

due to fear: **Mimulus**

due to indecisiveness: **Scleranthus**

due to bad experiences: **Star of Bethlehem**

When we cannot work though a devastating or traumatic experience, it continues to affect us internally and create insecurity.

caused by being too easily influenced: Walnut

Walnut is for people who are too easily made insecure and dissuaded from their plans or desires.

due to the lack of life goals: Wild Oat

Wild Oat helps us become confident and secure with respect to our long-term life goals.

insecurity caused by feelings of inferiority *5/19
insecurity caused by fear *5/20
insecurity caused by the fear of a guilty conscience *5/24
insecurity with indecisiveness *5/28
insecurity caused by a shocking experience *5/29
insecurity due to being too easily influenced *5/33
insecurity due to lack of an overall life concept *5/36

Insomnia

Insomnia has many possible causes. Next to organic causes (liver/gall, lungs, intestines, thyroid), psychic factors play an important role. The mind cannot relax as long as it's preoccupied with a serious problem; it's better to avoid these troubling thoughts in the night. When we wake up between 11 P.M. and 3 A.M., it's a sign that there is a problem in the liver/gallbladder system. If we wake up between 3 A.M. and 5 A.M., it's a sign of stress and worries.

due to problems kept secret: Agrimony
due to mulling over our worries: Elm
due to anger and rage: Holly
due to a general feeling of stress and overwork: Hornbeam
due to general restlessness and nervousness: Impatiens
due to fear: Mimulus
caused by depression: Mustard
caused by a weakness of the heart: Olive
caused by a guilt complex: Pine
caused by worrying about others: Red Chestnut
caused by mental overstimulation: White Chestnut
caused by bitterness and resentment: Willow

Instability

Instability should not be confused with flexibility. Flexibility means the ability to adapt appropriately to constantly changing life situations. Instability means drifting about like a boat in a stormy sea and being unable to navigate properly; we can find ourselves in situations we don't want to be in.

when our insecurity makes us continually seek advice: **Cerato**
when we have no endurance and give up at the first sign of difficulties: **Gentian**
when we do not dare to stand our ground because of a lack of self-confidence: **Larch**
when we are indecisive and too easily distracted: **Scleranthus**
when a traumatic experience causes us to lose our psychic stability: **Star of Bethlehem**
when we are too easily influenced: **Walnut**
when we don't know what we want and constantly change our plans: **Wild Oat**

Interest, lack of

due to an insufficient hunger for knowledge: **Chestnut Bud**
Chestnut Bud makes us more attentive and able to learn from our experiences.
lack of interest in the present due to dreams of the future: **Clematis**
When we are so caught up in dreams and fantasies of a wonderful future that we are not interested in the present, Clematis can turn our attention to reality.
due to persistent thoughts of the past: **Honeysuckle** (→ Homesickness → Grief → Loss)
Honeysuckle lets our memories fade until they assume the proper proportion so that they don't interfere with our view of the present.

Intestinal Conditions

diarrhea
Aspen (terrible, general), Mimulus (from a clear cause), or Rock Rose (panic) when due to fear
Star of Bethlehem when due to an unhappy life

constipation
   Agrimony when due to tension
   Aspen (terrible, general) Mimulus (clear cause) when due to fear
   Crab Apple for general purifying and cleansing
   Crab Apple + Mimulus when due to imposed morality and guilt feelings
   Oak when due to doggedness and stubbornness
   Olive + Wild Rose when due to weakness

Intolerance → Allergies

Intolerance can be reasonable and even necessary when we are in danger of losing our independence, but as soon as it becomes a habit, it can isolate us and even turn us into enemies. Allergies are a form of intolerance: the body simply can't abide certain substances. Mental intolerance can be inborn, or it can be the result of a psychic trauma that has led to a pathological change in attitudes. For example, overstimulated nerves can cause us to have an intolerance to noise, or, if we've been deceived by someone, we can develop an intolerance to dishonesty.

internalized and glossed over: **Beech**

Beech helps resolve intolerance that is deep-seated and integrated into our character. It is generally not a conscious phenomenon and is often masked by an exaggerated false tolerance. Beech should be taken for any form of intolerance or allergies, either alone or in combination with any of the following appropriate essences.

against oneself: **Rock Water**

People who impose strict discipline on themselves cannot stand certain qualities or characteristics about themselves. They try to suppress or overcome these characteristics by holding one-sided attitudes or maintaining extreme lifestyles. In doing this, they lose the "wholeness" of their being.

caused by missionary zeal: **Vervain**

Vervain is for people who are so sure of the "rightness" of their own convictions that they feel that everyone else will benefit from them. This is a diplomatic way of saying that they impose their ideas on others.

the closed-minded know-it-all: **Vine**

Vine is indicated when we can't listen to anyone's opinions but our own.

intolerance, total *3/32
intolerant behavior *31/32

Irrational Behavior → Obsession → Tension
irrational behavior due to fear *2/6

Irritability → Aggression
general: Holly
caused by impatience: Impatiens
irritated due to fear *15/20
irritated and impatient *15/28
irritable do-gooder *15/32

Isolation: Agrimony + Water Violet (→ Loneliness → Loner → Companionship)

Itching → Skin Conditions

Jealousy

Jealousy is a trait in humans and in animals. It is one of the basic reactions in nature and an instinctive reaction when our existence is threatened. We react jealously when something essential to our existence is taken from us or withheld from us. For an infant, it is a matter of survival to fight for its mother's essential love. For adults, it is threatening to their existence to lose the goodwill and attention of those on whom their material, spiritual, or emotional life depends; in such cases, we react aggressively and try to defend our rights. Despite this natural justification, jealousy can lose its lifesaving essence when it becomes excessive or arises for no reason. Inappropriate or excessive acquisitiveness or pathological anxiety often lead us to feel more threatened than we actually are—and this means that we become more jealous than we need to be, and we react more forcefully than is called for.

due to an excessive need for attention: Chicory
Chicory suppresses any pathological need for love that gives rise to jealousy at the sign of restrictions. Children often need Chicory, which can be favorably combined with Holly (8/15) or Willow (8/38).

aggressive: Holly

Anyone who manifests their jealousy aggressively needs Holly.

Joy, lack of → Depression

Joy means life. A lack of joy is dangerous—directly or indirectly—in the long term.

bad moods and depression: Mustard
guilt feelings: Pine
caused by worrying: Red Chestnut
caused by excessive self-discipline: Rock Water
due to a lack of meaning or purpose in life: Wild Oat

Kidney Conditions

Kidneys are primarily made up of arterial blood vessels, and, for this reason, every reaction of the blood vessels affects the kidneys as well. This is especially well known in the case of high blood pressure (→ Blood Pressure), which can cause and be caused by kidney problems. There is a definite connection between the kidneys and circulation; when one deteriorates, the other often does as well. Kidney conditions that can be caused by a cold are also related to the blood vessels. Psychic problems (especially stress and fear, which also increase the blood pressure) that are characterized by increased urine production are connected to the kidneys. In such conditions, it is notable that water (light urine) is produced not to excrete toxins, but to unload ballast and perhaps (in a biological sense) to "mark" territory.

The battle for territory and dominance in our sphere of influence is the cause of most work-related stress. Occasionally, stress-related tension is so strong that it can cause colic (abdominal pain). We use the same Bach flowers for kidney ailments that we use for stress that can overstimulate the kidneys and bladder. Sometimes mental or emotional stress is so strong that we feel we can't stand it. In general, the cause is a severe loss, which is akin to the body "losing" material through the kidneys. As a rule, the harshest and least bearable loss for humans is the loss of love or attention; many kidney ailments stem from human conflict. People who are dependent upon attention and recognition are especially susceptible to such ailments. Any Bach flower treatment that tries to treat kidney problems should have the goals of reducing stress (→ Stress → Blood Pressure) and restoring inner balance, minimizing our fears (→ Fear → Shock), and renewing human relationships (→ Partner Problems → Vanity). The appropriate essences are listed under the sections mentioned in parentheses. Crab Apple provides a general boost to kidney function and is effective in purifying the blood, and Olive strengthens the heart.

Know-it-all

with missionary zeal: Vervain
Vervain is for people who meddle in the lives of others and who think they know what's best for everyone.

petty and humorless: Vine

Learning Difficulties → Concentration, difficulties with → Forgetfulness

learning difficulties due to shirking *1/7
learning difficulties due to daydreaming *7/9
learning difficulties due to nostalgia *7/16
learning difficulties due to being too easily distracted *7/28
learning difficulties due to a lack of interest in life *7/37

Life, interest in, lacking, with learning difficulties *7/37

Life, meaning of, lacking → Purpose in Life

Life Change, postponed owing to discouragement *12/33 → New Beginnings

Life Crisis, with inner turmoil *28/36 → Crisis

Liver Conditions

Bach flower therapy is geared toward treating psychic symptoms, but because of the connection between body and spirit, they also have effects on the body. To treat ourselves properly, we should ask what purpose the illness is trying to achieve and what psychic equivalent a physical illness might have. The most common emotional causes of liver ailments are negative emotions, jealousy, greed, and stress (→ Illness).

due to humiliation: **Heather + Willow**

The liver has a certain connection to pride; humiliation will trigger an intense counterreaction, which consists primarily of infection or inflammation. This combination limits the craving for recognition and the tendency to take offense too easily.

with irritability due to anger, rage, or envy: **Holly**

When we are forced to deal with something we cannot cope with ("digest"), we can seethe with rage. This is commonly called a "choleric" reaction. The liver/gall system is geared to digesting heavy loads; when it is not successful, the result can be swelling, blockage, or irritation. The situation is similar with jealousy and greed; they correspond to a kind of psychic binge eating and can result in hyperactivity in the liver/gall system and produce the same blockages, infections, or stones. In unfavorable cases, a bile color or jaundice in the blood can develop so that, as the saying goes, we become green with envy or anger. Holly is the basic essence for treating all kinds of negative emotions.

due to being in a constant rush: **Impatiens**

Being in a constant rush leads to excessive activity in the liver/gall system and can result in tension, blockages, and infections. Impatiens can prevent these effects by making us calmer and more patient.

with depression: **Mustard**

Liver/gall ailments often trigger sad or depressive moods, which we also call melancholia (black, blocked gallbladder). Mustard can help reduce melancholic moods.

with exhaustion: **Olive + Wild Rose**

Liver ailments often cause abnormal fatigue, especially after eating. This combination gives us strength and minimizes the tendency to hang around aimlessly.

due to resentment and bitterness: **Willow**

Bitterness poisons our mood and the body as well, including the liver and gallbladder. (Bile is decidedly bitter!)

due to stress

Heavy foods and indigestible "psychic fodder" can cause stress and damage the liver. Most liver and gall problems are stress-related.

> Elm when functioning at our peak for too long puts us in danger of a total breakdown

Hornbeam when we do not feel up to the challenges and blows of daily life

Oak when we work grimly and thoughtlessly against ourselves

Vervain when we are too active and stressed

Loneliness → Loner → Contact Problems

Loneliness is caused by a lack of contact with living things—people, animals, or plants. The need can be very diverse. Introverted individuals seek only a few people to talk to while extroverts need many, and while one person perhaps needs only the company of his dog, another requires a whole community or circle of friends. Loneliness is less a question of the potential for contact than of the consequences of not being able to initiate and maintain contact with others. Even in society people can feel isolated and cast out because they cannot close the gap that separates them from those around them. When we are lonely, we should try to become acquainted with ourselves instead of merely feeling sorry for ourselves. Only when we understand ourselves can we begin to understand others and exchange thoughts and feelings with them.

due to a lack of openness: Agrimony

When we do not dare to show ourselves as we actually are and instead present only an artificial facade, we cannot have any true contact with other people. Despite superficial relationships, we become lonely and unhappy. Agrimony makes us more honest and natural and is often combined with Water Violet.

due to a craving for emotional relationships: Chicory

An excessive craving for emotional relationships has a repellent effect because it can be restrictive and confining and drives away the very people to whom we want to be close.

due to an excessive need for cleanliness: Crab Apple

Life is not a clean undertaking. Fanatical cleanliness can get on people's nerves and cause them to withdraw from us.

due to vanity: Heather

Pathological vanity or pompous behavior repels other people, and the result is that we are lonely.

due to distrust: Holly

When we do not trust others, we put them out of our lives and grow lonely.

due to sadness: **Honeysuckle**

When we mourn or miss anything that is past or lost, we are cut off from the present (where life is happening) and grow lonely.

due to impatience: **Impatiens**

Haste or impatience can make us lonely by disrupting our relationships with those slower than we are.

due to fear: **Mimulus**

Anxious people become lonely very easily because they try to distance themselves from "risky" life or "dangerous" people. Mimulus gives us the courage to put out our feelers again.

due to moodiness: **Mustard**

Bad moods and depression make us antisocial and repel other people.

due to exhaustion: **Olive**

Exhaustion restricts our ability to make and maintain contact with other people.

due to guilt feelings: **Pine**

Guilt feelings limit our human relationships, which makes us feel cast out and alone.

with total desperation: **Sweet Chestnut**

due to the need to be alone or the need for distance: **Water Violet**

loneliness caused by ambition *22/34

When we believe that we know everything and will listen to no one else's opinion, we need Vine.

Loner → Loneliness → Contact Problems

Being a "loner" is a natural quality of introverts. Because they internalize everything they see and experience, they need ample time and rest. When a serious mental or emotional trauma causes this behavior to increase such that they lose their ability to make contact with others, or when a sociable person begins to avoid other people, the situation is pathological and needs to be treated.

due to impatience or haste: **Impatiens**

Impatiens is for hasty people who feel that they are held up by slower people and therefore prefer to do everything alone.

for the goal of personal perfection: **Rock Water**

Rock Water makes us more sociable again when we excessively attempt to avoid anything and anyone we feel is harmful or corrupt.

with difficulties with human contact: **Water Violet**

Water Violet is helpful when the loss of our ability to approach other people causes us to become outsiders.

due to bitterness: **Willow**

People who become loners as the result of a disappointment or through bitterness, even though they had been sociable previously, will find their normal, conciliatory behavior restored. Willow is often combined with Water Violet.

Loss → Grief → Separation

We must work through a loss if we don't want to be destroyed by it. We must recognize that sheer nothingness doesn't exist, that emptiness is soon replaced by fullness, and that every loss that fate brings us will be replaced by a gift just as valuable. Because we determine the value of everything that we encounter, it's up to us to determine whether something makes us happy or not. Although an event may seem "objectively" negative, it is meant for us, tailored to our life. It is a part of us and therefore possesses a positive aspect, even though it might be a source of pain or even death for us. Losing something means receiving something new and, for the moment, something better. It is up to us to recognize this—which is an art that we can and must master if we don't want to be devastated by a great loss one day.

tendency toward: **Chicory**

People who have too great a need for possession often feel under constant threat of facing a loss, and Chicory can help them. If we don't have anything, we can't lose anything.

with grief: **Honeysuckle**

If we can't bring ourselves to part with what we've lost and constantly grieve, Honeysuckle can help.

causing psychic trauma: **Star of Bethlehem**

When we are not strong enough to bear a loss, it remains a painful wound in our spirit. Star of Bethlehem helps heal the wound.

as a cause of bitterness: **Willow**
loss of love causing sadness *8/16
loss causing depression *16/21

loss causing trauma *16/29
loss causing bitterness *16/38
loss of self-confidence from a mental or emotional trauma
  *19/29

Love, thoughts of, obsessive *8/35

Lung Conditions

Breathing is a decidedly vital, life-affirming phenomenon, and oxygen is one of our most important nutrients. Without the desire to breathe, the need for air and for life, the lungs can't remain healthy. Lung ailments have psychic causes, for the most part. Spiritual problems can weaken or damage the lungs and lead to such complications as bronchitis, pneumonia, tuberculosis, or a pulmonary embolism. The appropriate Bach flower treatment—as a supplement to medical treatment—speeds up the healing process and creates the conditions necessary for healing.

  asthma: **Rescue Remedy**
Asthma of the lungs (there is also asthma of the heart caused by a weakness of the heart) is generally a condition we're born with; it can appear in childhood as crusta lactea or eczema and later as an allergy (especially hay fever). Often there is inherited damage from tuberculosis. Asthma can often be triggered by suppressive allopathic treatment (such as corticosteroids or antibiotics) and also by chemicals, pollutants, and especially psychic problems. Animal hair can trigger a severe allergic reaction (→ Allergies). If homeopathic treatment is not successful, it should be followed by allopathic treatment. Bach flower treatment can be given to supplement medical treatment, with the goal of addressing the underlying psychic problems. In acute cases with panic, Rescue Remedy has proved to be effective: take three drops on the lips or tongue every five to ten minutes until the condition improves. For accompanying treatments, → *breathing difficulties* → Allergies.

  breathing difficulties: **Agrimony + Aspen + Mimulus**
It is difficult to breathe when we are afraid, because the tension blocks the diaphragm. Over the long term, this condition can affect the oxygen supply as well as the lungs' resistance. This combination helps minimize all sorts of fear.

chronic cough: **Crab Apple + Gentian + Heather + Larch + Star of Bethlehem + Walnut**

Chronic coughing often appears in connection with a lost territorial battle or some kind of discouragement (→ Compete, inability to). Crab Apple has a purifying effect, Gentian works against discouragement, Heather treats an excessive need for attention, Larch counters feelings of inferiority, Star of Bethlehem helps process unresolved trauma, and Walnut makes us internally stronger and more secure.

for an endangered constitution: **Impatiens + Wild Oat**

People who are rushed, impatient, or restless or who always need a change of pace are susceptible to lung conditions, especially tuberculosis. The physical constitution can be positively influenced by the following combinations.

tuberculosis (consumption)

Many lung conditions, especially tuberculosis, are cause by sadness and heartbreak. People who are sad, afraid, or without hope often cannot breathe properly. The following essences and combinations can help.

> Clematis + Wild Rose for a resigned attitude toward life and a latent death wish
>
> Gorse for hopelessness
>
> Honeysuckle for sadness associated with loss (especially→Homesickness) with a lack of interest in the present
>
> Red Chestnut for worry
>
> Mimulus for fear
>
> Mustard for inexplicable sadness or depression

pulmonary embolism: **Heather + Larch + Star of Bethlehem + Willow; Rescue Remedy**

Many supposed embolisms are, in fact, thromboses of the lung vessels that result from a humiliating experience. This combination (as a supplement to medical treatment) treats all the contributing factors: Heather helps temper an excessive craving for recognition, Larch helps lessen feelings of inferiority caused by a defeat or humiliation, Star of Bethlehem helps treat unprocessed shock, and Walnut helps lessen bitterness. In the acute phase, give Rescue Remedy (again in addition to proper medical treatment), two to three drops every hour.

Malice → Aggression → Bitterness → Rage

Mania: Cherry Plum + Impatiens + Mustard + Vervain + White Chestnut

We characterize someone as "manic" when they are excessively optimistic, active, and enthusiastic. Mania is the opposite of depression (in which everything comes to a standstill) and often alternates with it (manic-depressive condition). This combination can normalize the condition: Cherry Plum softens the emotions, Impatiens makes us calmer, Mustard prevents the condition from transforming into depression, Vervain makes us more restrained, and White Chestnut frees us.

Melancholia: Honeysuckle (→ Depression)

melancholic resignation *16/37

Memory

not good enough: Chestnut Bud
too good: Honeysuckle

A memory that is too good can make us sick when it focuses on painful, unresolved experiences. Normally, the psyche protects itself by forgetting and stores everything it cannot process in the subconscious for the day that it can be retrieved when needed. Honeysuckle helps us reach closure with the past. It can be combined with Star of Bethlehem (16/29).

obsessive memories *16/35

Menopause

In menopause, hormonal changes cause a woman to lose her fertility. This drastic loss, combined with the strain of beginning a new phase in life, are not always borne by women without complications. They will often experience such symptoms as hot flashes, heart palpitations, nervousness, and mucosal changes as well as emotional instability, depression, or psychoses. Some women find it difficult to accept their imagined sexual and social "devaluation." Women who have not led an active sexual life may try to overcompensate in the early phases of menopause.

due to suppression: Agrimony

Agrimony helps us come to terms with reality. It is useful for any woman who attempts to compensate for her advancing years by putting on a facade of exaggerated youth. Agrimony is often used in combination with Heather (1/14).

with hysteria or psychoses: **Cherry Plum**

A strong but suppressed sexuality can make a woman seem obsessed or "crazed." Cherry Plum reduces emotional pressure.

with hot flashes: **Cherry Plum + Impatiens + Rock Rose + Walnut**

Cherry Plum and Rock Rose are for uncontrollable vegetative reactions, Impatiens works against general restlessness, and Walnut restores the hormonal balance.

and feelings of inferiority: **Larch**

Larch helps women who feel devalued find renewed self-confidence and also helps prevent osteoporosis (→ Osteoporosis).

disruption in life flow: **Star of Bethlehem**

Unprocessed traumatic experiences can impede our mental and emotional development if they prevent us from expanding our consciousness. It is often fairly easy to locate the exact point in time that such an experience took place. Star of Bethlehem can help relieve the psychic blockade. It is often used for children who cannot accept the way things are because of their own unrealistic (and often learned) expectations and attitudes. It is often combined with Honeysuckle (16/29) or Willow (29/38).

general problems with adjusting: **Walnut**

Walnut should be used for any problems related to a new phase in physical or psychic development. It promotes inner order and helps us reorient ourselves.

Mental Anguish

secret: **Agrimony**
absolute: **Sweet Chestnut**

Mental Block, due to nebulous fears *2/35

Mental Illness → Absentmindedness → Obsession → Behavioral Problems

Misanthrope, irritable *15/34

Missionary Tendencies: Vervain

Vervain is for people who hold their convictions and ideas to be absolutely right and tend to impose them upon others.

Mistakes: Chestnut Bud (→ Learning Difficulties)

Chestnut Bud helps us to learn from our mistakes.

Mistreatment, consequences of → Shock

with general fear: Aspen
with a broken will: Centaury
with hate and feelings of revenge: Holly + Willow
with damage to the feeling of self-worth: Larch
with fear of repeating: Mimulus
with lingering effects: Star of Bethlehem

Mistrust

toward life: Aspen
toward our own instincts and feelings: Cerato
caused by a basic negative attitude: Holly
caused by a lack of self-confidence: Larch
due to fear: Mimulus
due to negative experiences: Star of Bethlehem

Modesty → Self-denial

True modesty means taking only what we need and never having the feeling that we are lacking anything. False modesty, on the other hand, is a form of denial; it is a type of hypocrisy, because secretly we are covetous.

due to an eagerness for self-denial: Centaury

Centaury is effective against any "modest" form of self-denial, which is really only the manifestation of a weakness in the personality.

instead of immoderation: Chicory

Chicory promotes true modesty by reducing greed and craving—especially for attention. It helps us be content with what we have.

due to underestimating oneself: Larch

Larch is appropriate if our modesty stems from a lack of self-confidence. This behavior is only a tactic, not a genuine form of modesty.

instead of indecisiveness: Scleranthus

Scleranthus helps us make sound decisions, which means deciding what is right for us. It is appropriate for anyone who has too many choices.

Moodiness

We often think that moodiness is just an undisciplined impertinence that can be overcome with willpower. Actually, it's the result of very complex emotional phenomena that cannot be easily dismissed. Sensitive people with intense emotions tend toward moodiness. When they can clearly see that their own inadequacy is the cause, they can begin to work on overcoming their moods or at least stop themselves from inflicting them on other people. We should also be aware that emotional instability can be the result of an illness (especially of the liver or heart or hormonal or intestinal problems). Sensitivity to the weather (→ Weather, sensitivity to) can be another important cause and can be a sign of a disruption of the vegetative nerve system.

due to the weather → **Weather, sensitivity to**

groundless bad moods: **Mustard**

Mustard works against depression and moodiness that can arise for no apparent reason.

frequent, changeable: **Scleranthus + Wild Oat**

This combination keeps changeable, unpredictable moods in balance, especially for people who are unsure how to behave or who are not sure of their purpose in life.

quick to take offense: **Willow**

People who seem to be looking for a reason to take offense need Willow. Taken in combination with Chicory (craving for love) or Heather (vanity), it can help avoid unpleasant moodiness.

Moods, bad → Depression → Moodiness

moodiness and depression *12/21

Mood Swings *21/28

Morals, obsessive Æ Conscience

Normally, we think of any learned or imposed rule or behavior that tries to maintain societal order as "moral." But there is also a more personal (and valid) form of morality—our inner voice, which tells us what is right for us and helps us act and think with the goal of making us happy and satisfied. Only this form of morality can make a person truly "good." Since it does not always jibe with the prevailing societal morality, this can often be a source of serious conflict or even put our lives in danger. In such cases, we must examine very carefully if we are prepared to endure the consequences of following our inner voice or if—at least for the moment—it might not be better to follow the pack until we are stronger.

due to the desire for purity: Crab Apple

Crab Apple can suppress an unnatural "moral" need for spiritual purity, which can lead to self-rejection.

with guilt: Pine

Pine is used by people whose morality is too severely dominated by a sense of guilt and motivated primarily by a fear of punishment. This type of morality does not make us better; it is imposed by education and a fear of punishment and results in a latent rejection of the self.

with self-denial: Rock Water

Rock Water helps us be more generous and lenient with ourselves and helps us question the moral rules we've imposed on ourselves.

moral compulsions making us unnaturally tolerant *3/24
morality and an obsession with cleanliness *10/24
feeling of moral inferiority *19/24

Morning Moodiness

due to feelings of stress and overwork: Hornbeam
due to a gloomy mood: Mustard

Mother Problems

The central position of the mother in every life has potential dangers that can only be avoided through a clear, honest definition of the mother's mission and roles. Too many children (and mothers as well) have become unhappy owing to a mother's immaturity, unrestrained emotions, and selfish behavior.

yieldingness, softness: Centaury

When a mother lets herself be used by her children, she's not doing them a bit of good. She's only preparing them for a life of selfishness and thoughtlessness.

doting mother: Chicory

The so-called doting mother, who does too much for her children, only serves to make them dependent on her and unable to deal with real life. Chicory can help free us to free our children.

worries: Red Chestnut

A mother's constant worrying is hardly a virtue but in truth a burden for all involved. Red Chestnut helps a mother let go and allow her children to lead more independent lives.

Muddleheaded, scatterbrained behavior → Concentration, difficulties with → Impatience

due to absentmindedness: Clematis
due to impatience: Impatiens
due to indecisiveness: Scleranthus
due to compulsive thoughts: White Chestnut

Naïveté → Influenced, too easily

Narrow-mindedness

Narrow-mindedness is useful when we want to reach a specific goal quickly, but it makes it difficult for us to react properly to the mutability of life or the wide range of experiences and interests of other people. Errors and unfairness are the inevitable results.

with purposefulness: Oak

Oak helps when we have latched too tightly on to an impossible plan and we can no longer see any alternatives.

with absolute conviction: Vervain

Vervain is useful when we monomaniacally try to convince other people of our ideas and attitudes.

with intolerant, arrogant, self-righteous behavior: Vine

Vine should be given to stubborn, dogmatic people who can take only their own opinions seriously.

Nausea: Crab Apple

Nausea can be a healthy instinctive reaction, or the result of oversensitivity; Crab Apple can help.

nausea, pathological *12/23

Nervous Behavior

due to overwhelming stress: Elm

caused by impatience and being rushed: Impatiens
due to a lack of self-confidence: Larch
caused by fear: Mimulus
caused by worries: Red Chestnut
due to a mental or emotional shock: Star of Bethlehem
due to contact problems: Water Violet

Water Violet improves the ability to communicate and makes us more able to bear the company of other people.

Nervous Collapse

for strong, suppressed emotions with the danger of a sudden irrational act or nervous breakdown: Cherry Plum
for excessive responsibility or a heavy load to bear: Elm
after a severe mental or emotional shock: Star of Bethlehem
for all emergencies where panic or shock is involved: Rescue Remedy
when we are absolutely desperate and see no way out: Sweet Chestnut

Neurodermatitis Æ Skin Conditions

Neuroses Æ Behavioral Problems

New Beginnings: Agrimony + Chicory + Gentian + Honeysuckle + Larch + Mimulus + Wild Oat (Æ Crisis)

Starting all over again is very difficult for many people. Many would rather stay in a familiar but unhappy situation out of fear, inflexibility, or possessiveness than dare to listen to their inner call for happiness or learn from their life experience and create a new life. These combinations are helpful and should be taken over the long term. Agrimony makes us more honest with ourselves. Chicory helps us let go. Gentian strengthens our will and our resolve so that we don't give up at the first sign of difficulties. Honeysuckle frees us from sentimental memories. Larch gives us self-confidence and allows us to believe in our success. Mimulus counters various fears. Wild Oat helps us recognize our new life goals. Willow frees us from negative emotional attachments.

Nightmares

Nightmares are dreamed fears, which are triggered by mental strain or physical disruptions (heavy meals, toxins, etc.). Generally they indicate the need for a life change.

caused by fear: **Aspen**

Aspen mitigates fears that can manifest in the form of nightmares and prevents our nightmares, in turn, from giving rise to further fears.

from feelings of guilt: **Pine**

Guilt is the moral alienation caused by the fear of punishment. Sometimes guilt even follows us into our dreams. The psyche wants to motivate us to behave in a better manner or bring us to the realization that we are not actually guilty.

from a terrible experience: **Star of Bethlehem**

Every experience—especially when it is traumatic—has a deep and personal meaning. If we cannot recognize this meaning, the psyche will not let go of it, and it will continue to surface in various forms.

through mental overexertion: **White Chestnut**

When certain problems or fears dominate our thoughts, they can also poison our dreams. White Chestnut can help us think clearly again and eliminate the thoughts that cause our fears.

Nostalgia

prohibiting a realistic attitude: **Honeysuckle**
nostalgia making us inattentive *7/16
nostalgic weakness *12/16

Obligation, excessive sense of → Perfectionism

Obsequiousness → Humility, false → Servility
obsequiousness caused by fear *4/20

Obsession → Rash Behavior → Irrational Behavior → Psychosis

When important emotions are suppressed or pushed out of our consciousness, they can, depending on their quality and intensity, dominate the psyche and terrorize our thoughts (psychosis) or provoke irrational behavior.

due to vague fears: **Aspen**

Suppressed, unclear emotions can elicit vague fears or a state of panic. Aspen can promote a healthy sense of judgment, clarify our feelings, and restore our inner balance and order.

psychotic: **Cherry Plum**

Cherry Plum is needed when we are in danger of going crazy or acting irrationally owing to strong, suppressed emotions. Sometimes it can help with an already existing psychosis and, at the very least, improves the effects of appropriate psychopharmaceuticals.

due to certain thoughts: **White Chestnut**

Certain thoughts can impose themselves and block our normal thoughts, especially when they are emotionally charged, until the underlying causes and issues are resolved. Generally, the cause is an important personal problem, the solution of which we (generally unconsciously) strive to avoid because it signifies a confrontation with embarrassments. Sometimes, however, the cause is only superficial thinking. In such cases, the psyche then allows us access only to certain thoughts in the deeper layers; these thoughts represent, so to speak, the eye of the needle through which we must pass. White Chestnut relieves these obsessions and returns our thinking to its natural, multileveled nature. (It is often combined with Cherry Plum → 6/35.)

obsessive thoughts *6/36

Offended, easily → Bitterness

due to a craving for emotional relationships: **Chicory**

When we want too much, we always have the feeling we aren't getting enough and are therefore easily disappointed. Chicory normalizes our need for attention (can be combined with Heather *8/14).

from an injured sense of vanity: **Heather**

Heather minimizes vanity or an excessive need for recognition so that we don't feel miffed (can be combined with Chicory *8/14).

due to problems with human contact: **Water Violet**

If we have broken off contact with someone owing to some insult or have withdrawn from the world, Water Violet helps us become open and approachable again. Only in this way can we hope to clear up misunderstandings (often combined with Willow).

with resentment or an unforgiving nature: **Willow**

Willow makes us more conciliatory with regard to the missteps of others. When we react with bitterness to an insult, we suffer twice as much.

Openness, excessive → Influenced, too easily

Having an open demeanor can make us well liked, but it can also have the danger of bringing us under the influence of other people, especially when we are enmeshed in personal problems and seek a new life path. Out of insecurity, we often cannot defend ourselves from a lot of "good advice" and more subtle forms of blackmail that friends, relatives, and acquaintances will try to inflict upon us to prevent us from setting out on the path to independence.

due to insecurity: Cerato

Cerato helps us trust our own instinct and become impervious to bad advice.

Opinionated: Vine (→ Dogmatism)

When we think we know the truth and demand that everyone listen to us, we need Vine.

Opposition, causing rage *15/32

Optimism, uncritical: Clematis

Optimism can be just as much a negative quality as pessimism if it is groundless. Clematis is used to treat groundless optimism and daydreaming.

Order, fanatical

People who suffer from fear and insecurity often tend to manifest these feelings in the form of a senseless (and ineffective) need for order. They attempt to impose external order while their internal life is characterized by disorder (insecurity or fear).

with obsessive cleanliness: **Crab Apple**

Crab Apple is for people who manifest their inner compulsions in the form of excessive cleanliness and order.

with excessive self-discipline: **Rock Water**

When order manifests itself only as compulsion, self-denial, and excessive self-discipline, Rock Water can help.

with others: Vine

People who feel compelled to force their inflexible opinions on others need Vine.

Osteoporosis → Spinal Problems

Outsider → Loner

Overwork

due to excessive perfectionism: Crab Apple + Rock Water
due to being rushed: Impatience
due to overactivity: Vervain

Pain

basic treatment: Agrimony

Pain is increased by tension and lessens with relaxation. Agrimony functions to decrease tension, and should be combined with the following essences, according to the condition.

for all emergencies: Rescue Remedy
if the pain is unbearable: Cherry Plum + Elm + White
   Chestnut
with a tendency toward self-pity: Chicory
with restlessness: Impatiens
after an injury: Star of Bethlehem
*with contrariness and an aversion to socializing and
   participating:* Water Violet

Panic → Rash Behavior

The more we avoid consciously facing our fear-related problems, the less we are able to deal with them; when we are confronted with them unexpectedly and directly, we lose the conscious control of our thoughts and actions. The ever present subconscious fear swells like a raging river after a thunderstorm, and it creates in us a primitive/animalistic instinct to flee, where we try to confront only the immediate threat. When this panicky, occasionally very aggressive impulse to flee confronts an equally strong inhibition related to societal taboos, the result is a severe inner conflict that negates all of our strength and makes us unable to act; we suffer paralysis from fear or horror, and let the disaster simply wash over us. Such catastrophes seldom come at us all at once with full force but rather by degrees; we can help defuse or avoid them by consciously facing the little everyday shocks and surprises and thus becoming aware of our weaknesses. This is where Bach flowers enter the picture. They can also often help when panic has already set in.

as a result of suppression: Agrimony
When we suppress anything that is unpleasant or causes anxiety, we run the risk of suddenly being overcome by it.

due to vague fears: Aspen
When we avoid our fears, we merely displace them. They remain indecipherable, morphing in our psyches, and they can often cause sudden, inexplicable, and severe panic that seems to come from out of the blue. Aspen can be used to prevent vague, anxious feelings and premonitions and also to treat sudden onset of panic and fear.

due to a traumatic experience: Rock Rose
While Aspen is used to treat panic due to internal causes, Rock Rose is helpful for panic that is triggered by external factors, such as a catastrophe. In combination with Star of Bethlehem, it can strengthen the psyche's defenses.

panic with the danger of going over the edge *6/26
panic with unconsciousness *9/26
panic due to stress *11/26
panicky hyperactivity *18/26
panic caused by fear *20/26
panicky worries *25/26
panic making us unable to act *26/28
panic due to psychic trauma *26/29
panicky fear leaving us desperate *26/30

Partner Problems → Distance → Contact Problems → Heartbreak

The term *partnership* is a traditional term for a sense of feeling or belonging together: it encompasses the terms *love, friendship,* or *marriage* and gives expression to the contemporary desire for more personal freedom and equality in relationships. The well-known problems of humans living together still exist, however, because people today struggle and compete for survival—perhaps in a more subtle form—and we, in principle, are no more mature or better equipped (in a spiritual sense) than our ancestors. The problems of interpersonal relationships have hardly changed because we are too seldom aware that we recognize ourselves only in other people and that we love or fight against the same things in those that we love as we do in ourselves. Thus, we end up unconsciously making the same mistakes again and again; leading to misjudgments, misunderstandings, and enmity. Moreover, we can't solve our problems because we are looking in the wrong place: we should look at ourselves. We also cannot keep the right measure of distance (→ Distance), which is the foundation of a harmonious relationship.

due to insincerity: Agrimony (→ Artificiality)

Honesty is the most important element in any relationship. Only honesty can bring about trust and freedom, and these, in turn, make it possible for us to open our hearts. It is a fundamental element of relationships and provides a stable foundation, but it is no law that can be followed by the letter. We don't need to burden our partners with every miserable petty detail or every minuscule problem; we don't need to point out to our partners their every personal weakness or trivial error. It's perfectly natural that we don't lay *all* our cards on the table (our partners are following suit). Another thing entirely, however, are the unnecessary, petty little lies and hypocrisy, false politeness, and poses that can lend a permanent air of artificiality to a relationship. Even if they are not done with malicious intent and are the result of old habits or childhood fears, they can sabotage an atmosphere of trust and intimacy, which is so essential to a loving partnership. The partners become actors, and the relationship develops into a comedy, drama, or tragedy. Agrimony will develop in us the desire (and the courage) for honest, natural behavior.

due to acquisitiveness or a craving for love: Chicory (→ Distance)

Excessive "love" is actually a form of greed or acquisitiveness, and it is repellent. When one partner tries to make the other dependent by excessive attention or doting, it often has the opposite of the intended effect; it triggers a more or less unconscious repulsion. Love can arise only voluntarily.

due to dreaminess: **Clematis, Honeysuckle**

A partnership takes place in the present. When we live in the past (Honeysuckle) or in the future, we don't pay sufficient attention to what's going on around us, and we endanger our relationship.

due to obsessive cleanliness: **Crab Apple**

Life is hardly a "clean" undertaking, and an excessive need for cleanliness can muck up any relationship. Furthermore, when sexuality is a cause of revulsion, we can never be content.

due to an excessive need for recognition: **Heather ($\rightarrow$ Egocentrism)**

When we use and abuse our partners in order to provoke their admiration, it is a serious detriment to relationships.

due to rage and irritability: **Holly**

As for abusive relationships, in which both partners can express only their aggressions, an unfriendly, irritating demeanor destroys every relationship over time.

due to impatience: **Impatiens**

Excessive impatience or haste prevents us from relating to our partners. Impatient people are often lonely.

due to feelings of inferiority: **Larch**

We accept each other at face value. To feel inferior to our partners is to undermine mutual respect, and to enjoy seeing our partners humiliated is a sign of immaturity. Larch can strengthen our feeling of self-worth and enable us to feel proud of ourselves regardless of our weaknesses and shortcomings.

due to exhaustion: **Olive**

We can't relate to our partners when we're exhausted. In the long term, the relationship becomes too strenuous because we're so exhausted that we can't even give ourselves the attention we need.

due to guilt feelings: **Pine**

Most bad partnerships continue because of the fear of a guilty conscience. We think that we'll be guilty if we try to free ourselves. This kind of guilty thinking is often used by those who stand to profit from it: by a partner, who uses it as a kind of emotional blackmail, and by society, which uses it to maintain order and the status quo. While this method can be effective in achieving a certain level of external, societal, or financial benefits, the people involved (and their ability to love) stand to lose the most: in the end, the results are guilt feelings and hate. In fact, more relationships are held together out of hate and guilt than out of friendship and love.

due to self-denial: Rock Water

People who concentrate on themselves, on disciplining or even denying themselves, are egocentric and mostly unable to devote attention to anyone else.

due to negative experiences: Star of Bethlehem

It's only natural that we have negative as well as positive experiences with other people. Such negative experiences can be learning experiences that bring us great insight, but they can also undermine our optimism and trust in other people—and our ability to engage in a harmonious partnership. Star of Bethlehem can restore our divine, trusting inner nature.

caused by missionary tendencies: Vervain

The habit of forcing our own thoughts on our partners, or of believing that what is good for us is good for our partners, is unpleasant and can drive the mate away. Each of us defends (even at the cost of unhappiness) his or her unique nature because it is what makes us at peace with ourselves and helps us find our own happiness.

due to intolerance: Vine

Love is not possible without tolerance. Tolerance means not just being forced to put up with our partner's faults but understanding them as a part of the whole—and if not understanding, at least accepting lovingly. Vine is for potential domestic tyrants who have difficulty doing this and who can tolerate in their partners only what they can accept from themselves.

due to loneliness: Water Violet

Excessive isolation inhibits the development of a relationship between partners. We don't need to spend every minute of every day in each other's company, but a certain amount of joy in spending time together is a prerequisite for a happy relationship.

due to frustration: Wild Oat

When we can't find any meaning in life, or when we don't know what we're after or which path we should take, we're often frustrated and are also unpleasant company. Some partnerships can be ruined in this situation. Water Violet helps us find our goals, sometimes even together with our partners.

due to lack of initiative or resignation: **Wild Rose**

Wild Rose helps when a partnership is threatened because we have no interest in life.

due to bitterness: **Willow**

A good partnership lives or dies based on our readiness to be understanding and forgiving of personal weaknesses. Willow prevents us from becoming too bitter when we're disappointed.

at the end of a partnership → **Separation**

Pedantry: Vine (→ Pettiness)

People who are absolutely convinced of the rightness of their opinions are unable to compromise in trivial matters. When everything does not meet their expectations down to the smallest details, they become frustrated or tyrannical.

Perfectionism

In the best sense, perfectionism means being able to do things properly, right down to the last detail; as long as this serves a purpose, it can be a meaningful, positive quality, especially in the areas of technology, science, or logic. But life, with its irrationality and uncertainty, is no place for perfectionism. We have limited insight and are not able to make everything "just so." Only nature and life itself are perfect; their examples can give us some insight into our own infallibility and, in so doing, allow us to try to become perfect and whole ourselves. When we are uncompromising in trying to realize our expectations down to the last detail, we have problems when we encounter reality, which seldom coincides with our expectations.

in matters of cleanliness: **Crab Apple**

Crab Apple can help people who have an excessive need for cleanliness or order. It puts us more at ease with our surroundings and with life in general.

due to principles: **Oak**

When we feel compelled to constantly behave perfectly, even when it is not within our abilities, we need Oak.

due to guilty thoughts: **Pine**

Pine is helpful when we strive for perfection not out of the joy of the thing itself but out of a fear of criticism. A guilty conscience can lead to no good.

due to self-denial: **Rock Water**

Rock Water helps us become more generous and forgiving with ourselves. It is helpful when we want to be better than we really are.

due to a high opinion of oneself: **Vine**

We need Vine when we always know exactly what is right and when we demand everyone to fulfill our expectations.

perfectionism, unyielding *22/24
perfectionism, obsessive *24/27

Pessimism → Depression → Hope, lack of

Pessimism is dangerous, and it often signals the beginning of the end; when we no longer have positive expectations, we are in no position to mobilize our strength when we need it. We all know that when we have the expectation of success, we are more likely to succeed than if we have negative expectations. Pessimism is just an external symptom with many causes. We must pay close attention to these causes if we want to overcome it. Often pessimism will accompany heart or liver/gall conditions, which should be treated appropriately.

due to fear: **Aspen, Mimulus**

Fear is a typical form of pessimism. Aspen helps resolve general fears, and Mimulus helps with specific ones.

due to stress and overwork: **Elm**

Elm helps us when we are confident and active, and then suddenly feel that we can't go on.

with a tendency to give up: **Gentian**

Gentian can help avoid pessimism that constantly threatens to overcome us and causes us to quit at the first sign of difficulties.

with hopelessness: **Gorse**

Gorse can help revive us if we are overcome with hopelessness and pessimism.

with gloominess: **Hornbeam**

Hornbeam can help if we are overcome with pessimism in the morning, and it is connected to our daily work.

due to a lack of self-confidence: **Larch**

Larch helps us look at our own abilities and prospects for success more optimistically.

due to exhaustion: Olive

Olive can help when fatigue and exhaustion are the root of our pessimism and negativity.

causing a mental block: White Chestnut

White Chestnut helps us find peace when we can think only of unhappiness and catastrophe.

due to bitterness: Willow

Bitter people have only negative expectations of the future; their bad experiences have poisoned their outlook. Willow helps us come to terms with the world.

Pettiness

related to cleanliness: Crab Apple
and guilt: Pine
in our personal convictions: Vine

"Piety," false

Good Christians often consider a person "holy" if he bases his life on self-denial. Normally, however, such people are just practicing false piety, a sort of playacting, which serves to satisfy a certain vanity, need for power, or neurotic guilt feelings. On the other hand, people who lead a life of genuine, unpretentious simplicity seldom consider themselves to be holy—it is not in their temperament.

caused by bearing suffering without complaint: Agrimony

Agrimony is for people who keep their problems and fears concealed and who even try to cheer up those around them. It seems as if they do this to help others, but actually they are afraid of facing their own problems.

caused by selflessness in service to others: Centaury

If we deny or suppress our own needs and put ourselves in the service of other people, we come very close to an ideal state of piety. Such individuals are more common than we might think. While a genuinely pious person will act this way out of a conscious, life-affirming choice to help others, people who need Centaury act "selflessly" because of their own weaknesses.

caused by a selfless concern or worry over others: Red Chestnut

People who worry only about the welfare of others and neglect their own well-being are often admired for their selflessness. In reality, however, they are just projecting their own fears. Their behavior often helps no one and often hurts the very people they are trying to help.

caused by extreme self-discipline: **Rock Water**

Self-denial is often incorrectly taken to be a form of piety or holiness. Except for a few cases in which it is actually a conscious attempt to learn our personal limits, it is really a sign of limited intelligence, unreflective force, or even a life-negating phenomenon. Life is by nature expansive and geared toward joy, not toward denial and negativity.

Pigheadedness → Dogmatism → Stubbornness

Pimples → Skin Conditions

Pity → Self-pity → Self-sacrifice

Sympathy is a special form of sorrow. Sorrow is a sign that something is not right. Normally, we regard pity as something of a virtue and believe that suffering shared is suffering halved. Actually, sharing our suffering with another only doubles the suffering. We should strive for something else, namely, compassion: the ability to take an interest in the suffering of another and, if needed and necessary, stand by that person. We are social creatures, and compassion provides the bridge that links us to other people. Above all, it helps lessen the world's suffering; we strive not to suffer ourselves and to ease the suffering of those around us.

with self-pity: **Chicory**
excessive: **Red Chestnut**

Poisoning, fear of: Aspen + Crab Apple

This combination is useful when compulsive cleanliness leads to a fear of being poisoned.

Posture, bad → Spinal Problems

Pregnancy → Birth

with vague fears of the future: **Aspen**
with daydreaming and losing touch with reality: **Clematis**
with a feeling of being overwhelmed: **Elm**

with clear, specific fears: Mimulus
with depression: Mustard
with general exhaustion: Olive
with anemia: Olive + Wild Rose
with worries for the child: Red Chestnut
for transition and self-discovery: Walnut

Prejudice → Dogmatism → Stubbornness

Prejudice is a product of the imagination; we can judge only when we have some idea what's going on. Prejudice is a sign of emotional immaturity and is often an expression of fear.

due to excessively strong missionary convictions: Vervain
Vervain is for people with the urgent desire to bring others to their own way of thinking. If they would admit that other people have just as much of a claim to the truth, their actions would lose their moral justification.

due to closed-mindedness: Vine
Vine is for the dogmatic know-it-all who takes only her own opinion seriously and feels justified in passing judgment without considering all the facts.

Premonitions and Foreboding, anxious: Aspen

Knowledge that is not conscious is often experienced in the form of premonitions. When we try to fight against this knowledge because we can't bear the potential consequences, we feel fear.

Presence of Mind, insufficient → Panic

Pressure, excessive emotional: Cherry Plum
pressure, excessive emotional, caused by repression *1/6

Pride → Arrogance

Pride can mean many things. It can be the expression of sheer happiness because of an accomplishment or a quality and, in this sense, is a perfectly healthy, self-affirming sign of a feeling of self-worth. It can also be a way of protecting us from people whom, for whatever reason, we cannot accept. Or it can be arrogance. The first form of pride can create happiness and bring us friends; the second helps us achieve a certain distance and prevents conflict with those different than we are; and the third creates enmity and can be a source of humiliation for other people. People who are proud of something in which they played no active role (such as inherited privilege) should not be proud; instead, they should be joyfully thankful, quietly and reflectively, for their unearned good fortune.

with a great need for recognition: **Heather**

Heather is for people who make themselves indispensable everywhere and find it important to be admired for their talents and merits. This can be very irritating to those around them.

with distance: **Water Violet (→ Isolation)**

Water Violet is for people who are loners by nature. They keep a natural distance, which is often taken as a sign of excessive pride.

Problems

Seeing more problems than actually exist is a sign of psychic imbalance. See the appropriate essences discussed under Pessimism.

avoiding: **Agrimony + Gentian**

Avoiding problems is absolutely natural and proper. Sometimes, however, we must face them and try to solve them, especially when we are in the position to take action and when they can have negative consequences. Avoiding them buys us only a temporary reprieve.

looking for: **Oak**

Oak can help people who tend to find a personal challenge in all problems. They always take the most difficult route and often stretch themselves beyond their limits. When difficulties seem unsolvable, Oak can make us more yielding and willing to compromise.

Psoriasis → Skin Conditions

Psychosis → Obsession → Rash Behavior

psychosis, impending, due to suppression *1/6
psychosis, impending, with restlessness *6/18
psychosis, impending, due to stress and overwork *6/22
psychosis as the result of severe self-suppression *6/27
psychosis due to an emotional or mental injury *6/29
psychotic rage *6/15

Puberty: Agrimony + Larch + Pine + Walnut (+ Water Violet) (→ Sexual Dysfunction)

During puberty, we become aware of our most important biological function. This decisive new orientation can bring about great problems: we must develop a healthy relationship to our new physical needs, and we must also define our new role in society. Agrimony helps us behave naturally; it helps counter the affected shame that often arises in connection with developing sexuality. Larch strengthens our feelings of self-worth, which now must take on a new dimension with our burgeoning sexual awareness and strength. Pine helps curb sexual guilt feelings that today indecently poison the growing person. Walnut is the most important essence for change and new beginnings and helps us transfer our internal order to external functions, allowing us to be and become our "true" selves. Water Violet can be given to a young person with human contact problems.

Purpose, lack of

when we give up too easily: **Gentian**
when we can't make decisions: **Scleranthus**
when we don't know what we want: **Wild Oat**

Purpose in Life, lacking or unrealistic

We need a purpose in life if we're to develop our joy, strength, and creativity. When we have no goals or when life seems meaningless, we become physically or psychically ill. Bach flower therapy can help us find our true character and our purpose in this life.

due to insecurity: **Cerato**

When we don't know what to do or when we don't trust our own instincts, we are unable to fulfill our personal mission in life. Cerato helps us understand our own inner "adviser" and makes us more confident with our own opinions.

due to a weak will: **Gentian**

When we are too easily discouraged and distracted from our goals, Gentian can help restore our strength of will and resolve.

due to a lack of self-confidence: **Larch**

Sometimes when we are faced with happiness, we feel that we are not up to it or that we haven't earned it. Larch can help strengthen our self-confidence.

leading to depression: Mustard

Many people are overcome again and again by a seemingly groundless depression. Actually, a lack of motivation or goals in life can be the cause.

due to pathological guilt: Pine

Pine helps us pursue our goals and desires when we feel that we are not deserving and that our lives must be filled with self-denial.

due to self-denial: Rock Water

Rock Water is useful when we believe that we can find meaning in life only through self-discipline and through eliminating our "worthless" or "superficial" qualities.

due to being too easily influenced: Walnut

We all have our own personality and our own life path. The more resolve we use in following it, the happier we'll be. The more we allow ourselves to be dissuaded from it, the more frustrating and meaningless life will seem.

due to a lack of clarity: Wild Oat

Wild Oat helps us in our search for goals or a purpose in life. It can open our eyes to our own personal talents and tendencies, but it must be taken over a long period of time.

lacking a purpose in life due to insecurity *5/36*
lacking a purpose in life because of inattentiveness *7/36*
lacking a purpose in life due to a lack of self-confidence
    19/36
false purpose in life due to self-castigation *27/36*
lacking a life goal *33/37*

Pushiness → Distance, emotional → Missionary Tendencies

pushy, insistent "helping" or concern for others: Chicory
from missionary zeal: Vervain
imposing one's will: Vine
pushiness in love or caring for others *8/22*
pushiness caused by a fear of loneliness *14/20*

Rage → Aggression → Cold Emotions → Hate → Bitterness

directly felt: Holly
internalized, with bitterness: Willow

rage, psychotic *6/15
rage caused by opposition or errors *15/32
rage and bitterness *15/38

Rash Behavior → Panic → Psychoses

When we are suddenly overcome by intense emotions, we can lose conscious control of our reactions and become absolutely numb or lose control.
due to the suppression of drives: **Cherry Plum**
with panic: **Rescue Remedy, Rock Rose**

Recognition, need for: Heather + Larch (→ Vanity → Inferiority, feelings of)

An extreme need for recognition is the result of strong feelings of inferiority (→ Inferiority, feelings of) combined with ambition (→ Ambition) or pronounced vanity (→Vanity). People who crave recognition try to gloss over their feelings of inferiority by trying to be acknowledged, admired, or honored. This is a major source of stress for them because they are in constant fear of being exposed and it tends to make them unpopular. It would be much better for them if instead of seeking approval from others, they paid more attention to themselves. That way, they wouldn't think so much about their (mostly imaginary) weaknesses but could concentrate on their strengths, which they possess just as anyone does. The value of all things is relative; it just depends on who the observer is—and the social worth of a person depends in large part on the company that person keeps. When we feel inferior, it's often because we're running with the wrong crowd, just as a plant will not thrive if it's not planted in the right location. We need to be in the right place, where our talents and qualities will be appreciated and where we can appreciate them ourselves. The combination described here makes us more discreet, modest, and self-confident. It can also be combined with Walnut.

Rejection, of other people (→ Self-denial)

Normally, rejecting unpleasant people is the expression of a natural instinct for self-preservation. It can, however, be the result of a psychic disruption or pathological insecurity; in such cases, it serves no use but only makes us tense or lonely.

because others are too slow: **Impatiens**

The need to do everything quickly makes us feel that slower people are a burden or an obstacle.

from fear: **Mimulus**

We avoid with excessive caution any human contact that might put us at risk.

due to a negative experience: **Star of Bethlehem**

A child learns to stay away from a fire once he has been burned; likewise, we avoid anyone who reminds us of a traumatic situation.

from the need to be alone: **Water Violet**

We don't want to be disturbed and take great pains to avoid human contact.

from disappointment or bitterness: **Willow**

> Willow helps us understand and forgive.

Relapse

into old habits: **Honeysuckle**

Honeysuckle helps us face the present instead of living in the past.

in the healing process: **Gentian**

When we suffer continued setbacks in the healing process, Gentian can help restore the body's resilience.

relapse during convalescence *12/28

Relationships, inability to initiate and maintain → Contact Problems

Relationships, fear of: **Water Violet**

Water Violet makes us more sociable and counters the pathological fear of human relationships. It cannot make a social butterfly out of a total loner, but it can free us from excessive isolation.

Remorse, excessive → Guilt Feelings

Renunciation → Self-sacrifice → Selflessness

It is better to give than to receive but only when the giving is voluntary and with positive intentions. Denial is essentially life-negating; the natural tendency of life is one of expansion and increase. Because life consists of soul as well as body, renunciation, if it leads to spiritual enrichment, can be more of a blessing than retention. This is the significance of the classic biblical victim who, with little cost, is able to achieve great rewards (the blessing of God). Renunciation doesn't have to be a self-negating phenomenon; but it can be an uplifting joy of giving. It is only "right" when we derive joy from giving, instead of the poison of guilt feelings, moralistic blackmail, or personal weakness. When our motives are pure, we need no thanks; the act of giving is its own reward. Purely motivated giving and renunciation help promote personal integrity and spiritual maturity. Normally we must work for a long time with great honesty to earn this ability.

caused by a weak personality: Centaury

People who act in the interests of others and neglect themselves because of psychic immaturity or weakness only strengthen the thoughtlessness of those who use them. It's common to see children who sacrifice themselves for their egotistical parents. They live like slaves and need Centaury to begin living their own lives.

due to despondency: Gentian

Gentian is for a weak will, which causes us to give up at the first sign of difficulties and makes us easy game for others willing to profit from our own weakness.

due to a lack of self-confidence: Larch

When we have no self-confidence, we tend toward unnecessary and premature self-denial and renunciation.

caused by exhaustion: Olive
due to self-castigation: Rock Water (→ Asceticism)

Resentment → Bitterness

Reserved: Water Violet

Water Violet is helpful when we suddenly become cold or antisocial or if we suddenly shun the company of others at the onset of or during an illness.

reserved, mentally *7/34

Reserved Behavior: Water Violet (→ Distance, emotional)

Resignation: Gorse + Wild Rose (→ Giving up → Interest, lack of → Hopelessness → Resignation to Fate)

When we have lost all hope and have no will to live, the life virtually goes out of the body. Resignation poses a danger that should be taken seriously, especially when an illness is involved. These combinations can reawaken our will to live.

resignation due to a weak personality *4/37
resignation and a longing for death *9/37
resignation and a weak will *12/37
total resignation *13/37
resignation with melancholic memories *16/37
resignation due to stress and overwork *17/37
resignation due to a lack of self-confidence *19/37
resignation due to depression *21/37
resignation due to exhaustion *23/37
resignation due to a mental or emotional trauma *29/37

Resignation to Fate

Fatalists, in the good sense of the word, truly know how to make the best of things. They try their best to achieve their plans and desires, but when they are confronted by insurmountable obstacles, they are prepared to give up. They realize that there is a divine, benevolent order working toward an unknown goal. They don't fall to pieces at every mishap, setback, disappointment, accident, or illness. Instead, they use these unexpected events as opportunities to extract the strength and the insight to further their personal development. They submit to fate without complaint, but that doesn't mean that they flutter around aimlessly like leaves on a tree. They are willing to follow the signs that life has given them.

with hopelessness: **Gorse**

Hopelessness signifies not just resignation but a rejection of fate.

with resignation: **Wild Rose**

People who are uninterested and let life pass them by need Wild Rose.

too little (resignation)

We suffer when blind ambition or mere contrariness makes us resist the inevitable.

> Oak is for people who don't know when to give up, even though the strain is too great

Sweet Chestnut helps us take life as it comes and not become desperate with each test of fate or misfortune

Willow makes us conciliatory, open, and willing to compromise

Resistance, mental and emotional, impaired owing to exhaustion *23/29

Resistance, to psychic trauma, too weak *29/33

Resolve, lack of

when we can't form our own opinions and constantly ask for advice: Cerato

when we have no staying power in resolving our problems and give up too easily: Gentian

when we cannot choose among several alternatives: Scleranthus

when we lack purpose and begin new projects before we complete existing ones: Wild Oat

Responsibility, excessive → Guilt Feelings → Unreliability

Being responsible means being accountable, either to ourselves (the psychological "superego") or to a higher authority (of a divine nature or a person). Responsibility engenders security, because it brings order to our behavior; it can either serve to constrain us when it obligates us or it can be a kind of distinction. Some people gladly accept responsibility because it brings a clarity and moral authority to their lives; others, on the other hand, fight against it because they feel their freedom is inhibited. Responsibility (apart from its function of providing social order) is a subjective matter; it's perfect for us when it's a source of happiness but totally inappropriate when it causes us to suffer.

compulsive: Oak

An excessive feeling of responsibility (compulsion from the superego) can cause us to lose sight of our own limits and harm ourselves in pursuit of a task or mission. Oak is for people who pursue their goals so ambitiously and uncompromisingly that they harm themselves.

due to guilt: **Pine**

Pine can free us from a compulsive sense of responsibility that stems from a latent guilt complex. It is useful when we act out of a sense of obligation and not out of joy.

to oneself: **Rock Water**

When we hear ourselves say, "It's my own fault," it's a sign that we are not free with ourselves. Rock Water is often used in combination with Pine.

avoiding: **Water Violet**

Responsibility helps maintain the social order and cannot be totally avoided. We should all undertake as much responsibility as is good for us. If we avoid it to the extent that we become alienated from society at large, we need Water Violet.

Restlessness, inner: Agrimony + Cherry Plum + Scleranthus + White Chestnut

This combination makes us more easygoing and more mature and brings us to a state of inner clarity.

Restraint → Distance, emotional

Revenge, lust for → Hate

revenge, unrelenting lust for *22/38

Rheumatism → Sciatica

Rheumatism describes any illnesses or painful changes of the bones, joints, muscles, or tendons. Bach flower treatment can bring a certain amount of improvement because character or behavior often play important roles in this condition.

general purification of the blood: **Crab Apple**

Rheumatic complaints are often caused by chronic infections that arise at various locations (especially the teeth, sinuses, gallbladder, lower body, or intestines). Crab Apple promotes the elimination of toxins and pathogens and should be used as a primary essence in the treatment of rheumatism.

with liver conditions: **Holly, Mustard, Willow, Water Violet**

Any essence that treats a bad mood is appropriate for liver conditions, including Holly (irritability), Mustard (melancholia), Willow (bitterness), and Water Violet (antisocial behavior).

with impatience, nervousness, restlessness: **Impatiens**

Impatiens can be used to strengthen the constitution when rheumatism is present, which appears in the framework of a tubercular predisposition (inherited weakness or a cured illness). Movement will bring improvement.

with inflexibility or unyieldingness: **Oak, Rock Water, Vine**

Mental or emotional rigidity mean stiffness and inflexibility in the body. Oak is for people who are unyielding, Rock Water for people who are too strict with themselves, Vine for mental inflexibility.

Rules, making: Vine

Vine is effective against the nasty habit of telling others what they should do; it's for people who always believe they know what's right.

Running Amok → Irrational Behavior

Rush and Stress *18/34

Sad Thoughts and Feelings: Cherry Plum + Mustard + White Chestnut

This combination helps us achieve an inner distance; it can be taken with Honeysuckle or Willow.

Sadness → Depression

Scatterbrained Behavior → Concentration, difficulties with → Impatience

due to thoughtlessness: **Clematis**
due to impatience: **Impatiens**
due to indecisiveness: **Scleranthus**
due to compulsive thoughts: **White Chestnut**

White Chestnut is called for when our concentration is disrupted because we can't shake certain thoughts or ideas.

Schizophrenia

Schizophrenia is the result of severe emotional conflict and inner turmoil and consists of a splitting up of the personality into various personalities or realities. Some Bach flowers treat the causes of this disruption and are appropriate as preventive or therapeutic treatments.

due to a "double life": Agrimony

People who act other than their true nature need Agrimony. They are split and live in a constant state of tension because they have no outlet for their potentially explosive emotions.

with fears and anxieties: Aspen + Mimulus + Rock Rose

When fear has no appropriate outlet, it can give rise to inner conflict, and this can be disastrous in people with a tendency toward schizophrenia. This combination treats fears of all kinds.

due to suppressed emotions: Cherry Plum

Emotions have a lot of energy: if they are suppressed and not allowed an outlet, they can create dangerous internal pressure, which can disrupt and split the consciousness.

due to unprocessed shock: Star of Bethlehem

Traumatic experiences that are not consciously processed and worked through can become permanent sources of emotional problems. Star of Bethlehem should be used whenever the mental and emotional faculties are disrupted, even when there is no evident source of trauma.

with compulsive thoughts: White Chestnut

People whose thoughts are dominated by the same ideas repeated over and over need White Chestnut.

Sciatica → Rheumatism → Spinal Problems

Here we refer to painful irritation or inflammation of the sciatic nerve, which stretches from the lumbar to the toes. The pain associated with this condition is often in the back side of the upper thighs. Sciatic problems can be triggered by a disc problem, infections, or sudden or irregular movements. Normally, they appear in relation to infections or kidney or abdominal problems. Psychic influences can play a role as well, by causing tension in the muscles around the spine, which can limit our flexible movements. A relaxed body and an "upright" mind and spirit are the best preventive measures for spinal complaints.

with a strain: Agrimony + Star of Bethlehem

To treat spinal strains and tension and to loosen up the spinal musculature.

due to aggravation and rage: **Holly**

Severe aggravation can affect the spine by causing our movements to become violent or aggressive, which can irritate the sciatic nerve. Holly can alleviate the tension and cause the irritation to subside.

due to stress: **Impatiens**

Impatiens is indicated when our movement becomes rushed, hasty, or impatient, which can lead to "dislocations" of the spine.

with excessive ambition or the need for accomplishment: **Oak**

Oak is indicated when our excessive ambition or desire for accomplishment causes too much tension in the body. This places an extreme strain on the spine.

Secrecy → Facade

Self-abuse → Asceticism

self-abuse due to fear *2/27
self-abuse due to mental and emotional dependence *5/27

Self-alienation

Only when we have an understanding of the deeper, fundamental factors of life and of our abilities, needs, and qualities can we mold them all into a unified whole and find a satisfying meaning in life. We can accomplish this in spite of the multifarious influences that can drive us to a sense of self-alienation: possessions, idle pleasure, honor, power, fear, and a system of education that has nothing to do with humanity and everything to do with making us useful and productive. Most of us spend our whole lives running from ourselves, until a meaningless death takes us away in fear. When we are at one with our true selves, we have no reason to fear life or death because we possess the fundamental knowledge that everything that happens is right and meaningful.

due to repression and hypocrisy: **Agrimony**

Agrimony is for people who do not dare to be themselves. They put up a front, play a role, and take pains to be anything but what they really are. They don't dare show their true natures to anyone, often even to themselves. Agrimony strengthens our desire to be and act as we really are, allowing our external life to jibe with our internal goals and needs. Agrimony helps remove this defense mechanism and can be combined with Walnut, which helps rebuild the true personality.

lack of clarity: **Wild Oat**

Anyone who feels that they don't know where to find the meaning in life or who is discontented because they feel that time is just slipping away uselessly can take Wild Oat to get back on track. It must be taken over a long period of time.

self-alienation, total *1/33

Self-assertiveness, insufficient → Compete, inability to

Self-awareness, lack of *1/36

Self-blame: Pine (→ Conscience → Guilt)

Blaming ourselves is both unnatural and dangerous because it disrupts our inner balance. It means accepting the values imposed upon us by others, and it is a sign of a lack of self-confidence and a deeply rooted fear of punishment. We are no longer aware of the reasons for our actions, which were appropriate at the time. We all make mistakes, but we generally realize this only when we are somewhat advanced in our development. Blaming ourselves after the fact is pointless, because it means applying our current awareness and knowledge to an earlier situation, which is impossible.

Self-castigation → Asceticism

self-castigation and retreat from the world *27/34
self-castigation as a replacement for a meaning in life *27/36

Self-confidence → Inferiority, feelings of

too little: **Larch + Walnut**
too much: **Oak, Water Violet**

    Oak when we don't know, or want to know, our own limits

    Water Violet when we believe that we don't need other people

self-confidence is suddenly lost *11/19
self-confidence, insufficient, with a weak will *12/19
self-confidence, insufficient, causing fear *19/20
self-confidence, insufficient, due to exhaustion *19/23
self-confidence, insufficient, due to a mental or emotional trauma *19/29

self-confidence, insufficient, causing us to be too easily influenced *19/33

self-confidence, insufficient, making a meaningful life impossible *19/36

self-confidence, insufficient, making us resigned *19/37

Self-confidence, insufficient

A healthy sense of self-confidence is essential because it gives us courage and strength in the struggle for survival. It means being aware of and being able to assess our strengths as well as our weaknesses, our abilities and our "disabilities," and being able to assess our position in society.

with a tendency toward self-denigration: Centaury

with feelings of inferiority: Walnut

Walnut gives us more clarity with respect to our needs and protects us from external influences.

Self-control (excessive)

when we hide our fears, suffering, and problems behind a carefree facade: Agrimony

when we don't know when to give up: Oak

when we don't allow ourselves to make any mistakes: Rock Water

Self-criticism → Self-blame

Self-deception → Modesty → Hypocrisy → Inferiority, feelings of

Self-deception is a form of lying. It is even found in nature (in various guises) and is a legitimate phenomenon as long as it's used for protection, but it has negative consequences when it's used for no good reason. Deceiving ourselves is a form of self-negation and can lead in the wrong direction in life because we are falsely judged by those around us and alienated from ourselves.

due to unnecessary deception: Agrimony

Agrimony is appropriate when we try to pass ourselves off as something other than we truly are and when our true essence and feelings are hidden behind a facade.

due to obsequiousness: Centaury

Centaury is helpful when we allow ourselves to be used by other people instead of living our own lives.

caused by a lack of self-confidence: Larch

When we feel that we are inferior, we tend (without good reason) to try to blend into the background.

Self-denial → Renunciation

caused by guilt feelings: Pine
with strict morality: Rock Rose

Self-discipline, severe, with a need for cleanliness *10/27

Self-love → Egocentrism

Self-negation → Self-deception

Self-pity: Chicory (→ Pity)

When we have pity for ourselves, we want it from others as well. Self-pity is just like a drug; it's great when we're weak but it does nothing to help us out of our misery. When we feel self-pity, we're portraying ourselves as poor, innocent victims who can do nothing about our own suffering. This is a crippling attitude, especially because it's usually untrue. If we say, however, "It's your own fault, so stop complaining and do something about it," we are ready and motivated to improve our situation. Taking responsibility for ourselves makes us free and strong; feeling sorry for ourselves makes us weak and a slave to misfortune. Chicory strengthens our independence and is often combined with Walnut.

Self-righteousness → Bitterness

Self-sacrifice → Selflessness

with a weak personality and weak will: Centaury

We selflessly put ourselves at the disposal of others but cannot assert ourselves.

with other motives: Chicory

Chicory is appropriate when we want to obligate other people with our selflessness.

out of a strong sense of responsibility and unyieldingness: **Oak**
self-sacrifice, simultaneously selfless and selfish *4/8
self-sacrifice due to guilt *4/24
self-sacrifice caused by resignation *4/37
self-sacrifice, total *8/25

Self-torment → Asceticism

due to useless worrying about others: **Red Chestnut**
due to being severely strict with ourselves: **Rock Water**
tormenting obsession to achieve *22/27

Selfish Self-sacrifice *4/8

self-suppression leading to psychosis *6/27
self-contempt due to feelings of being unclean *10/19

Selflessness, pathological → Self-sacrifice → Renunciation

Usually, we instinctively avoid any kind of self-denial. If we can't plant our own field, we can't share the harvest. Self-destructive selflessness serves no positive purpose. It serves only to feed the selfishness of the egotist and the addiction of the (emotional) blackmailer. True selflessness requires a healthy, stable psyche; only then can we hope to help those weaker than we are, and thereby enrich our own souls.

due to a weak personality: **Centaury**
Centaury helps people who achieve a false "selflessness" out of a lack of self-assertiveness, which serves only to strengthen the selfishness of others.

with worries: **Red Chestnut**
Red Chestnut can help anyone who thinks only of others and forgets about her own needs.

selflessness, worrisome *4/25

Sentimentality: Clematis + Honeysuckle

Sentimentality is an artificial, arbitrary state of mind. It causes us to be sentimental; we lose our grip on reality as well as the ability to feel true happiness and to overcome unhappiness. Clematis helps treat sentimental fantasies of the future, and Honeysuckle is appropriate for sentimental memories.

Separation → Partner Problems → Grief → Loss

Human relationships can never be severed. If the relationship is an enriching one or a damaging one, it is the expression of the spirit of each of the participants and changes all involved. Externally, a relationship may come to an end, but internally everything endures. When a partnership ends, we can tell if it was characterized by friendship and love or by psychic weaknesses and opportunism. If we have the luck to be able to hold on to the wonderful feelings that existed at the beginning of the relationship, then the end doesn't mean a devastating loss but is more like leafing through the pages of a good book; we retain what we've read in the previous pages and take that as a prelude of what's to come. Separation is just one step further in the ongoing process of widening our horizons.

due to dishonesty: **Agrimony**

Agrimony helps us stay honest with ourselves and with our partner. It can prevent a false, painful atmosphere from developing in the process of separation and becoming a black spot in our biography.

due to possessiveness: **Chicory**

When "love" becomes possessiveness or emotional dependence instead of free and joyful emotions, it's difficult to let go of someone. Chicory helps us let go, to become free ourselves, and to avoid self-pity.

due to hateful rage: **Holly**

Holly minimizes negative feelings; it makes it possible for us to behave in a loving, friendly manner.

due to feelings of loss: **Honeysuckle**

Honeysuckle helps us find closure with what is already past and direct our attention to the present.

with bitterness: **Willow**

If separation causes bitterness or resentment, or leads us to rail against fate, Willow is helpful.

Seriousness, excessive → Humorlessness

Servility: Centaury (→ Humility → Obsequiousness)

Serving something or someone is positive only when it is done out of a positive motivation. Our own happiness is the best motivation, which means that we put ourselves in the service of something that seems good to us or that we can make ourselves happy by some helping act. *Serving,* understood correctly, means wanting to act in a strong and positive manner in order to serve a higher good or value. If a weakness in our personality causes us to be put in a position of servility or to be subjugated when we normally would protect ourselves against it, we need Centaury to put an end to the degrading situation.

Sexual Dysfunction

Sexual dysfunction generally stems from psychic causes. Sexual relationships are characterized by especially intense, private contact with another person. Sexuality embraces procreation and also the possibility of experiencing profound emotions; it's no wonder, then, that practically all psychic problems can have a negative impact on it.

due to a lack of emotional investment: Agrimony

The more trust we place in our partners and the more enthusiasm for life we have, the more satisfying our sexual experiences will be. Agrimony helps when we hold back too much or when we're just going through the motions.

due to revulsion: Crab Apple

From a strictly biological point of view, sexuality is a primitive, animalistic phenomenon; there are some people who live in a sterile, artificial, antiseptic world and who see sex as filthy or revolting, which inhibits their enjoyment. Crab Apple helps minimize compulsive cleanliness.

leading to psychosis: Cherry Plum

At times, the sexual drive is one of the strongest powers we possess. When moral pressures inhibit this drive, a severe inner conflict can result, in which the inner balance is disrupted and we are in danger of a breakdown, hysteria, or psychosis. Cherry Plum helps relieve these pressures and resolve our inner conflict.

due to overarousal: Impatiens + Vervain

due to fear: Mimulus

Sexuality can be disrupted by all kinds of fear, some justified and some arising for absolutely no reason—for example, fear of becoming pregnant, fear of contracting an illness, fear of disgrace, or fear of damnation. Mimulus can help eliminate the ungrounded fears. It is often used for a first sexual experience. In the case of fear of failure, it can be combined with Larch.

due to exhaustion: Olive

due to moralistic pressures: **Pine**

Over the past few centuries, Christian culture has demonized sexuality to the extent that, even today, many people see it as a "sinful" experience. When we do something with a guilty conscience, we can't enjoy it and, in some circumstances, will try to avoid it.

due to negative experiences: **Star of Bethlehem**

Because of our great expectations and lack of experience, the fears and reservations associated with sex can develop into psychic trauma that is often difficult to work through owing to the complex nature of the topic. Such traumas can eventually lead to a kind of sexual block.

frigidity

Frigidity can be caused by a lack of emotional investment, fear, revulsion, moralistic compulsions, or previous negative experiences. See the appropriate sections for more information.

impotence

Impotence can be caused by overstimulation (Impatiens + Vervain), fear of failure (Larch), exhaustion (Olive), or negative experiences (Star of Bethlehem). See the appropriate sections for more information.

Shame

lack of: **Cherry Plum**

Shamelessness can be a way of venting emotional pressures.

excessive

Shame is the expression of taboos placed on the individual by society to promote "appropriate" behavior. These taboos are deeply embedded in the emotional structure through threats and punishment and can inhibit certain kinds of behavior. When shame is thoughtful and reflective and indicative of our finer emotions, it can serve a purpose. When it is unreflective, groundless, and forced upon us, however, it can inhibit the development of a healthy personality and lay the foundation for many psychic problems.

> Agrimony is used when we act falsely and are afraid to show our true nature
>
> Crab Apple can be taken when we have an excessive need for cleanliness and purity, especially with sexual behavior
>
> Larch helps when our shame stems from feelings of inferiority
>
> Pine is given when our shame is associated with guilt feelings

Shock

Shocks and traumas disrupt the existing order and clear the way for a better one. If we can transform a traumatic experience into a new form of knowledge or an important addition to our life experience, we become stronger, smarter, and more secure; otherwise, we will be eliminated from the "war games" of life. This happens when we cannot absorb a shock or trauma. It has something like the effect of a deep freeze on us: we lose our elasticity and flexibility and are easily shattered. It's good to use the little shocks of day-to-day life as a sort of practice for the larger, more devastating ones.

acute: **Clematis + Cherry Plum + Rock Rose; Rescue Remedy**
Clematis is for the tendency to faint, Cherry Plum is for falling to pieces, and Rock Rose works against panic. This combination constitutes part of Rescue Remedy.

consequences of: **Star of Bethlehem**
Star of Bethlehem helps relieve psychic numbness, which can arise as the result of a shock.

shock reaction, allergic *3/15
shocking experience leading to insecurity *5/29
shock causing unconsciousness *9/29

Showing off → Inferiority, feelings of
showing off owing to feelings of inferiority *14/19

Shyness → Conformity → Contact Problems

We all have feelings about other people and know whether they have our well-being at heart, and we all have a tendency to categorize everyone we know as "friends" or "enemies." When we feel strong, we fight to reach our goals, but when we feel defeated, we withdraw. This behavior can manifest itself as extreme shyness (especially when we are very sensitive or have suffered through negative experiences or are among people who do not understand us) and can seriously inhibit our ability to make contact with other people. Bach flower treatment or psychotherapy is needed in these circumstances, especially for children.

out of fear of showing who we are: **Agrimony**
due to fear: **Aspen, Mimulus**

Shyness is a fear of other people. It can be eased with Aspen when the cause is not entirely clear or with Mimulus when the cause is known. It can also be combined with Star of Bethlehem when the cause is an intimidating experience.

due to feelings of inferiority: Larch

When we avoid contact with other people because we feel we won't be noticed, Larch can help. When these feelings of inferiority arise from a discouraging experience, Larch can be combined with Star of Bethlehem (19/29).

due to pathological isolation: Water Violet

Some people are by nature reserved. Water Violet is needed only when their condition becomes a disadvantage or causes them unhappiness.

Skin Conditions

The skin is not just a protective layer but above all our largest excreting, reacting, and regulating organ. Skin conditions, such as eczema, abscesses, and allergies, are nearly always reactions to some inner disturbance and represent the organism's attempt to defuse the problem by drawing it out of the body. Any treatment of skin conditions must therefore first be directed at inner problems: when we merely shut off the body's "ventilation system," for example, with cortisone treatments, we are just making the skin unable to react properly and intensifying the inner problem. Depending on the severity of the problem, this can put the whole organism into danger.

neurodermatitis: Beech + Crab Apple + Holly + Impatiens + Larch + Willow

There are nutritional, environmental, and psychic factors that contribute to neurodermatitis and psoriasis. The more healthy our lifestyle (both physically and spiritually), the less often these conditions appear. Beech has positive effects on the allergic component. Crab Apple purifies the blood and promotes the skin's reactive abilities. Holly lessens extreme reactions and calms the disposition. Impatiens makes us calmer and more stable and lessens itching. Larch strengthens the feeling of self-worth when we are plagued by skin conditions and prevents us from feeling embarrassed. Willow works against negative attitudes that can cause skin reactions.

with pus or abscesses: Crab Apple

Pus is a function of blood purification. It is not an illness in itself, but a sign that the body is detoxifying itself. We should not try to eliminate or reduce pus, but instead allow it an outlet and support the body in its efforts, for example, by giving Crab Apple combined with Star of Bethlehem.

impurities: **Crab Apple, Larch**

Crab Apple is the most important of the essences for purifying the blood. It should be used as a basic treatment for skin conditions. Larch strengthens our feelings of self-worth, especially if we are plagued with acne.

acne: **Crab Apple + Larch + Walnut**

Crab Apple purifies the blood, Larch treats self-rejection, and Walnut restores hormonal balance and develops the personality.

with itching: **Impatiens**

Impatiens can have a positive influence on nervousness, itching, or tingling and can be diluted and applied directly to the skin.

psoriasis → neurodermatitis

Sluggishness → Apathy

Softness: Agrimony + Mimulus + Walnut

Agrimony is for the inability to deal with unpleasantness, Mimulus for timidity, and Walnut for insufficient inner resolve.

Spinal Problems

There is an inseparable bond between body and soul. Generally, we can recognize from afar what kind of mood someone is in or what kind of person he is. Continuous tension deforms the spine, as does obsequiousness, an inferiority complex, or stress. Proper posture is impossible without a straight spine.

osteoporosis **(Bechterev's syndrome, Scheuermann's syndrome): Centaury + Larch (Mimulus, Mustard)**

Osteoporosis is an abnormal, sometimes painful reduction of bone matter, which can lead to fractures of the bones and spine. Medical science has uncovered many fascinating details but has not devoted any attention to psychic factors. Medical treatment usually tries to rebuild bone matter, which brings a certain amount of improvement but can also have harmful side effects; complete recovery isn't possible unless treatment takes both body and soul into account. Allopathic treatment should be undertaken only in severe cases and only after other, natural forms of treatment have proved ineffective.

We should start by asking why the organism is reducing the amount of bone matter. The answer lies in the function of bone: it is a framework, which helps us go through life upright and with confidence. With weak bones or a weak spine, we can't stand up to difficulties, stand at the same level as other people, or even lift ourselves above them. Reduction of bone makes people, to some extent, like lowly reptiles, and it always occurs when we lack the strength to stand upright that comes from a healthy sense of self-confidence. When we feel that we are inferior, less able, or weaker than those around us, we simply can't approach them upright. Our posture and crooked back are signs of fear and submissiveness. The body reflects our inner state, and the frame loses its upright, resilient appearance. Scheuermann's syndrome can develop in children, Bechterev's syndrome in young adults, and osteoporosis in older people (especially menopausal women). This comes as no surprise, since many menopausal women feel socially and sexually inferior when they lose their reproductive capabilities. An unconscious consequence is that they can no longer bear themselves upright and with self-confidence, which leads to poor, bent posture and weakening of the spine. An example is the so-called widow's hump, which used to be quite common when widowhood meant a loss of social status. Osteoporosis in the thighs is also a common problem, distinguished by diminished walking ability and the typical and dangerous fractures of the femur in older people when they can no longer meet the demands of daily life. Any meaningful form of treatment (or prevention) must help restore or instill self-confidence. It is common knowledge that we are lost when we give up. The combination given here can help strengthen self-confidence and feelings of self-worth. It is also appropriate for older people who are having difficulty dealing with the loss of strength and abilities that accompany the aging process; it helps compensate with a corresponding increase in mental, spiritual, or human values and activities. Mimulus should also be given in cases of timidity and Mustard in cases of depression.

Stage Fright: Cherry Plum + Gentian + Heather + Hornbeam + Impatiens + Larch + Mimulus (+ Star of Bethlehem)

Cherry Plum works for inner tranquillity. Gentian is for inner confidence. Heather counters the fear of disgrace. Hornbeam fights feelings of inadequacy.

Impatiens alleviates nervousness. Larch instills more self-confidence. Mimulus minimizes timidity.

with negative experiences: Star of Bethlehem

Standoffishness Æ Pride Æ Distance

*standoffish with excessive tolerance *3/34*

Stomach Ailments

The connection between mind and body is especially clear in the stomach. It can become ill when it receives too much or too little or the wrong kinds of food. For the stomach, the world consists of food that must be processed and digested, just as the psyche must process and digest certain life situations and problems.

gastritis due to stress and overwork

When we are faced with a great challenge or responsibility, the stomach reacts just as if it had a load of food to digest. It responds by boosting the production of acids, which in turn eat away at the stomach's mucous lining. Essentially, it ends up digesting itself, and the result is heartburn and pain. In such cases, the causes of stress should be limited.

> Elm when we feel we've taken on too much and are afraid of failing
>
> Impatiens when we're always in a rush
>
> Mimulus when we're afraid of an upcoming responsibility or test (can be combined with Larch)
>
> Oak when we've taken on more than we can handle, but don't know when to give up

gastritis caused by envy or greed: Chicory + Holly

The feeling that we don't receive what we deserve is similar to the stomach's feeling of hunger. An empty stomach eats itself up, so to speak. We should try to be content with what we have. This combination helps suppress envy and anger.

gastritis and ulcers caused by anger and annoyance

Suppressed anger has the same effect as that of indigestible, inedible food. It eats away at the stomach. Over time, gastritis can become an ulcer (a wound in the stomach's mucous lining). In severe cases, it can even become cancer. Anger that arises from family situations can be especially devastating. It develops over a long period of time, and we try to keep it quiet so as not to rock the boat. If we cannot find a way of avoiding this anger (for example, by leaving the family), we must try to change our attitude.

Holly for long-term irritability or rage

Star of Bethlehem when we take things too seriously

Willow to enable us to forgive and forget

Strain → Tension

Strength, loss of → Exhaustion → Weakness

Stress

Theoretically, stress is caused by greed or a lack of discipline. It is a sign that we've passed the limits of what we can safely achieve. Long-term stress is harmful because it inhibits the body's normal processes of detoxification and regeneration. Short periods of stress can make us ill; long periods of stress can kill us.

due to secrecy or artificiality: **Agrimony**

When we try to disguise or hide our true nature, we are going against our own best interests and are also afraid of being found out.

due to suppressed drives and emotions: **Cherry Plum**

When we suppress important natural drives and emotions, we only create stress because this must be done forcefully.

with an acute sense of stress and overwork: **Elm**

Elm is useful when an important job or responsibility makes us feel so stressed that we're in danger of a collapse.

due to impatience: **Impatiens**

Hasty, impatient people often find themselves stressed when they are held up for any reason.

due to fear: **Mimulus**

due to unyieldingness or ambition: **Oak**

Oak is for people who put themselves under too much pressure.

due to excessive enthusiasm: **Vervain**

stress bringing us to the emotional breaking point *6/22

stress, emotional, leading to psychosis *6/30

addicted to love and popularity *8/14

stress causing panic *11/26

stress and haste *22/31*

stress due to an overbearing compulsion to achieve *22/31*

Stress and Overwork

on the verge of collapse: Elm

imagined: Hornbeam

Hornbeam is for people who believe that they are not up to a task, even though they are perfectly capable.

caused by a lack of self-confidence: Larch

We are quickly overwhelmed when we lack confidence.

stress and overwork caused by dependence *4/17*

stress and overwork leading to discouragement *11/12*

stress and overwork with hopelessness *11/13*

stress and overwork caused by a compulsion to achieve *11/22*

stress and overwork with desperation *11/30*

stress and overwork causing a retreat into the past *16/17*

stress and overwork caused by a lack of self-confidence *17/19*

stress and overwork causing resignation *17/37*

Strictness → Discipline

strict with oneself and unnaturally generous with others *3/27*

strict personality *27/32*

Stubbornness → Dogmatism → Habits and Routines → Tension

Stubbornness and inflexibility prevent us from acting quickly. This is a cause for concern, since life and growth are dynamic, expansive phenomena characterized by constant change. Tradition brings with its unchanging nature a certain amount of comfort and security, but it prevents the necessary process of renewal. Inflexibility means death, while flexibility means life. Inflexible people have a tendency toward tension (→ Tension), rheumatism (→ Rheumatism), and degeneration.

with unyieldingness: Oak

Oak is needed when we are too uncompromising.

with oneself: Rock Water

Rock Water is effective against obstinate self-discipline.

with others: **Vine**

Vine is helpful for people who are inflexible and intolerant.

Stuttering

Bach flowers can be effective for stuttering children when we keep in mind the underlying psychic causes. Treatment often involves combining several essences.

with persistence: **Gentian**

Gentian prevents us from giving up too easily when we can't form our words. Persistence will help us overcome the problem. It should be given frequently.

with an excessive need for recognition: **Heather**

Heather is for vain children who have an urgent need for recognition and temporarily lose the ability to speak freely and fluidly.

due to nervousness: **Impatiens**

due to fear: **Mimulus**

If we have ever stuttered, it's quite natural that we will be afraid that it might recur. Mimulus is effective against these fears of negative expectations.

caused by problems with muscular coordination: **Scleranthus**

Scleranthus enables the body to coordinate its efforts and allows us to properly articulate our words. It is a basic essence in the treatment of stuttering.

due to psychic trauma: **Star of Bethlehem**

Star of Bethlehem can help when stuttering has been caused by a psychic trauma.

trauma caused by a fear of punishment, unresolved *24/29

Suicide, danger of

Rescue Remedy should be used in any emergency, even a potential suicide situation.

due to mental anguish: **Agrimony**

When we try too hard to conceal our problems we suffer twice as much.

due to emotional pressure: **Cherry Plum**

Cherry Plum is helpful when we suppress our drives and emotions so severely and for so long that we lose our ability to act rationally and are on the verge of a nervous breakdown.

with a death wish: **Clematis**

We have no joy in life because we can't come to terms with it. Typically, we want to end it all.

due to total hopelessness: **Gorse**
due to depression: **Mustard**

Mustard is appropriate for any condition in which it seems as if our lives are covered by a black cloud that obscures the meaning of life from us.

due to desperation: **Sweet Chestnut**

Superficiality

due to forced, artificial behavior: **Agrimony**

Agrimony helps people who cannot bring themselves to face their problems and fears and seek refuge in superficial words and deeds.

in society: **Heather**

Heather helps people who do not seek deeper interpersonal relationships but who are concerned only with being regarded in a favorable light.

due to haste and impatience: **Impatiens**

People who need Impatiens are so driven that they have no time for deeper relationships or activities.

due to isolation: **Water Violet**

Water Violet helps bridge distance between people and fosters deeper human relationships.

Suppression: Agrimony

Suppressing the unpleasant is a natural and useful function of the psyche. It protects us from any mental or emotional influences that can overpower us. The suppressed material is stored in a kind of subconscious archive, where it can be retrieved when we are ready to deal with it. It then appears in the form of a "problem" and affords us no rest until we solve it. The attempt to suppress or ignore problems that have surfaced in our consciousness leads to severe inner conflict. Agrimony helps put an end to this running from ourselves and helps us tear down the facades we present to the world in an attempt to conceal the truth. The more willing we are to honestly confront the unpleasant questions the spirit asks us, the more content we will be. The soul can accept only the truth.

suppression of fears *1/2
suppression creating excessive psychic pressure *1/6

Talkativeness

to be popular and distract us from ourselves: Agrimony
Agrimony helps people who try to hide their problems and fears behind a flurry of cheerful chatter.

due to insecurity: Cerato
Cerato is helpful for anyone who needs to talk about all her problems and wants good advice.

psychotic: Cherry Plum
Cherry Plum is indicated for people who are under extreme emotional pressure and need solace and companionship to keep from going crazy.

due to a craving for recognition: Heather
Heather is for people who feel compelled to boast of their own talents and accomplishments.

due to missionary zeal: Vervain
Vervain diminishes the urge to convince everyone of our own ideas and convictions.

Teeth

jaw problems
The shape of the jaw and the type of "bite" can be divided into two categories: the overbite and the underbite. By looking at the bite, we can see the attitude with which a person relates to his environment—for example, if he tends to give up or dig in the heels and fight back when faced with difficulties. With an overbite, the lower jaw is less prominent than the upper, and the chin recedes. This type of bite doesn't have quite the same "dangerous" or "brutal" expression as an underbite, where the lower jaw protrudes farther than the upper. Between these extremes is a neutral position, in which the jaws are evenly aligned. Naturally, Bach flower essences can't change the shape or alignment of the jaw, but they can help the underlying personality conditions.

overbite
Overbite, characterized by a smaller lower jaw and teeth aligned to the rear, can be found in people who are overly sensitive and have difficulty asserting themselves. They tend to be introverts; everything first affects them internally

and must be mulled over before they can react appropriately. They tend to give up when faced with difficulties or to subordinate themselves or put themselves through agonizing inner struggles. When this characteristic is very pronounced, use any essence that strengthens courage and personal strength.

> Centaury for excessive cheerfulness and tractability or allowing oneself to be used
>
> Gentian for insufficient strength of will
>
> Hornbeam for stress and overwork and fear of failure
>
> Larch for underdeveloped self-confidence

underbite

Underbite occurs less frequently. The chin juts forward and gives the face an energetic expression. These people are usually easily provoked; they don't try to avoid difficulties but confront them directly. Essences that promote yieldingness, friendliness, and flexibility are appropriate.

> Holly for a tendency toward rage or violent outbursts of anger
>
> Oak for unyieldingness and unwillingness to compromise
>
> Vervain for excessive enthusiasm and hyperactivity
>
> Vine for a tendency toward self-righteousness

tooth decay, cavities, and receding gums

Cavities and receding gums have a variety of causes, many of which have yet to be fully understood. Improper dental care, bacteria, hereditary weakness, internal illness, or toxins can all be decisive factors, but psychic factors have been little noticed. In times of emotional stress, the force used in biting, chewing, and grinding can have devastating effects on teeth, roots, and gums.

> Agrimony for internal tension
>
> Elm for excessive stress
>
> Holly + Willow for anger and rage
>
> Oak for a tendency to struggle and fret through difficulties

grinding teeth: Agrimony + Holly + Oak + Vervain

This combination helps relax the jaw muscles. Agrimony works generally against tension, Holly helps counter aggression, Oak suppresses emotions, Vervain minimizes hyperactivity. Willow should be added to curb bitterness, and Cherry Plum to help resolve bottled-up emotions.

children's teeth: **Walnut**

Walnut helps body and soul make the transition to a new life phase. It helps everything run smoothly and exactly as planned.

    debilitating guilt complex *23/24

    debilitating worries *23/25

Temperament

too soft

    Centaury for yieldingness

    Gentian for a weak will

    Larch for lack of assertiveness

too hard

    Holly for aggressiveness

    Vervain for a hot temper

    Vine for intolerance

Tension → Stress

Pathological inner tension arises when we take on or expect of ourselves more than we are able to achieve. Tension can assist the development of certain abilities, but it is harmful when we don't allow ourselves periods of rest.

due to artificiality: **Agrimony**

The attempt to seem to be something that we are not creates a severe inner tension because our real self must be forcefully kept in check. Generally, we can recognize inner tension in our movements, posture, and artificial or phony facial expressions.

caused by unyieldingness: **Oak**

When we demand more of ourselves than we are able to accomplish, we must allow ourselves a rest if we are to continue. In the long term, nothing good can come of the situation.

due to excessive self-discipline: **Rock Water**

Self-discipline is often motivated by the desire to suppress certain qualities, but since these qualities are integral parts of the personality, they resist this suppression.

due to overzealousness: **Vervain**

Tension, inner: **Cherry Plum**

Cherry Plum is helpful when we are under such severe internal pressure that we are in danger of acting irrationally or of psychosis.

Terrible Emotions: Aspen

Thoughtlessness → Egotism

toward others: Holly, Impatiens

Holly minimizes aggressive behavior, while Impatiens works against impatience, which causes thoughtless behavior.

toward ourselves: Oak, Red Chestnut

Oak is for people who are so obsessed with reaching their goals that they forget about their other needs until they are at the limits of their endurance. Red Chestnut is effective against the senseless habit of worrying intensely about other people and forgetting about ourselves.

Thyroid Problems

The thyroid transfers emotions into bodily functions. We become ill when this does not happen successfully.

hyperactive thyroid, with glassy eyes, nervousness, restlessness, shaking, thinness

> Cherry Plum for strong, suppressed emotions and sexual drives
> Impatiens + Vervain for severe nervousness and hyperactivity
> Oak when we are grim and put too much pressure on ourselves

hypoactive thyroid, characterized by reduced activity with slowness, lethargy, weakness

> Clematis + Wild Rose for lack of enthusiasm and drive, drowsiness, and a lack of interest in life
> Hornbeam for weakness and a permanent feeling of stress and overwork

Timidity → Fear

Tolerance → Intolerance → Chapter 1: Beech, Vine

True tolerance stems from the knowledge that everything is justified in its existence and that we should all learn to live and let live. If we are to be tolerated by other people, we must be willing to tolerate them as well. This can happen only when we learn to tolerate all of our own inconsistencies and shortcomings; any quality that we disapprove of in ourselves, we are certain to disapprove of in other people. The more openly and honestly we can face our own shortcomings, the more tolerant and understanding we will be with other people. We are not all tolerant by nature. There are people who are intolerant and struggle against everything with which they are not familiar. When they try to hide their intolerance and pass themselves off as tolerant and understanding, they become confused by their own lies. It's better if they simply learn to recognize and acknowledge their intolerance—their eternal criticizing and struggling will at least have a note of honesty, which will be more tolerable for other people.

hypocritical: **Agrimony**

Agrimony is useful for people who try to pass themselves off as tolerant and positive to distance themselves from their true nature and to be popular.

apparent: **Beech**

When we appear to be tolerant but deep inside we are actually intolerant, we need Beech. This openness and understanding has an artificial air and prevents us from facing reality honestly.

due to a lack of interest: **Wild Rose**

When we have lost our interest in life, nothing really matters anymore. This "tolerance" is the sign of a spiritual illness and is by no means an indication of virtue.

tolerance, artificial or excessive *1/3
tolerance, opportunistic *3/14
tolerance, due to a lack of self-confidence *3/19
tolerance, due to timidity *3/20
tolerance, unnatural and moralistic *3/24
tolerance, excessive, and emotional distance *3/34

Trauma, psychic → Injury

trauma leading to hopelessness *13/29
trauma caused by humiliation *14/29
trauma due to a loss *16/29
trauma undermining self-confidence *19/29
trauma creating timidity *20/29
trauma causing depression *21/29
traumatic experiences causing excessive worry *25/29
trauma weakening the psychic defenses *29/33
trauma causing human contact problems *29/34
traumatic thoughts *29/35
trauma causing resignation *29/37
trauma causing bitterness *29/38

Tuberculosis → Lung Conditions

Turmoil, inner

due to insecurity: **Cerato**

When we are too afraid of making mistakes, we tend to ask everyone for advice; the problem is that we end up exactly where we started because we don't have a clue whose advice is correct. Cerato improves our ability to act on our own impulses.

due to indecisiveness: **Scleranthus**

Scleranthus helps when we waver among several alternatives and simply can't make a decision.

caused by lacking direction in life: **Wild Oat**

Wild Oat is useful when we want to do something sensible and meaningful but we don't know what and we undertake many things halfheartedly.

turmoil, inner, and life crisis → 28/36

Ulcer, duodenal → Stomach Ailments

Unbearable Life Situations

due to placing oneself under extreme pressure: **Cherry Plum**

The more strongly we suppress important needs or drives, the greater is our distress. Cherry Plum is useful when we feel we can't stand the pressure anymore and are about to do something terrible.

due to insufficient mental and psychic strength: **Star of Bethlehem**

Star of Bethlehem helps us work through traumatic, devastating situations.

due to inner inflexibility: **Sweet Chestnut**

When we are too strong and refuse to bend to fate, we can create an unbearable inner pressure from which there seems to be no release. Sweet Chestnut can help defuse or prevent such situations.

Uncleanliness Causes Fear *10/20 (→ Cleanliness)

Uncompromising → Stubbornness

Unconsciousness: Clematis

Clematis is a preventive measure when we have a tendency to lose consciousness. For emergencies (→ Emergencies), use Rescue Remedy, which contains Clematis.

*unconsciousness with panic *9/26*
*unconsciousness caused by a shocking experience *9/29*

Understanding, excessive: Beech (→ Tolerance)

Uneasiness → Restlessness

due to secret worries: **Agrimony**

Agrimony is for people who try to conceal their true inner condition. This causes a constant strain. Although they try to appear carefree, they are somehow driven and restless.

due to insecurity: **Cerato**

When we want things to be just fine with everyone but don't know how to make them so, we lose our inner peace and never find ourselves.

with nervous chatter and showing off: **Heather**

Heather is for people who become restless when they don't receive enough attention; they constantly draw attention to themselves and put themselves in the spotlight.

with impatience and nervousness: **Impatiens**

Impatiens is the basic essence for all conditions related to haste or restlessness and uneasiness.

due to guilt feelings: **Pine**

We can never find inner peace when we have a bad conscience.

due to excessive worrying about others: **Red Chestnut**
*restlessness and danger of psychosis *6/18*
*restlessness with fear *18/20*
*restlessness caused by worries *18/25*
*restlessness with a tendency toward panic *18/26*

Unforgiving: Chicory + Willow (→ Bitterness)

Unforgiving people are, above all, emotional and demanding. They invest their emotions heavily in their expectations and tend to become deeply disappointed when these expectations are not met. Sometimes they can feel a need for revenge as well. Chicory helps diminish these intensive emotional demands, and Willow counters the tendency to react bitterly. We can come to terms with the supposed injustice and become more conciliatory.

Ungratefulness

due to never being satisfied: Chicory

Chicory is for people who can never seem to have enough.

due to bitterness: Willow

When resentment or denial of a desire causes us to forget everything that we do have, we need Willow.

Unhappiness → Depression

Unreliability

caused by an inability to make decisions: Scleranthus

People who have difficulty making decisions jump from one choice to the next. It often seems that they are being pressured to reverse their decisions, and they appear to be unreliable.

due to being too easily influenced: Walnut

When we are too easily influenced, we are not reliable and can often not even trust ourselves. Walnut helps us stay true to ourselves and hold our own course.

caused by distraction: Wild Oat

When we don't know what we want, it's easy to be distracted from our goals or to be interrupted from a task that we've started. Wild Oat helps us recognize what's important and what's right.

Unsociable, due to exhaustion *23/34

Unyielding → Stubbornness

*unyieldingness with perfectionism *22/24*

Used, allowing oneself to be → Good naturedness

Validation, need for: Cerato

We try desperately to avoid mistakes by asking others for their opinion, which makes us even more insecure.

Vanity: Heather (→ Inferiority, feelings of)

It is a healthy function of the psyche to want to be beautiful, adored, or important. Such desires motivate us to positive social behavior. When this behavior makes people unhappy because it is excessive or unrealistic, or becomes compulsive out of the fear of being rejected by society, or endangers our being able to get along with other people, it takes on a negative character. Heather can bring our need for recognition and popularity to tolerable (for ourselves and others) levels and reduce our fear of disgrace and humiliation.

vain youth *14/16
compulsive vanity *14/35

Vices, secret: Agrimony (→ Drug Abuse → Facade)

Victim → Self-sacrifice → Used, allowing oneself to be

Violence → Aggression

Vision Problems → Eye Conditions

Vocation, unsure of: Wild Oat

Wild Oat helps us rediscover meaning in our lives—either consciously or unconsciously, intellectually or practically. We can be happy only if we find our true calling.

Washing, compulsive: Crab Apple

Weak Personality

We are all blessed with a variety of talents and abilities, which form our personality. The more fully and purely this occurs, the more decisively we can strike out on our path in life. The strength of a personality consists of an inner aspect (how we treat ourselves) and an outer aspect (our relationships with others). People with stronger personalities are sure of themselves and behave correctly and confidently take their proper place in society. Whether they have a low or high social standing, they give the impression that they are confident in themselves and that they have a unified, whole personality. Weak personalities, on the other hand, cannot come to terms with themselves, with other people, or with life itself. They often give the impression that they are somehow underdeveloped or that something is missing. Bach flowers can help remedy these deficits.

with fear of the truth: Agrimony

Agrimony awakens within us the desire to be as we truly are. When we do not dare face the truth about ourselves, or when fear of other people causes us to be other than we are, we become weak and unstable and must constantly blind ourselves to important aspects of reality. We cannot develop a strong personality in such a state.

due to a lack of self-confidence: Centaury (→ Servility)

Only people who are psychically weak and defeated let themselves be used and deceive themselves. Centaury will help them become more aware of their rights and obligations and enable them to stand up to emotional blackmail and free them from a position of servitude. Naturally, this has nothing to do with people who serve others out of an inner sense of freedom and strength: they will not be used or blackmailed but act only out of a sense of inner joy.

with insecurity and mistrust of our instincts: Cerato

To help ensure our survival, nature endowed us with instincts and our critical faculties. Cerato helps us when we constantly seek the advice of others instead of finding the important answers for ourselves.

due to vanity: Heather

Vanity is not just compulsive cleanliness but has to do with the image we want to project to others as well. It is essentially a personal weakness because we depend upon the recognition, praise, or admiration of others and become dependent on trying to please them. Heather is especially suitable for treating that special form of vanity that is characterized by showing off and annoying boasting.

due to feelings of inferiority: Larch

Larch helps build self-confidence. It is helpful when we don't pay attention to ourselves or don't believe in ourselves and are therefore not taken seriously.

due to guilty thoughts: Pine

When we judge ourselves, we make ourselves weaker. A significant sign of a strong personality is self-reconciliation. If we carefully examine our guilty conscience, we realize that in very large measure it arises out of a fear of punishment and—taking all factors into account—that we acted the best we could under the circumstances. It's senseless to judge ourselves, and the result is that we are voluntarily acting in a juvenile, obsequious manner. It makes more sense to get to know ourselves better and to learn to improve our actions from one day to the next.

due to indecisiveness: **Scleranthus**
The ability to make clear, thoughtful decisions is the sign of a strong personality. Scleranthus helps us when we let all of our divergent tendencies get the better of us.

due to psychic trauma: **Star of Bethlehem**
Being able to survive a severe mental or emotional trauma is an important factor of a strong, healthy personality. Star of Bethlehem helps restore our inner balance and maintain our mental and emotional resilience.

from being too easily influenced: **Walnut**
Staying true to oneself is one of the most important measures of a strong personality. It means the unity of being and doing and of internal and external life; without this unity, there is no contentment.

weak personality with dependence *4/5
weak will and personality *4/12

Weakness → Exhaustion
weakness with nostalgic tendencies *12/16

Weather, sensitivity to
Sensitivity to the weather signifies an instability of the vegetative nerve system, which can be caused by either a hereditary illness or hidden infections or can be a sign of a developing illness, which Bach essences can often help prevent.

with ominous feelings: **Aspen**
with fatigue: **Elm + Olive**
with irritability: **Holly**
with restlessness or fidgetiness: **Impatiens**
with moodiness or depression: **Mustard**
with the need for quiet and distance: **Water Violet**

Weepy → Hypersensitivity

Will, strong

A strength can become a weakness if it can't be controlled or damages us.

makes us inflexible: Oak
as a cause of self-abuse: Rock Water
in the form of missionary pushiness: Vervain
with stubborn self-righteousness: Vine

Will, weak → Giving up

when we let ourselves be used too much: Centaury
when we give up too early when we encounter difficulties:
  Gentian
weak will and a weak personality *4/12
weak will and inattentiveness *7/12
weak will and hopelessness *12/13
weak will and daydreaming *12/16
weak will and a lack of self-confidence *12/19
weak will caused by psychic trauma *12/29
compliance due to hopelessness *4/13

Worries

hidden: Agrimony
fearful: Aspen
caused by a desire to possess: Chicory
about others: Red Chestnut
dominating the thoughts: White Chestnut
worries, secret *1/25
worries, vague and dominated by fear *2/25
worries, inducing rage *6/25
worrisome restlessness *18/25
worries, with fear *20/25
worrisome depression *21/25
worries, debilitating *23/25
worries, due to a bad conscience *24/25
worries causing panic *25/26
worries caused by negative experiences *25/29
worrisome thoughts *25/35

Wounds, mental and spiritual behind a happy
  facade *1/29

Yieldingness → Conformity → Compete, inability to

Zealous Convert → Know-it-all → Missionary
  Tendencies

We need Oak if we cannot give up once we have a goal in mind.

RESOURCES

The original Bach Flower Remedies are still collected at the same sites used by Dr. Edward Bach and are prepared according to his method. These original flower essences can be purchased individually or as a complete set from the following suppliers:

North America

Nelson Bach USA
100 Research Drive
Wilmington, MA 01887
Phone: (978) 988-3833
Fax (978) 988-0233

England

Bach Flower Remedies Ltd.
Dr. Edward Bach Center
Mount Vernon
Sotwell, Wallingford
Oxfordshire OX10 0PZ

Healing Health Ltd.
P.O. Box 65
GB-Hereford HR2 0UW

Australia

The Pharmaceutical Plant Company
P.O. Box 68
Bayswater, Victoria 3153
Phone: 03-762 8577/8522

Martin & Pleasance Wholesale Pty Ltd.
P.O. Box 4
Collingwood, Victoria 3066
Phone: 03-419 9733

FURTHER READING

Bach, E. *Collected Writings*. Ed. J. Barnard. Hereford, England: Flower Remedy Programme, 1987.

Bach, E., and F. J. Wheeler. *The Bach Flower Remedies*. New Canaan, CT: Keats, 1979.

Barnard, J. *Patterns of Life Force*. Hereford, England: Flower Remedy Programme, 1987.

Barnard, J., and M. Barnard. *The Healing Herbs of Edward Bach: An Illustrated Guide to the Flower Remedies*. Bath, England: Ashgrove, 1988.

Chancellor, Philip. *The Handbook of the Bach Flower Remedies*. New Canaan, CT: Keats, 1980.

Cunningham, D. *Flower Remedies Handbook*. New York: Sterling, 1992.

Damian, Peter. *The Twelve Healers of the Zodiac: The Astrology Handbook of the Bach Flower Remedies*. York Beach, ME: Weiser, 1986.

Kaminski, P. *Flower Essence Repertory*. Nevada City, CA: Flower Essence Society, 1994.

Krämer, Dietmar. *New Bach Flower Therapies: Theory and Practice*. Rochester, VT: Healing Arts Press, 1995.

———. *New Bach Flower Body Maps*. Rochester, VT: Healing Arts Press, 1996.

Lo Rito, D. Iridotherapy. In *Iridology Review*, Vol. 1(3), 1992.

———. *Bach Flower Massage*. Rochester, VT: Healing Arts Press, 1997.

Mazzarella, Barbara. *Bach Flower Remedies for Children*. Rochester, VT: Healing Arts Press, 1997.

Scheffer, Mechthild. *Bach Flower Therapy: Theory and Practice*. Rochester, VT: Healing Arts Press, 1988.

———. *Mastering Bach Flower Therapies*. Rochester, VT: Healing Arts Press, 1996.

Vlamis, Gregory. *Bach Flower Remedies to the Rescue*. Rochester, VT: Healing Arts Press, 1990.

Weeks, Nora. *The Medical Discoveries of Edward Bach, Physician*. New Canaan, CT: Keats, 1979.

Healing Arts Press books may be ordered by calling 1-800-371-3174.

INDEX

bed-wetting, 239
beech *(fagus sylvatica)*, 5
    meaning and use of, 19–22
    see also allergies; generosity;
        intolerance
behavior problems, 128, 239–40
    see also compulsions; irrational
        behavior
beliefs, strength of, 241
birth
    as life change, 144–46
    pregnancy, emotions of, 329–30
    stages of, 241–42
bitterness
    compulsive, 155, 233, 242
    depression caused by, 167, 221,
        242, 259
    offended easily, 319–20
    in willow syndrome, 164–67, 240
    see also aggressiveness; cold
        emotions; resentment;
        self-righteousness;
        unforgiving behavior
bitterness, causes of
    dependence/lack of freedom, 232
    disappointment, 164–67, 209, 260,
        335
    ingratitude, 43, 192, 242
    intolerance, 242
    loss, 211, 242
    rage/hate, 69, 167, 242, 334
    rejection, 43, 192, 242
    unprocessed trauma, 131, 242
blackmail, emotional, 41, 43, 165–66,
    242–43
blood pressure, 243–44
    hypertension, 53, 78, 97, 137, 141,
        143, 291
    hypotension, 291
blood purification, 49, 236, 253, 279
breakdown,
    in old age, 175
    psychotic, 32–33
    verge of, 144, 168, 184, 197, 198, 247

breakdown, causes of
    panic, 115, 173, 244
    stress/overwork, 35, 51–52, 185
    suppression, 170, 244
    trauma, 131, 199

cancer, 60, 116, 128, 203, 244–45
carelessness, 31, 36, 39, 45, 181, 187, 245
caring, excessive, 40, 111–14, 245
centaury *(centaurium umbellatum)*, 5
    meaning and use of, 23–27, 162
    see also cheerfulness; selflessness;
        servility
cerato *(ceratostigma willmottiana)*, 5
    meaning and use of, 19–22, 28–31
    see also dependence; insecurity;
        uncertainty
cheerfulness, 14, 23–25, 240
cherry plum *(prunus cerasifera)*, 5
    meaning and use of, 32–35
    see also hysteria; obsession; psychosis
chestnut bud *(aesculus hippocastanum)*, 5
    meaning and use of, 36–39
    see also inattentiveness; learning
        difficulties
chicory *(cichorium intybus)*, 5
    meaning and use of, 40–43
    see also jealousy; love, conditional;
        mothering
Christianity, 26, 29–30, 106–9
circulatory problems, 97, 112, 120,
    141, 143, 162
cleanliness, compulsive, 345
    consequences of, 196, 306, 324
    in crab apple syndrome, 48–50,
        240, 328
    fanatical, 196, 246, 274, 320
    on moral grounds, 195, 196, 315
    and perfectionism, 326
    see also filth aversion
clematis *(clematis vitalba)*, 5
    meaning and use of, 44–47
    see also death wish; fantasies;
        unconsciousness

with suicide danger, 357
dejection, 90, 256
delusions, 256
    see also psychosis
dependence, 41
    on authority, 105–9, 238
    causes of, 144–45, 178, 256, 257
    consequences of, 182, 232, 342
    and influenceability, 27, 144, 147,
        180, 256, 257
    and insecurity, 28 30, 257
    and stress/overwork, 27, 179, 256
depression, 257–59
    anxious, 95, 219, 276
    endogenous, 56, 90–95, 258
    hidden, 12
    with moodiness, 128, 201, 314
    in mustard syndrome, 90–95, 240
    with other factors, 220, 221, 250, 258
    reactive, 55
    see also hopelessness; pessimism;
        sadness
depression, causes of, 257–59
    bitterness, 221, 242, 259
    fear of failure, 75, 258
    guilt feelings, 219, 259, 283
    heartbreak, 287
    hopelessness, 203
    loss, 156–57, 210, 259, 308
    meaninglessness, 156–57, 220–21,
        259
    psychic trauma, 128, 220, 259, 363
    purposelessness, 220–21, 258, 333
    rejection/loneliness, 206, 259
    self-denial, 24, 257
desperation, 259
    causes of, 54, 186, 199, 202, 227,
        229, 307
    hopeless, 61, 135, 204, 259, 289
    with stress/overwork, 35, 186, 199,
        356
    in sweet chestnut syndrome,
        132–35, 240
    see also breakdown; depression

developmental difficulties, 259–60
    see also learning difficulties
diet/exercise, 119, 120, 174
disappointment
    with bitterness, 164–67, 209, 260, 335
    due to failure, 260
    illness caused by, 293
    in love, 128
    and rejection of others, 150, 335
discipline, toward others, 228, 261
    see also self-discipline
discontent, 261
    due to repression, 13–14
    frustration, 74, 124, 145, 156–58
    ungratefulness, 366
    discouragement, 55–57, 201, 240,
        261, 270
    see also exhaustion; giving up
dishonesty
    in agrimony syndrome, 13, 239
    lying, 13, 344
    see also artificiality; facade
disloyalty, 261
disorder, 249, 261–62
distance, emotional, 262
    with apparent tolerance, 178
    with contact problems, 220, 253
    due to pride, 149, 331
    inhibitions, 252–53, 297
    reserved behavior, 149, 336
    and tolerance, 178, 363
    see also loner; missionary zeal
distracted behavior, 36, 123, 188, 250,
        262
distress, 262
dogma, 138, 241, 263–64
dogmatic compulsive thoughts, 119,
        121, 155, 231, 264
dogmatism, 263–64
    closed-mindedness, 97, 140–43,
        188, 238, 240
    opinionated thought, 320
    pigheadedness, 96, 97, 132
    prejudice, 330

stubbornness, 96–97, 356–57, 364
in vine syndrome, 140–43, 240
see also fanaticism; obsession
do-gooder, 136–37, 207, 231, 262–3, 302
domination, 41, 136, 140–3, 162, 264
dreaminess, 70–72, 192, 324
dreams. *see* daydreaming; nightmares
drive, lack of, 264–5
with depression, 91, 265
reasons for, 212, 216, 225, 233
see also weakness
drives, suppressed, 170, 334, 355
drowsiness. *see* resignation
drug abuse. *see* substance abuse

ear/hearing problems, 265
eating disorders, 12, 237–38, 255
education/upbringing, 94–95, 106–8, 162
egocentrism, 266–67
in heather syndrome, 62–63, 65
self-centeredness, 37
egotism, 266–67, 268, 362
excessive, 40–42, 206, 267
insufficient, 267
with selflessness, 191
see also greed; jealousy; thoughtlessness; vanity
elm *(ulmus procera)*, 5
meaning and use of, 51–54
see also achievement; illness;
stress/overwork
embarrassment, 267
emergencies
accidents, 127, 128
injuries, 150, 168, 298, 321
leadership qualities in, 142
responses to, 184, 193, 204, 227, 229
in rock rose syndrome, 115–18
see also breakdown; Rescue Remedy
endurance, 55, 184, 268
enthusiasm, lack of
in children, 188, 189
and depression, 90–91, 268
in wild rose syndrome, 160–63, 240

see also discontent; moodiness;
resignation
envy, 66, 68, 268
see also egotism; jealousy
epilepsy, 193, 268
erratic behavior, 123–24, 269
see also unreliability
excitement, 269
exemplary behavior, 269
exhaustion
causes of, 99, 198, 219, 224, 269–70
and discouragement, 214, 261, 270
and noncompetitiveness, 248
in olive syndrome, 101–4, 240
see also discouragement; weakness
exhaustion, consequences of, 270
absentmindedness, 192, 270
concentration difficulties, 192, 250
depression, 104, 219, 270
drive, lack of, 225, 265
flight into past, 210, 270
hopelessness, 60, 104, 270
influenceability, 147, 224
resistance, weakened, 131, 224
unsociability, 224, 270, 366
expectations
creating fear, 87, 270
negative, 103, 106, 111, 113–14
positive, 161, 165, 204
see also fantasies
extortion. *see* blackmail, emotional
eye conditions, 270–71, 280
cataracts, 271
conjunctivitis, 271
glaucoma, 271, 280
poor eyesight, 271

facade
artificiality, 10–14, 238, 239
carefree, 170–71, 245
courage to remove, 272
hiding psychic wounds, 14, 371
tolerant, 20, 169
see also artificiality

causing in others, 165–66, 283
conscience, guilty, 105–9, 182, 251, 283
debilitating, 223, 283
and education/upbringing, 106–8
fear of, 89, 109, 217, 277
guilty compulsive thoughts, 195, 226, 283
and moral inferiority, 215
in pine syndrome, 76, 105–10, 240
remorse, 335
self-blame, 226, 343, 344
see also remorse; responsibility, excessive
guilt feelings, consequences of, 283
depression, 219, 259, 283
perfectionism, 225
self-sacrifice, 29, 180, 283
worries, 225, 283, 365

habits, 144, 145, 283–84
hallucinations, 47, 104, 192, 284
Hamer, R. G., 128
happiness, pursuit of, 93–95
harshness, against self, 284
haste, 77–79, 213–14, 284, 307, 356
hate, 284–85
with bitterness, 209, 285
due to abuse by others, 313
see also aggressiveness; bitterness; rage; revenge
headaches, 152–53, 285
heart conditions, 63
arrhythmia, 286
due to fears, 173, 285
heart attack, 168, 285
palpitations, 286
weak heart, 101–2, 258, 286, 299
heartbreak, 286–88, 322
heather (calluna vulgaris), 5
meaning and use of, 62–65
see also egotism; recognition; showing off
helpfulness, 179, 265, 296, 333

helplessness, 28, 31, 134, 245, 257, 288, 294
hesitation, 288
holly (ilex aquifolium), 5
meaning and use of, 66–69
see also aggressiveness; unfriendliness
homeopathic treatment, 3, 8, 134
homesickness, 70–72, 188, 200, 240, 288
see also memory; nostalgia
honeysuckle (lonicera caprifolium), 5
meaning and use of, 70–73
see also dreaminess; grieving; home-sickness
hopelessness, 288–89
causes of, 93, 197, 203–4, 288–89
consequences of, 179, 203, 289
in gorse syndrome, 59–61, 240
and weak will, 58, 200, 289
see also depression; giving up; resignation
hormone system, 145
hornbeam (capinus betulus), 5
meaning and use of, 74–76
see also perfectionism; stress/overwork
horror, 289
humiliation, 63, 65, 206, 289
humility, false, 289–90
see also servility
humorlessness, 222, 290
joy, lack of, 90–91, 119, 210, 303
seriousness, 99
hyperactivity, 290, 291
physical. see allergies
see also impatience; obsession
hypocrisy, 291, 344
piety, false, 328–29
see also artificiality; facade; self-deception
hysteria, 32–34, 35, 240, 291–92

I Ching (Wilhelm), 25
idealism, 292
consequences of, 76, 136–37, 215, 251, 296

morality-based, 105
in rock water syndrome, 119–22
in vervain syndrome, 136–39
illness, 292–94
acute, 51–52, 196
aggressive, 67, 292
causes of, 63, 74–76, 97, 145,
292–93
with changeable symptoms, 123
chronic, 293–94
with death wish, 60, 194, 292
with fear/panic, 86, 292
with hopelessness, 60, 292
as life change, 145, 150
needing attention/sympathy, 63, 292
psychosomatic, 2–3, 92, 129
with resignation, 92–3, 161, 162, 293
and tendency to withdraw, 149,
150, 293, 336
see also specific illness
illusions, 128, 187, 294
imagination, 15, 112, 275
immodesty, 294
impatience, 294
with aggression, 235
cause of concentration difficulties,
78, 250
and flightiness, 279, 294
in impatiens syndrome, 77–79, 140
and irritability, 69, 206, 294
with rheumatism, 340
and scatterbrained behavior, 213, 316
see also hyperactivity; restlessness
impatiens (impatiens glandulifera), 5
meaning and use of, 77–79
see also impatience; restlessness
imposition of will, 30, 136–38,
140–43, 294
see also domination
impurity, 48, 50, 83, 194, 196, 294
inattentiveness, 26–37, 39, 189, 240,
288, 294–95
inconsistency, 123, 145, 295
indecisiveness, 295–96

and changeability, 245
and concentration problems,
123–24, 250
in scleranthus syndrome, 123–26,
240
indecisiveness, causes of, 295–96
clarity, lack of, 156, 246, 295
daydreaming, 126, 193
fears, 126, 174–75, 217–18, 296
self-confidence, poor, 182–83, 295
indifference, 296
infallibility. see dogmatism
infection, 49, 91, 145, 296
inferiority, feelings of, 296–97
due to idealism, 76, 215, 296
in larch syndrome, 80–84, 240
and uncleanness, 194–95, 296
see also self-confidence
inferiority complex, effect of
excessive helpfulness, 179, 296
recognition, need for, 62–64, 296
showing off, 205, 296
inflexibility, 97, 132–34, 136, 140–43,
228, 279, 297
see also unyieldingness
influenceability, 297
contradicting wants/needs, 49–50,
108, 297
and dependence, 144, 180, 256, 297
in walnut syndrome, 144–47, 240
with weak personality, 127, 172, 297
influenceability, causes of
anxiety, 218, 297
excessive openness, 320
exhaustion, 147, 224, 297
insecurity, 29–30, 299, 320
self-confidence, poor, 80, 215–16,
297
see also naïveté
inhibitions, 297
initiative, insufficient, 160–63, 194,
297–98
injuries, 150, 168, 298, 321
see also emergencies

coughing, 254, 310
pulmonary thrombosis, 310
tuberculosis, 310, 364
see also asthma, bronchial
lymph system, 145

melancholia, 70–72, 90–95, 211, 248, 311
see also grieving; moodiness
memory, 70–72, 127 30, 211, 311
see also nostalgia; past
menopause, 81, 144–46, 291, 311–12
mental block, 312
mimulus *(mimulus guttatus)*, 5
meaning and use of, 85–89
see also anxiety; fear; timidity
missionary zeal, 136–39, 238, 240, 312
see also do-gooder; know-it-all
mistakes, 187–88, 313
learning from, 187, 189, 313
mistreatment, 162, 209, 313
mistrust, 16–18, 66, 175, 182, 313
modesty, 74, 80–84, 313
moodiness, 314
and depression, 128, 201, 314
frequent, changeable, 220, 314
morning, 315
morality, 48, 112, 137
imposed by others, 34, 217
personal, 50, 119
morals, obsessive, 196, 215, 314–15
mothering, 17, 40–43, 112, 240, 264, 315–16
see also relationships
musculature, problems with, 120
mustard *(sinapis arvensis)*, 5
meaning and use of, 90–95
see also depression; melancholia

naïveté, 62, 145, 146, 241, 316
see also influenceability
narrow-mindedness, 140–41, 316
naturopathic treatment, 8
nausea, 50, 316

nervous behavior, causes of, 77–79, 112, 316
see also haste; stress; tension
nervous collapse, 247, 317
nervous system, 137
neuroses, 127–28, 239 40, 317
nightmares, 127–28, 318
noncompetitiveness, 247–48, 371
nostalgia, 58, 70–72, 188, 192, 200, 318
see also memory; past
nutrition, 79, 101, 129, 161
oak *(quercus robur)*, 5
meaning and use of, 96–100
see also ambition; uncompromising behavior
obsequiousness. *see* servility
obsession, 318–19
conspiracy fears, 251
fixations, 152–55, 231, 278
and missionary zeal, 137
with possessions/power, 125, 370
see also compulsions; fanaticism
obsessive thoughts, 319
with aggression, 208
anxious, 112, 155, 218–19, 277
with bitterness, 233
concentration problems caused by, 152, 188–89, 250
of future, 194, 249
guilty, 155, 226
of love, 155, 191, 249
mental overactivity, 187, 214
offended, easily, 164–66, 319–20
olive *(olea europea)*, 5
meaning and use of, 101–4, 162
see also exhaustion; weakness
openness, excessive, 320
see also influenceability
opinionated thought, 320
optimism, 171, 320
order, fanatical, 141, 320–21
osteoporosis, 81, 352
outsider. *see* loner
oversensitivity. *see* sensitivity

overwork, 199, 321
see also stress/overwork

pain, physical, 321
panic, causes of, 199, 213, 277, 322
panic, feeling of, 321–22
   and driven behavior, 213
   effects of, 171, 227, 235, 322
   horror, 289
   panicky worries, 217, 226, 322
   with psychic trauma, 227, 322
   with rash behavior, 334
   in rock rose syndrome, 115–18, 240
   with unconsciousness, 118, 193,
      322, 365
   see also fear; psychosis; shock
panic attacks, 168
   and breakdown, verge of, 115, 173,
      185, 244, 322
   with fear, 15–16, 174
partner problems, 322–26
   heartbreak, 286–87
   separation, 282, 308, 347
   see also relationships
past, reasons for escape into
   exhaustion, 210, 270
   fear of future, 277
   inferiority complex, 296
   self-confidence, poor, 72, 209
   stress/overwork, 72, 209, 278, 356
   timidity, 210
perfectionism, 74–76, 249, 326–27
perfectionism, causes of, 326–27
   ambition, 100, 221
   guilty thoughts, 105–9, 225, 326
pessimism, 327–28
   anxious, 219
   with gloominess, 90, 327
   in gorse syndrome, 59–60
   with tendency to give up, 55, 56,
      58, 200, 327
pessimism, causes of, 74–76, 113–14,
   327–28
   pettiness, 49–50, 177, 326, 328

pigheadedness, 96, 97, 132
   see also dogmatism; stubbornness
pine *(pinus sylvestris)*, 5
   meaning and use of, 105–10
   see also guilt feelings; perfectionism
pity, 41, 43, 329, 345
poisoning, fear of, 48, 256, 329
pregnancy, emotions of, 329–330
   see also birth
prejudice. *see* dogmatism
premonitions, 238, 289, 330
pressure, emotional, 32–35
   from computer games, 79
   excessive, 14, 86, 171, 184, 330
   self-imposed, 184, 185, 186, 198
   see also obsession; psychosis
pride, 238, 330–31
   with distancing, 148, 149, 331, 354
   see also arrogance; distance
psychosis
   causes of, 35, 173, 186, 331
   in cherry plum syndrome, 32–34
psychotic obsession, 319
psychotic rage, 331
psychotherapy, 12, 14, 81, 103, 172
puberty, 144–46, 332
purpose in life, lack of, 332–33
   and changeability, 246
   depression caused by, 220–21, 258,
      333
   and lack of drive, 233
purposelessness, causes of, 156–59,
   232, 246, 332–33
pushiness, 65, 136, 205, 277, 333

rage, 333–34
   with bitterness, 209, 333, 334
   caused by opposition, 69, 143, 208,
      320, 334
   psychotic, 34, 331, 334
   uncontrollable, 35, 184
   see also aggressiveness; hate
rash behavior. *see* irrational behavior
reality

Scheuermann's disease, 81
schizophrenia, 340–41
sciatica, 339–40, 341–42
    see also rheumatism
scleranthus (scleranthus annuus), 5
    meaning and use of, 123–26
    see also flightiness; indecisiveness
secrecy. see facade
self-abuse, 342
    due to dependence, 182, 342
    due to fear, 174, 342
    in rock water syndrome, 119–22, 240
    self-torment, 119–20, 346
    see also asceticism
self-alienation, 342–43
    due to repression, 172, 342
    and lack of clarity, 156, 343
    in walnut syndrome, 144–47, 240
    see also intolerance, against oneself
self-awareness, 14, 69, 172–73, 343
self-castigation. see asceticism
self-centeredness. see egocentrism
self-confidence, insufficient
    consequences of, 209, 211, 214,
        267, 343–44
    due to emotional trauma, 343
    and influenceability, 28–29,
        144–46, 344
    and noncompetitiveness, 248
    with weak will, 83, 197, 343
    see also inferiority, feelings of
self-deception, 23, 26, 344–45
self-denial, 345
    depression caused by, 24, 257
    due to guilt feelings, 107, 108, 180,
        345
    pathological, 56, 59, 80, 81
    rejection of others, 334–35
    with timidity, 201
    see also modesty; renunciation;
        selflessness
self-discipline, 260
    moderation in, 69, 260
    severe, 119–21, 194–96, 284, 345

strictness, 119–21, 174, 177, 346, 356
    see also asceticism
selflessness
    and being used, 169, 366, 367
    in centaury syndrome, 23–25
    pathological, 25–26, 112
    with worry, 180, 346
    see also renunciation; self-sacrifice;
        victim
self-love. see egocentrism
self-pity, 40–43, 321, 329, 345
    see also pity; self-sacrifice
self-righteousness, 141, 165, 345
    see also bitterness
self-sacrifice, 345–46
    due to guilt, 180, 346
    selfish, 27, 40, 41, 43, 178, 346
    total, 43, 191, 346
    with weak will, 24, 345
    see also selflessness
sensitivity, 369
    excessive, 54, 85–88, 111–12, 115
    as trait, 10–12, 15–16, 127–31, 240
    to weather, 369
    see also offended, easily
sentimentality, 346
    see also daydreaming
separation, 282, 308, 347
    see also grieving; loss
seriousness. see humorlessness
servility, 23–26, 180, 276, 318, 347–48
    see also humility
sexual dysfunction, 348–49
    due to disinterest, 162
    due to exhaustion, 103, 348
    due to moralistic pressures, 106,
        108, 120, 349
    due to revulsion, 49, 324, 348
    impotence/frigidity, 349
shame, 349
shock, 350
    acute, 115–17, 127–30, 150, 350
    distress, 262
    horror, 289

386   INDEX

violence, 66, 67, 116, 367
  see also aggressiveness

walnut *(juglans regia),* 6
  meaning and use of, 144–47
  see also influenceability;
    self-alienation
water violet *(hottonia palustris),* 6
  meaning and use of, 148–51
  see also contact problems; loner
weak personality, 367–69
  causes of, 83, 144, 368–69
  with dependence, 23–24, 27, 369
  resignation caused by, 27, 181
weak will, 370
  avoidance of difficulties, 170, 192,
    370
  causes of, 162, 202, 313, 370
  confidence, lack of, 200–201, 370
  in gentian syndrome, 55–58, 240
  hopelessness with, 200, 370
  noncompetitiveness with, 248
  with weak personality, 23–24, 27,
    144, 369
weakness, 101–4, 264–65, 355, 369
weather, sensitivity to, 369
weepy, 369
  see also sensitivity
white chestnut *(aesculus
    hippocastanum),* 6

meaning and use of, 152–55
  see also compulsive thoughts
wild oat *(bromus ramosus),* 6
  meaning and use of, 8, 156–59
  see also goals, lack of; restlessness
wild rose *(rosa canina),* 6
  meaning and use of, 160–63
  see also enthusiasm, lack of;
    resignation
Wilhelm, R., 25
willow *(salix vitellina),* 6
  meaning and use of, 164–67
  see also bitterness; unforgiving
worries, 370
  concern, excessive, 111–14, 240
  debilitating, 103, 223–24, 293
  about others, 174, 180, 217, 225,
    277, 370
  with panic, 217, 226, 322, 370
  in red chestnut syndrome, 111–14,
    240
  and restlessness, 114, 365, 370
  secret, 14, 114, 171, 370
  thoughts dominated by, 152, 370
worries, causes of, 370
  bad conscience, 110, 225, 370
  desire to possess, 370
  guilt feelings, 225, 283, 365
  heartbreak, 287
  negative experiences, 226, 370

BOOKS OF RELATED INTEREST